ABO-incompatible Organ Transplantation

Yi Wang
Editor

ABO-incompatible Organ Transplantation

Springer

Editor
Yi Wang
The Second Affiliated Hospital of Hainan Medical University
Haikou, Hainan
China

The Second Affiliated Hospital
University of South China
Hengyang, Hunan
China

ISBN 978-981-13-3398-9 ISBN 978-981-13-3399-6 (eBook)
https://doi.org/10.1007/978-981-13-3399-6

Library of Congress Control Number: 2018968536

This Springer imprint is published by the registered company Springer Nature Singapore Pte Ltd.
The registered company address is: 152 Beach Road, #21-01/04 Gateway East, Singapore 189721, Singapore

Foreword

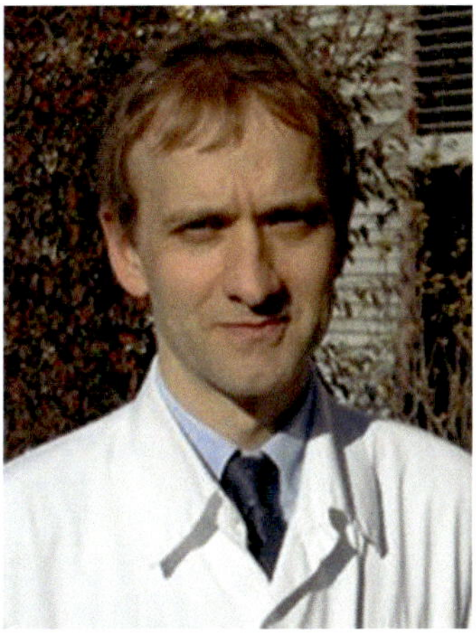

Organ transplantation has been a major milestone of progress in the recent history of medicine, and this strategy is currently curing many patients with various end-stage organ failures all around the world. Unfortunately, organ donor shortage limits the future development of organ transplantation, and it is increasingly necessary to include marginal organ donors with higher risks of post-transplant failure and complications. ABO incompatibility was initially seen as an impossible barrier to cross, with immediate humoral destruction of the grafted organ. This barrier has been progressively studied using experimental models, and the complex mechanisms leading to acute organ rejection have come to be understood. Through precise and careful research, ABO incompatibility is no longer an absolute barrier for specific cases of patients in need of kidney grafts, although clinical application requires highly prepared and trained teams of nephrologists, surgeons, and nurses. Only with careful preparation are such difficult transplants possible. Pr. Yi Wang has successfully introduced ABO-incompatible kidney transplantation in China and has gained strong experience and leadership. His new book will certainly allow new transplant centers to launch ABO-incompatible organ transplantation programs in China and lead to the treatment of numerous patients.

Furthermore, ABO incompatibility is somewhat similar to xenotransplantation, which is still perceived as an impossible barrier for clinical application. However, intensive research might also allow us to fully understand the mechanisms that lead to organ xenograft rejection and overcome these hurdles by using new genetic modifications of donor animals and the development of new immunosuppressive agents. One day, xenotransplantation perhaps will be seen like ABO-incompatible organ transplantation was some years ago. Therefore, the introduction of ABO-incompatible organ transplantation programs will eventually enhance the field of xenotransplantation.

I congratulate Pr. Wang for his achievements and strongly advise any center considering the launch of an ABO-incompatible organ transplantation program to use his experience.

Geneva, Switzerland Leo Buhler

Foreword

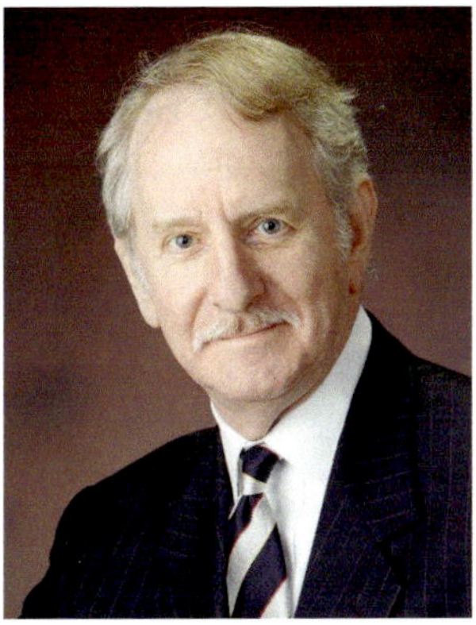

Organ transplantation across the blood group barrier has grown immensely in clinical importance since kidney transplant surgeons—Maurice Slapak, Guy Alexandre, and others—made their initial independent attempts to overcome this barrier in the mid-1980s [1–4]. That hyperacute rejection could occur when the ABO barrier was crossed had been discovered inadvertently by Hume [5], Starzl [6], and others during their pioneering efforts to establish kidney transplantation in the 1950s and 1960s. Thereafter, surgeons took pains to avoid ABO incompatibility.

The topic proved important not only in kidney transplantation but also in the transplantation of other organs [7, 8], with the possible exception of the liver [9, 10]. Indeed, the first heart transplant might have been carried out by Richard Lower and his colleagues at the Medical College of Virginia before that by Christiaan Barnard in Cape Town, but the opportunity was declined because the donor was found to be ABO incompatible with the recipient (Lower R, personal communication 1991).

During the past two decades, however, great efforts have been made to overcome this barrier, largely by (1) reducing the blood level of existing antibodies directed against the donor AB blood type and (2) suppressing production of new anti-AB antibodies [11]. These efforts have proved immensely successful, and although there remains perhaps a higher risk of early graft loss, today organ transplantation across this barrier is carried out with long-term results comparable to those of ABO-compatible transplantation.

From these studies, the concept of 'accommodation' was developed [12–14], and evidence was put forward by West and her colleagues for the development of B-cell tolerance in infants with ABO-incompatible heart grafts [15, 16]. These studies also stimulated research on the structure of the ABO oligosaccharide antigens [17, 18] and their distribution in the major organs [19, 20].

It is to these efforts that this book is primarily directed. The editor, Professor Yi Wang, is himself a pioneer in China of the techniques involved in overcoming the ABO barrier and so is ideally suited to edit such a book. The contributors to the book have covered the field comprehensively, presenting an overview of all aspects of the topic from the history of its pioneering efforts and its pathobiology to all aspects of its clinical status today. The chapters explore the topic from a general scientific perspective to in-depth discussions of how it impacts transplantation of each of the major organs.

Today, with the increasing use of living kidney and liver donors who may be ABO incompatible with the intended recipient, the management of ABO incompatibility is a subject that all transplant surgeons and physicians and allied staff need to understand. The publication of this book, therefore, is timely as it will provide all those involved with organ transplantation with knowledge of this increasingly important subject. I congratulate Professor Wang on making so much information available to the transplant community.

References

1. Slapak M, Naik RB, Lee HA. Renal transplant in a patient with major donor-recipient blood group incompatibility: reversal of acute rejection by the use of modified plasmapheresis. Transplantation. 1981;31:4–7.
2. Alexandre GPJ, Squifflet JP, De Bruyere M, Latinne D, Moriau M, Ikabu N. Splenectomy as a prerequisite for successful human ABO-incompatible renal transplantation. Transplant Proc. 1985;17:138–43.
3. Alexandre GP, Squifflet JP, De Bruyere M, Latinne D, Reding R, Gianello P, Carlier M, Pirson Y. Present experiences in a series of 26 ABO-incompatible living donor renal allografts. Transplant Proc. 1987;19:4538–42.
4. Bannett AD, McAlack RF, Raja R, Baquero A, Morris M. Experiences with known ABO-mismatched renal transplants. Transplant Proc. 1987;19:4543–6.
5. Hume DM, Merrill JP, Miller BF, Thorn GW. Experiences with renal homotransplantation in the human: report of nine cases. J Clin Invest. 1955;34:327–82.
6. Starzl TE, Marchioro TL, Holmes JH, Hermann G, Brittain RS, Stonington OH, Talmage DW, Waddell WR. Renal homografts in patients with major donor-recipient blood group incompatibilities. Surgery (St. Louis). 1964;55:195–200.
7. Cooper DK. Clinical survey of heart transplantation between ABO blood group-incompatible recipients and donors. J Heart Transplant. 1990;9:376–81.
8. Egawa H, Teramukai S, Haga H, Tanabe M, Mori A, Ikegami T, Kawagishi N, Ohdan H, Kasahara M, Umeshita K. Impact of rituximab desensitization on

blood-type-incompatible adult living donor liver transplantation: a Japanese multicenter study. Am J Transplant. 2014;14:102–14.
9. Gordon RD, Iwatsuki S, Esquivel CO, Todo S, Makowka L, Tzakis A, Marsh JW, Starzl TE. Experience with primary liver transplantation across ABO blood groups. Transplant Proc. 1987;19:4575–9.
10. Egawa H, Teramukai S, Haga H, Tanabe M, Fukushima M, Shimazu M. Present status of ABO-incompatible living donor liver transplantation in Japan. Hepatology. 2008;47:143–52.
11. Montgomery JR, Berger JC, Warren DS, James NT, Montgomery RA, Segev DL. Outcomes of ABO-incompatible kidney transplantation in the United States. Transplantation. 2012;93:603–9.
12. Chopek MW, Simmons RL, Platt JL. ABO-incompatible kidney transplantation: initial immunopathologic evaluation. Transplant Proc. 1987;19:4553–7.
13. Bach FH, Platt JL, Cooper DKC. Accommodation—the role of natural antibody and complement in discordant xenograft rejection. In: Cooper DKC, Reemtsma K, White DJG, editors. Xenotransplantation: the transplantation of organs and tissues between species. Heidelberg: Springer; 1991a. p. 81–99.
14. Bach FH, Turman MA, Vercellotti GM, Platt JL, Dalmasso AP. Accommodation: a working paradigm for progressing toward clinical discordant xenografting. Transplant Proc. 1991b;23:205–7.
15. West LJ, Pollock-Barziv SM, Dipchand AI, Lee KJ, Cardella CJ, Benson LN, Rebeyka IM, Coles JG. ABO-incompatible heart transplantation in infants. N Engl J Med. 2001;344:793–800.
16. West LJ. B-cell tolerance following ABO-incompatible infant heart transplantation. Transplantation. 2006;81:301–7.
17. Schacter H, Tilley CA. In: Manners DJ, editor. Biochemistry of carbohydrates, vol. II. Baltimore: University Park Press; 1978. p. 209.
18. Clausen H, Hakomori S. ABH and related histo-blood group antigens; immunochemical differences in carrier isotypes and their distribution. Vox Sang. 1989;56:1–20.
19. Paul LC, van Es LA, Riviere GB, Eernisse G, de Graeff J. Blood group B antigen on renal endothelium as the target for rejection in an ABO-incompatible recipient. Transplantation. 1978;26:268–71.
20. Bariety J, Oriol R, Hinglais N, Zanetti M, Bretton R, Dalix AM, Mandet C. Distribution of blood group antigen A in normal and pathologic human kidneys. Kidney Int. 1980;17:820–6.

Pittsburgh, PA, USA
(For Chinese Version in 2016)

David K. C. Cooper

Preface

ABO blood group incompatibility kidney transplantation(ABOi-KT) started in the 1980s. The country which has accumulated a wealth of experience is Japan. In the early days, to implement of this kind of transplant, the doctors were working to remove the native preexisting antibodies and decrease the number of B cells in the body; more obvious results have been achieved. In the twenty-first century, all have not only have accumulated valuable experience because of the removal of blood type antibody, high risk in infection, bleeding and clotting dysfunctions, and many other complications of treatment, but also in overcoming hyperacute rejection, and obtaining comparable or better long-term survival in ABO-incompatible than in ABO-compatible transplantation, thus leading to more and more doctors in the world able to carry out incompatible organ transplantation.

In China, ABO-incompatible kidney transplantation (ABOi-KT) began in December 2006. China was one of the earliest countries in the world to do this work. The first case was a man with blood type O. Five years after this patient received renal transplantation, his new kidney lost function. His PRA (plasma renin assay) antibodies were higher: class I was 47.9% and class II was 27.3%, and because of long-term hemodialysis, his peripheral vascular system was extremely difficult to puncture. As a specific recipient, his father (with blood type A) wished to donate a kidney to save his child, and this operation was performed at the urging of the patient and his family. After almost 12 years, the recipient and donor are surviving well, with very good renal function. The successful implementation of this surgery has accumulated valuable experience for ABO blood group incompatibility organ transplantation in China. In recent years, West China Hospital, Sichuan University, The First Affiliated Hospital of Sun Yat-sen University, Beijing Chaoyang Hospital, Zhongshan Hospital, Fudan University, and a number of transplant units in China have carried out kidney transplantation with ABO incompatibility, providing the opportunity for surgery for more specific recipients, and satisfactory results are achieved now also.

Compared with ABOi-KT, when ABO incompatibility liver transplantation was implemented earlier in China, it was mainly to provide patients a short but important time when in a very dangerous situation and waiting for a ABO-compatible donor, because at that time preoperative atempts to remove ABO blood type antibodies of recipients mostly failed. In recent years, with the continuous improvement of plasma processing technology, there are more and more units planning to do

ABO-incompatible liver transplantation, and the functional survival rate is constantly increasing.

There are not many centers in the world that can carry out ABO-incompatible heart transplantation and ABO-incompatible lung transplantation independently. China does not have complete records about these kinds of recipients so far, and therefore the most relevant experience described in this book has come from abroad.

For this reason, this book covers the history of ABO incompatibility organ transplant, ABO blood group antigens, ABO blood group antibodies, pathology, pathophysiology, and related basic theory and knowledge to share the clinical experience of heart, liver, lung, and kidney transplant, the four major substantive ABO-incompatible organ transplants. Doctors and related staff not only learn from a more comprehensive and systematic method in ABO-incompatible organ transplantation that can be used for reference, but also from early schemes, that now seem inappropriate treatment, which we retain intact to provide to you, so that the readers can understand the hard and not easy task of the explorers.

This book is informative and readable and is one of the best reference books for transplant colleagues and related workers.

Because of both lack of knowledge of some editors and the rapid update of knowledge in this field, it is hard to avoid omissions or even fallacies. I hope you will give me advice so that I can revise these errors in the reprint.

In the process of writing this book, The Chinese Society of Organ Transplantation, Hokkaido University, Japan, Sun yat-sen University, Beijing Chaoyang Hospital, Beijing Friendship Hospital, Wuxi People's Hospital, Zhongshan Hospital, Fudan University, Tongji Hospital, Huazhong University of Science and Technology, the Nanjing General Hospital of PLA, 309 Hospital of PLA, Tianjin Medical University, and the Nagoya Daini Red Cross Hospital gave the preparation of this book high importance and strong support. Here, I wish to express my appreciation for all.

Haikou, China Yi Wang

Acknowledgments

I would like to express my gratitude to the many people who have taken time to help me during the process of writing this book; to all those who provided support, talked things over, read, wrote, offered comments, allowed me to quote their remarks, and assisted in the editing, proofreading, and design.

We wish to give a special thanks to Pr. David K.C. Cooper, MD, PhD, FRCS, University of Alabama at Birmingham (UAB) Co-Director, Xenotransplantation Program Department of Surgery, from 2009, when he worked in the Thomas E. Starzl Transplantation Institute, University of Pittsburgh, who has been supportive of my career goals and who worked actively to provide me with the protected academic time to pursue those goals. As my teacher and mentor, he has taught me more than I could ever give him credit for here.

I am also immensely grateful to Pr. Leo Buhler, President of the International Xenotransplantation Association, Head of the Surgery University Hospital, Geneva, Switzerland, for the foreword, comments, and for sharing pearls of wisdom with us during the process of writing this book.

We thank Ms. Kripa Guruprasad, Project Co-ordinator (Books) for Springer Nature, for overseeing the seamless integration of our text and for organizing and checking all the chapters.

This book would not have been possible without the efforts of many, many people. We are grateful to the talented colleagues with whom we have had the pleasure of working, at the following facilities:

- Xiaopeng Hu, Beijing Chao-Yang Hospital, Capital Medical University
- Jiang Qiu, The First Affiliated Hospital, Sun Yat-Sen University
- Jiqiu Wen, Nanjing General Hospital, PLA
- Chunbai Mo, Tianjin First Center Hospital
- Zhiqiang Liu, Tianjin Medical University
- Daiki Iwami, Hokkaido University Hospital
- Ming Cai, The 309th Hospital of Chinese People's Liberation Army
- Haihao Wang, Tongji Hospital, Tongji Medical College of HUST
- Lin Wei, Beijing Friendship Hospital, Capital Medical University
- Bo Wu, Wuxi People's Hospital

- Gang Chen, Tongji Hospital, Tongji Medical College of HUST
- Ruiming Rong, Zhongshan Hospital, Fudan University
- Tchomte Romeo Martial, The Second Affiliated Hospital of Hainan Medical University

These colleagues provided insight and expertise that greatly assisted me during the process of writing this book.

Nobody has been more important to me in the pursuit of this project than my parents, who are over 85 years old, and whose love and guidance are with me in whatever I pursue. I would like to thank them here. They are the ultimate role models. Most importantly, I thank my loving and supportive wife Ruibing Liu, and my wonderful daughter Lingxiao Wang, for inspiring me and for granting me the time it takes to work on such a book.

Last and not least: I beg forgiveness of all those who have been with me over the course of the years and whose names I have failed to mention.

Contents

Editor-in-Chief

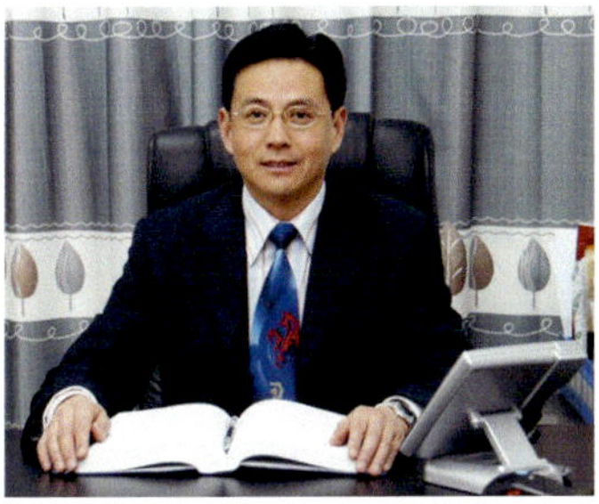

Yi Wang, M.D., Ph.D. Professor at National Level II, Doctoral Supervisor, Member of the Chinese Society of Organ Transplantation, Committee Member of the Chinese Academy of Research Hospital Transplantation Medicine, Committee Member of All-China Federation of Returned Oversea Chinese of Distinguished Experts.

Dr. Wang handled the first case of ABO-incompatible donor kidney transplantation and ABO/Rh-incompatible donor kidney transplantation in China, and now is in charge of several research grants including some from the National Natural Science Foundation of China.

Deputy Editors

Zhiqiang Liu, M.D., Ph.D.
Department of Physiology and Pathophysiology
School of Basic Science, Tianjin Medical University,
Tianjin, China

Jiqiu Wen, M.D., Ph.D.
Kidney Transplant Center, National Clinical Research Center of Kidney Diseases,
Jinling Hospital, Nanjing University School of Medicine,
Nanjing, China

Introduction 1

Yi Wang, Hongtao Jiang, and Luogeng Liu

Abstract
ABO-incompatible organ transplantation has experienced a long and tortuous development. In this chapter, we would have a short review of the major breakthroughs in the history of organ transplantation and efforts of medical scientists to overcome the blood barriers and briefly introduce some important organ transplantation concepts.

Keywords
Blood barriers · Organ transplantation · Historical events

Thousands of years ago, mankind has sprouted a dream of organ transplantation. But this dream didn't come true until 1954, when Murry, an American doctor, successfully performed the first kidney transplantation for a pair of twin brothers. What followed was the problem of organ sources and immune rejection. The tissue compatibility and the blood compatibility are the main reasons for onset of the severity of immune rejection. In 1985, Alexander and his colleagues successfully performed the ABO-incompatible kidney transplantation, which successfully overcame the blood barriers, and expanded the organ sources. In this chapter, we would have a brief review of the key progress in the history of organ transplantation, together with mankind's efforts to overcome the blood barriers and make a brief illustration on some organ transplantation concepts.

Y. Wang (✉)
The Second Affiliated Hospital of Hainan Medical University,
Haikou City, Hainan Province, China

The Second Affiliated Hospital, University of South China,
Hengyang City, Hunan Province, China
e-mail: wy@usc.edu.cn

H. Jiang · L. Liu
Zhengxiang District, 35 Jiefang Ave, Hengyang City, Hunan Provience 421001, China

Y. Wang (ed.), *ABO-incompatible Organ Transplantation*,
https://doi.org/10.1007/978-981-13-3399-6_1

1 The History of ABO-Incompatible Organ Transplantation

1.1 The Basis for the Development of Organ Transplantation

Review of the medical history of organ transplantation shows that the clinical surgical vascular anastomosis, organ preservation technology and the discovery of immunosuppressive drugs and reasonable application, and the development of the diagnosis and treatment of host rejection have promoted the steady development of organ transplantation and laid a solid foundation for ABO-incompatible organ transplantation as well.

For vascular anastomosis in organ transplantation, improperly chosen suture material and technique cause vascular stenosis, resulting in slow blood flow; and the presence of the suture as foreign bodies, having undermined the integrity of the vascular endothelium, leads to the abnormal activation in human body blood coagulation mechanism. The cause of these reactions is infection and thrombosis. Vascular obstruction occurs again, and the graft will turn into inactivity, even necrosis, due to insufficient blood supply, and the patients may even suffer more serious consequences. For the ABO blood group incompatibility organ transplantation, blood purification treatment such as plasma exchange will be adopted before operation. After the patient's blood being processed, coagulation factor will be greatly reduced. In the process of transplantation, inappropriate vascular anastomosis may lead to anastomotic bleeding or even massive hemorrhage. Therefore, vascular anastomosis is very important in organ transplantation, which has promoted the development of organ transplantation to some extent.

The history of vascular anastomosis dated back to as early as 1762. The famous doctor, Lambert, stitched a rupture of brachial artery, and completed the first case of human blood vessel suture technique, which is a historic progress, because doctors could only treat broken blood vessels with ligation before. And the earliest for vascular anastomosis is Nicolai Eck. In 1877, he anastomosed the inferior vena cava and portal vein with side-to-side stapled anastomosis, and then interrupted the suture, and finally anastomosed the inferior vena cava and portal vein with end-to-side anastomosis technique. In 1899, Kummell made the first human artery end-to-end anastomosis. On the basis of these practices, many scholars conducted vascular suture technology researches, including continuous suture and interrupted suture, simple suture and cotton-padded mattress suture, and so on. Until 1902, Carrel invented the "three-point method" vascular anastomosis from the fixed burst of fabric before embroidery, as shown in Fig. 1.1a, b. The three-point method is to match the ends of the cross-sectional vessels taking three vertices of an equilateral triangle as fixed. So after a little pull, anastomosis operation becomes the operation of the three identical planes. After a lot of trial and error, Carrel improved vascular anastomosis. He sutured a father's artery with his daughter's leg veins, achieving "the first modern blood transfusion," and anastomosed the artery and vein in the operation successfully. In the same year, Swedish Karolinska Institute awarded Carrel the

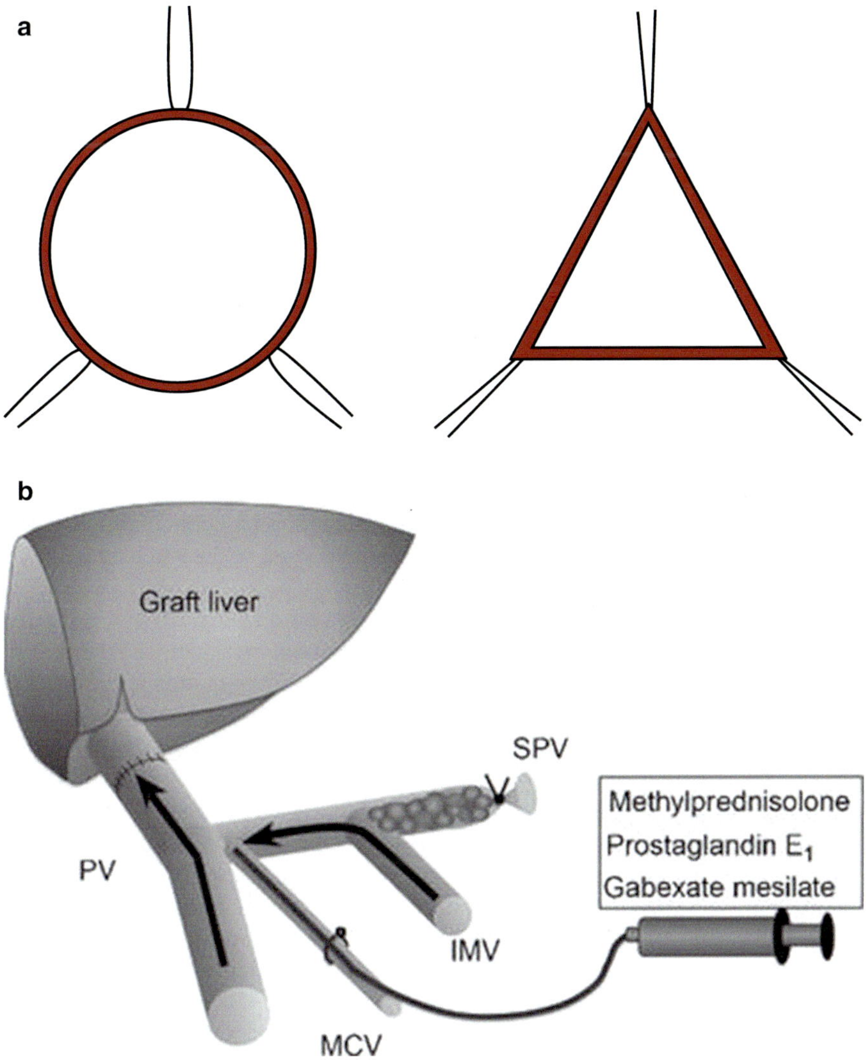

Fig. 1.1 (**a**, **b**) "Three-point method" vascular anastomosis

Nobel Prize in Physiology and Medicine for his invention of the anastomosis technique and thus validated the possibility of organ transplantation. The three-point method of vascular anastomosis not only broke through the bottleneck of vascular anastomosis but also laid the basic principles of modern vascular anastomosis, promoting the development of organ transplantation.

1.1.1 The Development of Organ Preservation Technology

Organ preservation means keeping the isolated organ alive. Organ preservation is one of the three pillars of organ implantology. To save the organ safely and effectively is the prerequisite of organ transplantation. The purpose of organ preservation is to minimize the damages caused by ischemia, and maintain viability of the isolated tissues or organs, so as to complete the delivery of tissues and organs, match of tissue types, preparations for surgery, and rapid recovery of its physiological function after the blood supply, reducing the graft function delays and no function, to ensure long-term graft survival.

For organ preservation, there are two methods to extend the life of isolated organs in principle. One method is to reduce the demand for the required material of maintaining cell metabolism or increase their tolerance as far as possible; the other method is to constantly supply the minimum necessary nutrients to sustain the activity of cells. The former needs the low temperature and the latter a continuous perfusion of preservation solution. But the practical effective method is the integrated use of the two principles above.

Organ preservation technology started in the early 1950s. In the next 20 years, cold storage has been regarded as the first method to extend the life of isolated organs by inhibiting cell metabolism in low temperature. The original method is to put the isolated organ in cold solution, which is called surface cooling. But the cooling of the deeper part in the center of the organs is poorer, so the whole organ can't be cooling uniformly.

Later cold lavage (0–4 °C) is adopted. Pouring cold lavage (0–4 °C) into the artery of the isolated organ for a short flush can not only wash down the harmful substances of intravascular residues but also drop the temperature in the center of the organ evenly below 10 °C (15 °C is the highest limit), and then the organ is saved in a solution of 1–4 °C, until the start of vascular reconstruction of the organ. This is called simple hypothermia irrigation preservation. Cold saline or electrolyte solution resembling extracellular fluid such as Ringer's solution or lactated Ringer's solution is often used for the sake of irrigation and conservation. The preservation time for the kidney is only 5 h. But such a short time for an organ preservation time was far from enough to meet the clinical need. Collins created intracellular-type solution in 1969 and successfully preserved a dog's kidney for 30 h, which also achieved good effect in the clinic. Collins made a landmark improvement in cold storage, ending the history of using extracellular-type solution to preserve isolated organs. In 1967, Belzar et al. used the machine continuous perfusion method to save the dog's kidney for 24–72 h, making the preservation time significantly longer than cold storage. But it still can't meet the need of organ transplantation. Subsequently, Belzar et al. created a new organ preservation solution, named the UW preservation solution (the University of Wisconsin solution, UW) [1]. Its composition is lactose potash, KH2PO4, MgSO4, cotton candy, adenosine, glutathione, insulin, penicillin, dexamethasone, allopurinol, hydroxyethyl starch, etc. The preservation solution can continuously cold-hold the pancreas and the kidneys for up to 72 h and the liver for up to 30 h or longer, which is a breakthrough in the history of the development of preservation solution, promoting the development of organ transplantation to some extent.

1.1.2 The Discovery of Immunosuppressive Drugs and Reasonable Applications

In recent years, the success rate of organ transplantation has increased year by year due to the discovery of immunosuppressive drugs and reasonable application in organ transplantation. Throughout the history of immunosuppressive drugs, its development course, although not long, plays a very important role in the development of organ transplantation.

In 1949, Philip S. Hench found the glucocorticoid and illustrated its structure and biological effect. In 1954, Hume firstly used glucocorticoid after organ transplants and achieved good effects. The glucocorticoid is mainly used for induction and maintenance stages of immunosuppressive therapy, which have stronger inhibitory effect on mononuclear macrophages and neutrophils, T lymphocytes, and B lymphocytes. Glucocorticoid can effectively reduce the rejection when used in combination with other immune inhibitors. In the case of acute rejection, the impact of large dose of glucocorticoid therapy may reverse most of the acute rejection reaction. In spite of the fast development of the immune inhibitors, glucocorticoid is still the important drug in basic immune suppression scheme.

In 1953, American doctor Robert S. Schwartz and British doctor Roy Calne successively used 6-mercaptopurine in the dog's kidney transplantation. Although its use was stopped later due to the side effects in clinical application, in 1962, Robert S. Schwartz and Roy Calne again used the derivatives of mercaptopurine and azathioprine, in organ transplantation, and made a major breakthrough in increasing the success rate of kidney transplantation, so azathioprine as a normal immune inhibitor later has been continuously used ever since.

In 1978, Swiss Borel extracted a circular polypeptide containing 11 amino acids from fungi glycolysis products, named ring spore A (CsA), and used it in the clinical organ transplantation as the first immune inhibitor target to calmodulin. CsA can achieve effective specific inhibition of lymphocyte responses and hyperplasia, especially in T cells at different stages, such as selective inhibition of Th cells. As a specific T cell proliferation inhibitor, CsA has obtained the good curative effect in the treatment of the graft rejection and earned many transplantation patients' longer life. The emergence of CsA also makes heart-lung transplantation and pancreas, bone, and marrow transplantation come true and ushers into a new era of organ transplantation as the most important second-generation immunosuppressor.

In 1985, Japanese Kino et al. discovered a new drug FK506 (tacrolimus), which can prevent a variety of graft rejections. The mechanism is similar to CsA, but the effect of antirejection is 10–100 times greater than CsA. In 1989, Starzl firstly used the drug in liver and kidney transplantation. He found that, compared with the CsA, the biggest characteristic is that tacrolimus can reverse the treatment outcome of "refractory acute rejection" that conventional immunosuppressive therapy fails to do, thus saving a large number of patients and organs and reducing the second transplantation greatly and, moreover, having less cytotoxicity than other immunosuppressants. So tacrolimus now has widely been used in liver, kidney, heart, pancreas, lung, and other solid organ transplantation.

In the late 1980s, five or six kinds of new drugs were developed one after another with different mechanisms, and their effects on inhibiting immune rejection were proved to be remarkable in the animal experiments, including mycophenolate mofetil, rapamycin, brequinar, deoxyspergualin, and mizoribine. But all immunosuppressants in application or trial have negative impacts on the human body in specific or nonspecific immune defense function and only differ in the severity and demonstrations. If used properly, they can appropriately reduce the body's immune reactivity of transplanted organs, and help to avoid or reduce rejection, so that the transplanted organ can perform its corresponding function continuously. As a result, the recipients can have their life maintained or even live a normal life.

1.1.3 The Development in Monitoring and Diagnosis of Graft Rejection

The graft rejection including severe antibody-mediated rejection, acute rejection, chronic rejection, and the acute rejection is one of the most important factors to the transplanted organ dysfunction. It is also an important factor affecting the long-term survival and the function. For all kinds of different organ transplantations, graft rejection has different clinical manifestations, and diagnosis methods are also different. Next, as an example, we will introduce the development of kidney transplantation rejection monitoring and diagnosis.

When the kidney transplantation rejection occurs, transplant renal biopsy is commonly used to confirm it. AR is mainly characterized by fever, weight gain, high blood pressure, reduced urine, elevated serum creatinine, proteinuria, erythrocytosis, and hemoglobin decline. Color Doppler ultrasound shows increased artery blood flow resistance index. At this point, transplant renal biopsy can diagnose AR and perform pathological classification according to Banff standard.

At present, with the wide application of the new immunosuppressants, clinical manifestations of AR are not typical, and refractory ratio is increased. However, early diagnosis of AR is helpful for the treatment of patients and reduces rejection of physical injury and even death. Therefore, early diagnosis of AR is especially important in organ transplantation. The early diagnosis of AR is mainly manifested in the postoperative immune detection. The established immune detection methods include the percentage of lymphocyte subgroup and functional testing, immune function test, immune molecule level test, DC subgroup detection, etc. Still the detection needs to be combined with graft living tissue pathologic examination, serum biochemical measures, radiology examination, and the clinical manifestations of the patients to have a comprehensive observation. We will introduce the determination of immune molecule level as an example.

Cytokines

When the graft enters the body, the immune cells of the body are sensitized to HLA antigen and produce cytokines, such as interleukin (IL)-2, IL-4, IL-5, IL-6, IL-10, interferon (IFN)-y, tumor necrosis factor (TNF), etc., which often act as indicators of the early diagnosis of AR.

Perforin, Granular Enzyme B, Fas/Fas Ligand, and Particle Lysine

When AR occurs, once cytotoxic T cells are activated, perforin/particle enzyme will directly lead to B cell swelling, rupture, dissolution, and apoptosis caused by Fas/Fas ligand and attack target cells. Monitoring of the transplant recipients of peripheral blood lymphocyte perforin/granular enzyme B mRNA expression denotes that the two indicators increase significantly, when recipients have AR, and become lower after hormone treatment. Thus, perforin/particle enzyme B mRNA expression is a noninvasive and sensitive early predictor of AR and helps to understand antirejection effect at the same time.

CD Molecules

CD30 is one of the TNF superfamilies, regulating Thl/Th2 response. CD30 mainly expresses on the surface of the T cells that secrete Th2 cytokines. After the $CD30^+$ T cell activation, its extracellular part is released into the blood by protease hydrolysis, the formation of serum-soluble CD30 (sCD30). The expression level of sCD30 protein in serum with AR is significantly higher than those without AR. Monitoring the expression of sCD30 is helpful to predict the AR.

Chemokines

Chemokines IFN-γ-inducible protein 10 (IP-10 CXCL10) can rapidly express in endothelial cells of donor organs after transplantation and promote NK cells' and T cells' gathering, activation, and expression of the corresponding receptor CXCR3. Fractalkine is one of the family members of CX3C and has the function of adhesion and chemotaxis to the IL-2, NK, and $CD8^+$ T cell. Peng *et al.* found that transplant recipients urine fractalkine mRNA continuously express high, and eventually AR occurs. Therefore, monitoring organ transplantation urine fractalkine mRNA level is of great significance in AR prediction and early treatment.

C4d

C4 is one of the complement proteins in the patient's blood complement system, hydrolyzed as C4a and C4b by C1, and then split to C4d and big fragment C4c; C4d has the activated sulfhydryl. In 1993, Feucht et al. first reported the relationship between graft capillary endothelial surface complement fragments' C4d precipitation and the graft loss, and the histological indexes can be used as the indicators of humoral rejection. So the clinical monitoring of C4d has significant meaning to the recipients.

The existing rejection monitoring technology is not ideal enough. In the future we need to establish a kind of AR-associated molecular monitoring system characterized by less technical complication, lower cost, noninvasion, integration, and higher sensitivity, which can provide AR early warning information, so that a definite diagnosis, as early as possible, can be made to reduce the inactivation caused by rejection and graft function.

1.2 The Development of ABO Blood Group Incompatibility Organ Transplantation

In general, organ transplants are performed only when donor and recipient blood types are compatible. However, in order to effectively solve the shortage of organ donors, and to provide new hope for more patients on the waiting list, some transplant centers have also started trying ABO-incompatible organ transplantation, and made the corresponding breakthrough, including the ABO-incompatible kidney transplantation, ABO-incompatible liver transplantation, ABO-incompatible heart transplantation, etc. And ABO-incompatible kidney transplantation is the forerunner and motivation of other organ transplantations.

1.2.1 The Development of ABO-Incompatible Kidney Transplantation

The ABO system was discovered by Austrian Karl Landsteiner, a prominent pathologist and physiologist at the University of Vienna, at the beginning of the twentieth century. This achievement also earned him the Nobel Prize in Physiology or Medicine in 1930.

In 1952, Hume and his partners performed the world's first case of ABO -incompatible kidney transplantation. Sadly the transplanted kidney failed to restore its function, and the operation failed.

In 1964, Starzl performed ABO-incompatible kidney transplantation for two patients, one of whom with incompatible type B blood achieved long-term graft survival.

In 1965, the Japanese Inou, Ota, and their colleagues completed an unfettered kidney transplantation, but the graft had a repulsive reaction.

In 1967, Sonoda and his colleagues completed a case of ABO-incompatible kidney transplantation accidentally without special treatment before operation but obtained long-term survival.

In the same year, Gleason and Murray reorganized the materials about ABO-incompatible transplantation. The report indicated that the surgeries have not yielded satisfactory results. After the report, ABO-incompatible kidney transplantation almost stopped.

In 1981, because of mismatch in the process of kidney transplant, acute rejection occurred in Slapak's patients, but this unintentional medical accident led him to introduce an important concept—plasma exchange. Plasma exchange can effectively reduce the incidence of acute rejection after organ transplantation due to the donation from cadaveric donors or blood group-incompatible transplantation caused by procedural errors. This is the first report that clearly demonstrates the effect of plasma exchange on handling the rejection of ABO-incompatible organs.

Since then, ABO-incompatible transplantation has enjoyed the rapid development, and a variety of methods are adopted to reduce recipients' anti-A/anti-B antibodies and suppress the activity of immune cells, such as removal of plasma, plasma exchange, splenectomy, and a series of immunosuppressive drugs, immune adsorbent, etc.

In 1985, Alexandre [2] used plasma exchange therapy to remove anti-A/anti-B antibodies for ABO-incompatible kidney transplantation patients before operation and particularly emphasized on the importance of splenectomy to realize long-term graft attrition and had a clinical observation of the postoperative graft survival condition. In 1987, Cardella's findings also supported this conclusion and also carried out the plasma exchange treatment for the patients of ABO blood group incompatibility renal transplantation postoperatively.

In 1987, Bannett and his colleagues from the United States used immune adsorbent selective removal of pre-existing antibodies in the blood plasma and put particular emphasis on the importance of splenectomy to realize long-term graft attrition and observed the postoperative graft survival condition.

In 1989, Japanese Takahashi and his colleagues, by using double-plasma purification filter before transplant, in combination with immune adsorption to remove the antibodies in the serum and the spleen excision surgery, successfully achieved long-term graft survival after surgery.

Later, from January 1989 to December 1995, 67 cases of ABO-incompatible renal transplantation were performed in Tokyo Nephrology Center of Women's Medical Center, Japan. The survival rate of transplant kidney compared with ABO-compatible kidney transplant is basically identical [3].

Internationally, Japan established the association of ABO blood group incompatibility renal transplantations in 1998 and, in 2001, established the ABO blood group incompatibility kidney transplant research center and made breakthroughs in renal transplantation research afterwards [4].

In China, ABO blood group incompatibility transplantation set out relatively late. On December 14, 2006, in the second affiliated hospital of South China University, Professor Wang Yi et al. completed the first ABO blood group incompatibility of kidney transplantation in mainland China, and the patient acquired long-term survival under the condition of preserving the spleen.

Up to now, on the basis of blood purification and immunosuppressive treatment, ABO-incompatible kidney transplantation has had better curative effect than ABO-compatible kidney transplantation and has not increased the risk of rejection or infection in the recipients of ABO blood group-incompatible transplantation.

1.2.2 The Development of ABO-Incompatible Liver Transplantation

On March 1, 1963, Starzl implemented the first cases of human liver transplantation. The patient is a 3-year-old child who suffered from congenital biliary atresia but died soon after operation. In Starzl's words "the operation began with a confident, but ended in disaster. The child only survived for 4 hours." Two months later, Thomas, who was known as the father of liver transplantation later, completed a second liver transplant surgery, which was very successful. Unfortunately, 22 days later, the patient died of pulmonary embolism, but the liver was in good condition.

In the 1960s and 1970s, because of the low survival rate after liver transplantation, liver transplantation has been in the stage of clinical research rather than a clinical treatment widely used. The advent of CSA completely changed the stagnant situation of liver transplantation, becoming an important milestone in the history of liver transplantation.

Both at home and abroad existed the serious lack of donor liver. Some of the patients with severe liver disease, due to a long wait for a suitable donor liver, had more serious complications and eventually died. In order to alleviate the contradiction of the lack of cadaveric donor liver, living donor liver transplantation has been maturely developed in foreign countries. It has also started in our country. But in clinical application, the liver donor and receptor ABO blood group inconsistent phenomenon often happens. Even parents and their children have about 10% possibility of different ABO blood groups. Therefore, in the case of an emergency or shortage of donor liver, ABO blood group incompatibility can be carried out for the receptor of liver transplantation.

In 1985, the French chirurgie pediatrique had an earlier report of the ABO blood group incompatibility liver transplantation [5]. Afterwards, it has been increasing worldwide and has made great strides, but there still exists a lot of controversy.

Early in the twentieth century (1980s–1990s), in Japan, a series of ABO blood group incompatibility liver transplantation experiments found that serious postoperative rejection, hepatic artery thrombosis, and refractory intrahepatic bile duct injury were likely to happen after operation. Demetris et al. also recorded the graft characteristic pathologic results of the transplant failure, including the hepatic sinus tubules and small artery endothelial immune complex deposition and hepatic parenchymal hemorrhage and necrosis [6].

In the early 1990s, the accumulated experience of living liver transplantation enabled ABO blood group incompatibility liver transplantation to grow. But the results of early ABO blood group incompatibility living donor liver transplantation are poorer, especially in older children and adults [7, 8].

In 1998, in Japan the hepatic portal vein infusion (Fig. 1.2) [9, 10] was first introduced to treat adult living ABO blood group incompatibility of liver transplantation and achieved great success. Partial graft infusion treatment has overcome the barrier of the ABO blood group, which is a crucial breakthrough in the development of ABO blood group incompatibility liver transplantation.

In 2003, using Rituxan infusion in local graft significantly raised the survival rate of the patients of ABO blood group incompatibility liver transplantation, and further perfected the ABO blood group incompatibility liver transplantation technique, which began to be widely applied in clinical practice.

The ABO blood group incompatibility of liver transplantation in our country is started rather late. In 2004, Professor Zhi-Hai Peng, in the first people's hospital affiliated to Shanghai Jiao Tong University, successfully carried out an emergency blood group incompatibility liver transplantation surgery in the treatment of acute liver failure.

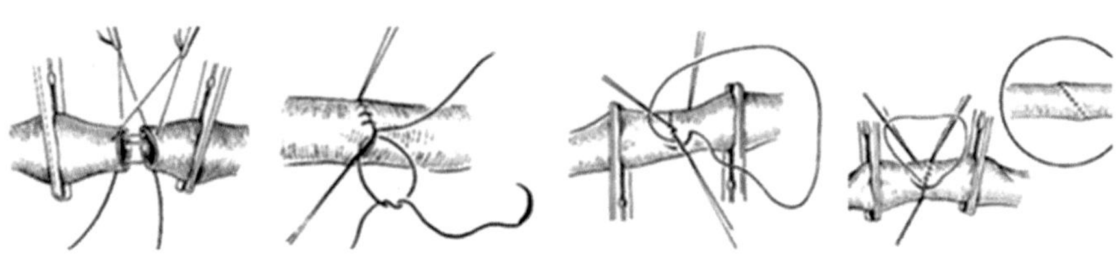

Fig. 1.2 Hepatic portal vein infusion

At present, for ABO-incompatible liver transplantation, the younger, the better effect; 5-year survival rate of babies less than 1 year old, children from 1 to 7 years old, children 8–15 and 16 years old, and adults are 76%, 68%, 53%, and 76%, respectively. So, until the latest, the adult of ABO-incompatible liver transplantation has a poorer curative effect and even is viewed as relatively contraindicated or as a final treatment for adult liver failure [10, 11]. In contrast, the effect of ABO-incompatible liver transplantation in infants is excellent and comparable to that of ABO-matched allografts and will even be better in the near future.

1.2.3 The Development of ABO-Incompatible Heart Transplantation

Heart transplantation is a surgical transplant mainly for advanced congestive heart failure and severe coronary artery disease. Until 2013, the most common surgical procedure is to take out the successfully matched human heart of a brain death completely and implant it into the receptor's chest, which is called allogeneic transplant. The receptor's own heart can be removed (called orthotopic heart transplantation) or retained to support the donor heart (called heterotopic heart transplantation). The heart transplant is not the conventional treatment of heart disease but one way to save life of end-stage heart disease patients and improve their life quality.

In December 1967, Cape Town, South Africa, Doctor Barnard [12] successfully performed the world's first orthotopic heart transplantation, although the patient only lived for 18 days after the operation due to pulmonary infection, but the success of this operation has attracted people's attention to heart transplantation in the world. His second heart transplant patient survived for 20 months. Soon after the first heart transplant in the world, Shumway and his colleagues completed their first heart transplants after full preparation. However, because of a series of problems, such as organ rejection after transplantation and selection criteria for receptors, which cannot be well solved, and the influence of traditional culture and religion, the development of heart transplantation has been stagnant for a long time afterwards.

With more liberation from traditional culture and religion, and the development of the heart transplant technology, in 1984, heart transplantation began to be widely used clinically. Since then the heart transplant has been leaping forward. Now each year, about 3500 people around the world undergo a heart transplant, and about 50,000 heart transplants have been completed globally. The increasing number of heart transplantation brings about the situation of a lack of donors. To solve the problem of donor deficiency, the advanced heart transplant centers in some countries begin to take ABO-incompatible cardiac transplantation into consideration, so that more patients waiting for heart transplant will avoid the occurrence of more serious complications and even death, which will give the patient new hope of life.

From 1996 to 2000, Lori J. West et al. [12] selected ten babies of 4 h to 14 months after birth with cardiomyopathy or congenital heart disease and other diseases and performed the ABO-incompatible heart transplantation for them, testing serum kin hemagglutinin drop degree before and after transplantation, using plasma exchange in extracorporeal circulation to remove the antibody in vivo, using standardized immunosuppressive therapy, and monitoring transplantation rejection through myocardial endometrial biopsy. Subsequently, the ten ABO-incompatible heart transplant patients were followed up from 11 months to 4.6 years, whose total survival rate was 80%. It was found that the premature death of two patients has nothing to do with the ABO incompatibility. The newborn does not produce antibody A and antibody B, and the same RBC lectins and antibody concentration in serum usually remain low until 12–14 months [13]; in addition, for a small baby, the complement system is not perfect [14]. Therefore, no early super acute rejection exists. Due to ABO-incompatible heart transplantation, the death rate of children waiting for a heart transplant decreased from 58 to 7%.

Since the middle and late 1990s, after the ABO blood group incompatibility heart transplantation for infants and young children, the number of ABO blood group incompatibility heart transplantation has been increasing. It definitely provides a new hope for infants and young children, who needed heart transplantation and whose immune system was not completely developed. In addition, it may also benefit the elderly patients and those patients who have the same red blood cell lectin-specific blood type antibody.

In 2009, Tyden G et al. [15] chose 6 relatively appropriate recipients from 13 patients who were suffering from heart disease and needed heart transplantation and carried out the ABO blood group incompatibility heart transplants at the Karolinska University Hospital in Sweden. The antibodies A and B in patients' body had been removed through plasma exchange treatment before operation, the IgG antibody drop degree of the patients decreased, and a series of immunosuppressive therapy were also conducted after operation. During postoperative 1-year follow-up, two patients survived. ABO-incompatible heart transplantation may be considered to have a certain feasibility for adults who need heart transplantation, although the efficacy has a certain gap compared to ABO blood group compatible heart transplantation, but there are a lot of rooms to grow.

So far, ABO-incompatible heart transplantation has been widely applied for infant patients who need heart transplants and has good curative effect. According to reports of many ABO blood group incompatibility heart transplants, the curative effect is better than the blood compatibility of heart transplantation. But applications in adult patients remain to be further developed.

1.2.4 The Development of ABO Blood Group Incompatibility Lung Transplantation

In 1963, James Hardy performed the first human lung transplantation surgery at the University of Mississippi for the 58-year-old man who suffered squamous cell carcinomas on the left side of the lung and pulmonary emphysema in the contralateral side. After surviving for 18 days, the patient died of kidney failure and malnutrition [16].

In 1983, Cooper performed the right lung transplant operation for a 58-year-old male patient with end-stage pulmonary fibrosis. The patient recovered and came back to normal life after a few weeks. Unfortunately he died of kidney failure after six and a half years. From 1983 to 1985, the lung transplantation group in Toronto led by Cooper has reported a total of seven cases of single lung transplantation, among which five cases survived [17], which further promoted the work of lung transplantation.

With the success of many lung transplants, people began to accept the surgery. Clinically, lung transplant is developed actively, and this technology has been more and more mature and become one of the effective methods to treat end-stage lung function failure. But with the wider use of lung transplantation in the clinic, and more and more patients on the waiting list, there exists shortage of donors. However, ABO-incompatible lung transplantation, which can effectively relieve the donor shortage situation, began to be carried out in some countries and transplant centers.

In 2003, James Jaggers et al. carried out the world's first case of ABO blood group incompatibility heart-lung transplantation for a 17-year-old girl, implementing the related immune therapy before and after surgery, but the patient finally died of transplant rejection and only survived for 4 days. Although the operation failed, it's a good beginning, which paved the way for ABO blood group incompatibility lung transplantation.

In 2008, M. Struber et al. [18] reported a case of a 21-year-old female patient who was cured after the ABO-incompatible lung transplantation. The patient received plasma replacement, immunosorbent, rituxan, and a series of immunosuppression before and after surgery. Nine months later, the patients completely recovered and were discharged from the hospital. The success of this operation shows that the ABO-incompatible lung transplantation is feasible clinically, and a series of immunosuppressive therapies are effective. With the technology development, the effect of ABO-incompatible lung transplantation can be comparable to ABO-compatible lung transplantation or even surpass it so as to be widely implemented in clinical application.

1.3 The Breakthroughs in the History of ABO-Incompatible Organ Transplantation

One of the main current problems facing ABO-incompatible organ transplantation is the rejection. Since 1981 when Slapak made the first report of using plasma exchange therapy to treat the transplant renal acute rejection caused by the ABO blood group wrong match, clinically plasma exchange has been used to remove A and B antigens of preoperative patients. Later, a series of clinical cases confirmed that blood purification plays an important role in the development of ABO-incompatible organ transplantation, which was a breakthrough in the history of ABO-incompatible organ transplantation. Blood purification scheme includes plasma exchange singly, double filtration plasmapheresis, immune adsorption, plasma exchange and double filtration plasmapheresis, plasma exchange and static note immunoglobulin (IVIG), plasma exchange/double filtration plasmapheresis, and CMV immunoglobulin (CMVIg).

1.3.1 Plasma Exchange (PE)

Plasma exchange (PE) is the process of taking out the patient's blood, applying membrane filtration separation or centrifugal separation method, separating blood plasma and cell composition, removing pathogenic factors in the plasma or the plasma, and infusing the cells and other components and equal amount of displacement fluid to the plasma lost back into the patient's body, so as to clear pathological substances and treat various diseases where general therapies are invalid. Its indications are myasthenia gravis, kidney diseases in the nervous system diseases of acute progressive glomerulonephritis, the blood disease of thrombotic thrombocytopenic purpura severe hepatitis, liver diseases, immune diseases caused by rheumatoid arthritis, certain drug overdose poisoning, etc.

In ABO-incompatible organ transplantation, the treatment theory of PE is as follows: take out the patient's blood, isolate the plasma from whole blood of patients through membrane plasma separation method, abandon the plasma, and then add the same amount of fresh frozen plasma or blood albumin displacement fluid to remove the A or B antibodies, so that the rejection of the ABO blood group-incompatible organ transplantation can be alleviated.

Advantages of plasma exchange are the following: (1) it can remove small molecules, the molecules, and macromolecular substances and especially has significant effect on toxin combined with protein; (2) it has certain effect on correcting common electrolyte imbalance and acid-base balance disorders in liver failure; (3) it can add substances necessary for human such as protein and blood coagulation factor; (4) it is suitable for all kinds of severe hepatitis patients; and (5) it gives priority to fresh frozen plasma (FFP) and can add some substitute such as low molecular dextran, hydroxyethyl starch, etc.

The shortcomings of plasma exchange are the following: (1) plasma purification is much less effective than the hemodialysis and hemofiltration; (2) it's unable to improve the condition of water overload; and (3) a large number of plasma needed, and a large number of inputs, such as blood plasma adjuvant therapies for many times, are exposed to all kinds of infections, especially new virus infection.

1.3.2 Immunoadsorption (IA)

Immunosorbent (immunoadsorption, IA) is the technique of treating diseases by extracorporeal circulation, using antigen-antibody immune response to remove pathogenic factors in the plasma or using adsorption materials to remove the pathogenic factors related to immunity. Immunoadsorption indications are very extensive, including the following:

1. A variety of rheumatic autoimmune disease, especially in systemic lupus erythematosus (SLE), systemic vasculitis, etc.
2. *Skin diesease associated with immune dysfunctions*
3. Kidney disease associated with immune nephritis, including purpura kidney and IgA nephropathy
4. The digestive system diseases, such as fulminant hepatic failure, primary biliary cirrhosis, obstructive jaundice, etc.
5. The nervous system diseases, such as Guillain-Barré syndrome, myasthenia gravis, frequent demyelinating neuropathy, etc.

6. Blood system diseases, such as cryoglobulinemia, macroglobulinemia, autoimmune hemolytic anemia, multiple myeloma, etc.
7. Endocrine metabolic disease, such as hyperlipidemia, hyperthyroidism crisis, type Idiabetes, and obesity
8. Poisoning, such as organophosphate poisoning

In ABO blood group incompatibility transplantation, the treatment principle of IA is using highly specific antigen and adsorption materials (carrier) in the selective removal of specific antibodies of blood cells in plasma so as to reduce postoperative rejection of transplantation. For ABO blood group-incompatible organ transplantation, preoperative immunosorbent to receptors every other day can reduce the drop degree resistance to blood type antibody (1:8 below average or lower than 1:2 compared with the donor cells), and for patients of highly allergic immunity, it can quickly remove the HLA antibodies, and turn cross match to negative, reducing the incidence of acute rejection.

Immunoadsorption therapy is a new technology developed on the basis of the plasma exchange. Compared with the commonly used plasma exchange in the past, immunosorbent has obvious advantages in the efficacy, safety, etc. First of all, the adsorption removal of pathogenic immune antibody is relatively complete. Second, the input of the patients' own plasma reduces the loss of useful components both in scope and number, and needs no supplement exogenous plasma and the displacement fluid, which can effectively prevent the spread of infectious diseases. Finally, the patients' own plasma back to the body can avoid more common problems in the plasma exchange such as citrate salt poisoning, abnormal blood clotting mechanism, allergic reactions, low blood pressure, hypokalemia, etc. In addition, the immune adsorption, with high selectivity and specificity, does not affect the drug treatment at the same time, consumes less materials, and costs less.

Adverse reactions of immune adsorption are mainly related to extracorporeal circulation process, and the use of the replacement of fluid and anticoagulants, which must be closely observed and given correct treatment. Common complications include hypotension, hypocalcemia, arrhythmia, allergic reaction, infection, hemolysis, and bleeding or clotting disorders.

1.3.3 Double Filtration Plasmapheresis (DFPP)

Double filtration plasmapheresis (DFPP) is a kind of selective plasma separation method, which uses two filtration membranes of different apertures, one for the plasma separator and the other for plasma filtration device. Because the plasma filtration membrane pore size is different, the albumin repression rate is also different, so treatment should choose different apertures of hemofiltration based on the molecular weight of pathogenic substances both to ensure the complete elimination of pathogenic matters and to minimize the loss of albumin. The application principle of double filtration plasmapheresis in ABO blood group incompatibility organ transplantation is that after primary separation of patient's blood, the plasma undergoes secondary separation to have the A and B antibodies removed, and then the plasma without A and B antibodies and blood visible part are returned to the body, so that the patients have lower antibody concentration in the body to meet preoperative indicators of antibody concentration.

DFPP is a new technology developed on the technique of membrane plasma separation. At present, it is widely used in the treatment of myasthenia gravis in the nervous system diseases, kidney diseases accelerated glomerulonephritis, the severe hepatitis of liver diseases, and immune diseases such as rheumatoid arthritis. Here we want to focus on its application in organ transplantation. In the ABO blood group incompatibility renal transplantation, DFPP is a reliable way to remove A and B antibodies. In the meantime, DFPP can also remove anti-HLA antibodies in patients with positive panel-reactive antibodies.

DFPP as a safe and effective treatment method, compared with the pure plasma exchange (PE) effect, has no obvious difference, but has the following advantages:

1. Loss of the plasma volume is relatively small. Every separation of 3–4 L of plasma loses about 500–600 mL of plasma and has kept most of albumin, namely, minimizing the loss of albumin.
2. Cross infection is reduced. DFPP uses albumin replacement fluid and has relatively less PE complications such as infections.

DFPP also has its own disadvantages:

1. DFPP cannot specifically remove pathogens. During the process of removing pathogenic substances, macromolecular substances were removed too. But immunoadsorption (IA) therapy can choose different adsorbers to remove pathogenic substances specifically in the plasma according to the different diseases. In terms of specificity, DFPP is not so good as IA.
2. Plasma filter has a certain repression of albumin, so there will be inevitably a small amount of loss. DFPP can rapidly reduce the concentration of these pathogenic factors in plasma, but cannot stop its production, so DFPP is not the root treatment and cannot completely replace the treatment of immunosuppression; it must be combined with immunosuppressive agents and other treatment programs to be more effective.

In addition, in the development of ABO-incompatible organ transplantation, application of splenectomy and Rituxan is also an important progress. The spleen is a peripheral immune organ. So early researches, which advocate conventional splenectomy in the ABO blood group-incompatible organ transplantation, suggest that splenectomy can effectively reduce the A and B antibody titers, reduce the number of B lymphocytes which produce antibodies, and improve the success rate of ABO blood group-incompatible organ transplantation. But the spleen surgery increases the risk of severe infection and sepsis in recipients and triggers immune deficiency of children under the age of 3. Recent researches show that there are a lot of memory B lymphocytes in the bone marrow, and spleen resection is invalid in this case. At present, most scholars recommended Rituxan (anti-CD20 monoclonal antibody) induction therapy in replacement of splenectomy. This can be regarded as a sort of temporary splenectomy but avoids the long-term risk of infection caused by splenectomy. Also some scholars advocate the splenectomy as salvage treatment measures of acute antibody-mediated rejection.

1.4 The Current Status of ABO-Incompatible Organ Transplantation

The success rate of ABO-incompatible organ transplantation has been increased more than ever, and now many patients with organ failure can be treated this way. Especially, both the short-term and long-term survival rates of kidney and liver transplantation have been greatly improved. On the other hand, ABO-incompatible organ transplantation costs no more than ABO-compatible organ transplantation but differs in the curative effect on different organs. For example, the effect of ABO -incompatible kidney transplantation is as good as or even better than ABO -compatible kidney transplantation. The curative effect of ABO-incompatible liver transplantation is basically identical with ABO-compatible liver transplantation. The effect of ABO-incompatible heart transplantation is even better than ABO-compatible transplantation for the younger children, but for the adult, it's far less satisfactory. So, in some cases, ABO-incompatible organ transplantation is only performed when patients are in critical condition and there is an absence of ABO-compatible donors. The success rate of ABO-incompatible organ transplantation is associated with many factors, such as age, patients' condition preoperative, etc. At present, although there are many ways to restrain the complications such as hyperacute rejection and acute rejection in ABO-incompatible organ transplantation, most of these drugs can cause various adverse reactions [19].

Infections are common complications due to immunosuppressive treatment pre- and post-renal transplantation. Only when the infection is controlled could we perform transplantation. Posttransplantation infections should also be given due caution. In addition, it is difficult to draw a unified standard because each organ transplant center has different treatment schemes and also differs in pretransplantation antibody levels. What's more, due to technical limitations, is that different transplant centers also have different opinions on the monitoring of antibody level after transplantation.

In conclusion, ABO-incompatible organ transplantation has made great strides in the short half a century, especially the past 20 years, but there are many problems to be solved toward the goal of more extensive application.

2 Basic Concepts of ABO-Incompatible Organ Transplantation

2.1 ABO-Incompatible Organ Transplantation

ABO-incompatible organ transplantation refers to the transplantation between the two blood group incompatibility individuals, during which an individual's healthy organ is transplanted to the other one and restores its function quickly. Its purpose is to replace the organ loss of function due to fatal diseases and enable the transplanted individuals to have the corresponding organs again, which will work normally. Now the ABO-incompatibility organ transplantation often carried out includes the kidney, heart, liver, lung, small intestine, bone marrow, etc. So far, in the face of the shortage of donor organs, ABO-incompatible organ transplantation has already become the most effective treatment for end-stage organ failure. Since 1954, when the renal transplantation succeeded in the United States in Boston, human beings have been able to transplant almost all the important tissues and organs except the brain. Individuals providing organs are known as donors (also called supplier); and individuals accepting graft are receptors (also known as the hosts, recipients); the transplanted cells, tissues, or organs are known as graft (transplant).

2.2 The Classifications of the Transplantation

2.2.1 Classifications According to the Genetic Differences of Donors and Recipients

Autologous Transplantation

Cells, tissues, and organs are getting access to themselves and implanted in their own body, namely, the organ donors and recipients are the same. No rejection occurs, and the organ can survive permanently, such as in situ implant (also called replantation, such as limb reattachment).

Isogeneic Transplantation

The donor and receptor are not the same individual, but they have identical genes. The receptor receives graft from the same gene donor and will have no rejection, such as the transplantation between the identical twin in the clinical application.

Allogeneic Transplantation

The donor and receptor are the same species, but their genes are different. It is the most widely used transplantation currently, and transplant rejection occurs. For example, kidney transplant and liver transplant between different individuals all belong to allogeneic transplantation.

Heterogeneous Transplantation
It refers to transplant between different individual species, which can cause very strong rejection after transplantation, such as the transplant of chimpanzee heart or baboon liver to human beings.

2.2.2 Classifications According to the Anatomical Position Classification

1. *Orthotopic transplantation* refers to the removal of the original diseased organs, and the transplant of the new organ to its original anatomical location, such as orthotopic liver transplantation and orthotopic heart transplantation.
2. *Heterotopic transplantation or auxiliary transplantation* refers to the transplant of the new organ to the part different from the original anatomical location, such as the vast majority of normal kidney and pancreas transplantation. In general, ectopic transplantation can proceed without removal of the original organ.
3. *Paratopic transplantation* refers to the transplant of the organ to the position close to the original organ, without resection or partial resection, such as paratopic pancreas transplantation.

2.2.3 Classifications According to Different Transplant Technologies

1. *Vascularized transplantation or vascular anastomosis transplantation* refers to blood vessels of the graft being cut off completely from the donor and anastomosed to the recipients, when transplanted, to establish effective blood circulation and restore blood supply immediately. Most of the substantial clinical organ transplantation, such as heart transplantation and liver transplantation and so on, all belong to this category.
2. *Pedicled transplantation* refers to the graft still having the pedicle of major blood vessels and lymphatic vessels or nerves connected with the donor, and the rest are separated in order to be transferred to the other parts needed, and blood is still in supply during the procedure. After the grafts set up the new blood circulation, the peduncle will be separated. Such transplants are all autologous transplantation, such as all kinds of skin flap transplantation.
3. *Dissociated transplantation* refers to the graft completely separated from the donor, without vascular anastomosis when transplanted. The establishment of the blood supply of grafts relies on the new blood vessels of recipients' surrounding tissues and the gradual growth into the graft, such as the dissociated flap skin grafting.
4. *Infused transplantation* refers to making the graft into dynamic cell or tissue suspension, which will then be inputted or injected into the recipients' body through various approaches, such as blood transfusion and bone marrow transplant.

In addition, according to the graft donor sources, there are classifications into cadaveric donor transplantation, embryo donor transplantation, living donor transplantation, expanding standard donor transplantation, domino organ transplant donor transplantation, and graft reusing donor transplantation. According to the nature of graft, it can be divided into cell transplantation and tissue transplantation, composite tissue transplantation, organ transplantation, multiple organ transplantation, and organ cluster transplantation.

In clinical application, in order to accurately describe the transplantation of some organs, the classifications and terminologies above are usually integrated, such as corpse orthotopic liver transplantation (OLT), living relative same ectopic kidney transplantation, vascular anastomosis of fetal parathyroid heterotopic transplantation, etc.

2.3 Related Terms of ABO-Incompatible Organ Transplantation

1. *Antigen* refers to substance that stimulates the body producing specific immune response and can be combined with immune response product (antibodies) and sensitized lymphocytes in vivo and in vitro and exerts immune effect.
2. *Antibody* is an important effect molecule mediating humoral immunity, is a glycoprotein produced by plasma cells which is from proliferation of B cells after accepting antigen stimulation, mainly exists in the serum and other body fluids, and produces humoral immune function in combination with the corresponding antigen specificity.
3. *Innate immunity or nonspecific immunity* refers to the natural immune defense function formed in the process of germ line development and evolution, namely, the nonspecific defense function immediately after birth.
4. *Specific immunity or acquired immunity* refers to the antigen-specific T/B lymphocyte antigen stimulation after its activation, proliferation, and differentiation, as effector cells, the whole process of a series of biological effects.
5. *Histocompatibility antigens* refer to specific antigen existing on the graft that can combine with specific antibody in the body of recipients and cause the body to produce rejection in organ transplantation.
6. *Major histocompatibility complex* (MHC) is formed by a group of closely chained genes, located on a particular area of the chromosome in animals or people, and is highly polymorphic. Its coding molecules are expressed in different cell surfaces, participating in antigen present and restricting the mutual recognition between cells and inducing immune response.
7. *Human leukocyte antigen* (HLA) refers to the major histocompatibility complex coding gene product in the human body. The antigen is close to rejection after organ transplantation and is also called the organ transplantation antigens.
8. *Panel reactive antibodies* (PRA) refer to the HLA antibodies in the body of recipients. Taking common HLA alleles as antigen in a particular crowd, the recipients' plasma reaction rate of this group of antigen is observed. Lower than

10% of HLA reaction is called not sensitization, and higher than 40% means high sensitization. PRA are important indicators of sensitized recipients preoperative of all kinds of tissue organ transplantation, closely related with transplant rejection and survival.

9. *Donor-specific antibody* (DSA). A portion of PRA antibodies are against donor organs, or after recipients accept the organ transplant, the body produces antibodies against the organ, called DSA.
10. *Allograft rejection* (AR) refers to the immune response in recipients induced by the alloantigens carried in the transplanted organs, which are the humoral immune response and cellular immune response. According to the onset time, allograft rejection can be divided into hyperacute rejection, accelerated rejection, acute rejection, and chronic rejection.
11. *Hyperacute rejection* (HAR) refers to the rejection occurring within a few minutes to 24 h after the transplanted organ blood vessels and recipients are switched on, and often mediated by native persisting antibody, which can be seen in patients who have a history of repeated blood transfusion, multiple pregnancies, repeated blood transfusion, multiple pregnancies, long-term hemodialysis, or retransplantation. Once HAR occurs, it is irreversible.
12. *Accelerated rejection* or vascular rejection or delayed super acute rejection, refers to the accelerate rejection in 2–5 days after transplantation. Accelerated acute rejection may have relations with cellular and humoral rejection. It can be reversed after the measures of the plasma exchange treatment.
13. *Acute rejection* (AR). Graft antigens released from endothelia a few days after transplantation stimulate the lymphoid tissue of recipients, and cause immune response, which leads to graft rejection. AR is the most common type of allogeneic organ transplantation and generally occurs in a month after the transplantation.
14. *Chronic rejection* (CR) mainly occurs by the cycle of low levels of specific antibody immune response causing inflammation around the blood vessels, which resulted in continued low degree of graft endothelial damage, accompanied by vascular smooth muscle cell hyperplasia blocking blood vessels, and graft function gradually declines. CR, which is often slow and occult, mainly occurs in months or years after surgery or after acute rejection.
15. *Immunological tolerance* refers to the T cells and B cells not being activated under the stimulation of antigen and producing no specific immune effector cells and specific antibodies and thus performing no immune response. Immune tolerance includes natural immune tolerance and induced immune tolerance.
16. *Immune accommodation* is based on Alexandre and Chopek's successful attempt on human ABO-incompatible kidney transplantation in the 1980s. In order to avoid humoral rejection caused by stored blood type antibody, recipients accept preoperative plasma exchange treatment many times, so that body blood type antibody concentration in recipients is relatively low on the day of surgery and early postoperation period. Though recipients' blood type antibody can be restored to normal levels after stopping plasma exchange treatment, the body's blood type antibody can be restored to normal levels, but the researchers found that 80% of the patients didn't have rejection as expected. This phenomenon indicates that it has some other biological mechanisms, which are different from

immune tolerance. This phenomenon that grafts survive without rejection reaction when the recipients are under the condition of existing graft antibodies and normal complement is called immune accommodation, which has a very important research and clinical value in overcoming the homograft humoral rejection and in the field of xenograft.

References

1. De Boer J, De Meester J, Smits JM, et al. Eurotransplant randomized multicenter kidney graft preservation study comparing HTK with UW and euro-collins. Transpl Int. 1999;12:447–53.
2. Alexandre GP, De Bruyere M, Squifflet JP, et al. Human abo-incompatible living donor renal homografts. Neth J Med. 1985;28:231–4.
3. Tanabe K, Takahashi K, Sonda K, et al. Long-term results of abo-incompatible living kidney transplantation: a single-center experience. Transplantation. 1998;65:224–8.
4. Hatakeyama S, Fujita T, Murakami R, et al. Outcome comparison of abo-incompatible kidney transplantation with low-dose rituximab and abo-compatible kidney transplantation: a single-center experience. Transplant Proc. 2014;46:445–8.
5. Muiesan P, Vergani D, Mieli-Vergani G. Liver transplantation in children. J Hepatol. 2007;46:340–8.
6. Demetris AJ, Jaffe R, Tzakis A, et al. Antibody-mediated rejection of human orthotopic liver allografts. A study of liver transplantation across abo blood group barriers. Am J Pathol. 1988;132:489–502.
7. Gugenheim J, Samuel D, Reynes M, et al. Liver transplantation across abo blood group barriers. Lancet. 1990;336:519–23.
8. Farges O, Kalil AN, Samuel D, et al. The use of abo-incompatible grafts in liver transplantation: a life-saving procedure in highly selected patients. Transplantation. 1995;59:1124–33.
9. Toso C, Al-Qahtani M, Alsaif FA, et al. Abo-incompatible liver transplantation for critically ill adult patients. Transpl Int. 2007;20:675–81.
10. Tanabe M, Kawachi S, Obara H, et al. Current progress in abo-incompatible liver transplantation. Eur J Clin Investig. 2010;40:943–9.
11. Pratschke J, Tullius SG. Promising recent data on abo incompatible liver transplantation: restrictions may apply. Transpl Int. 2007;20:647–8.
12. West LJ, Pollock-Barziv SM, Dipchand AI, et al. Abo-incompatible heart transplantation in infants. N Engl J Med. 2001;344:793–800.
13. Nguyen TC, Kiss JE, Goldman JR, et al. The role of plasmapheresis in critical illness. Crit Care Clin. 2012;28(3):453–68.
14. Schumacher KR, Gajarski RJ, Urschel S. Pediatric coronary allograft vasculopathy—a review of pathogenesis and risk factors. Congenit Heart Dis. 2012;7:312–23.
15. Tyden G, Hagerman I, Grinnemo KH, et al. Intentional abo-incompatible heart transplantation: a case report of 2 adult patients. J Heart Lung Transplant. 2012;31:1307–10.
16. Hardy JD, Webb WR, Dalton ML, et al. Lung homotransplantation in man. JAMA. 1963;186:1065–74.
17. Cooper JD, Pearson FG, Patterson GA, et al. Technique of successful lung transplantation in humans. J Thorac Cardiovasc Surg. 1987;93:173–81.
18. Struber M, Warnecke G, Hafer C, et al. Intentional abo-incompatible lung transplantation. Am J Transplant. 2008;8:2476–8.
19. Hanto DW, Fecteau AH, Alonso MH, et al. Abo-incompatible liver transplantation with no immunological graft losses using total plasma exchange, splenectomy and quadruple immunosuppression: evidence for accommodation. Liver Transpl. 2003;9:22–30.

The RBC Blood Group Antigen System

2

Xiaopeng Hu, Zijian Zhang, and Song Zeng

Abstract

In this chapter, some of the human blood group systems and their specific antigens are discussed. The human blood group system is classified by erythrocyte antigens, and the antigenic determinant of erythrocyte can cause an immune response. The immune responses in blood type incompatible organ transplantation are mainly caused by the ABO antigen expression in the surface of tissue cell, so the ABO blood group antigens are considered in more detail. Rh, Duffy, Kell, and MN systems will also be described in this chapter.

Keywords

Blood group system · Rh blood system · Erythrocyte antigen · Hemagglutinin Glycoproteins · Allele gene

Introduction: The human blood group system is classified according to the erythrocyte surface antigens in different individuals. The antigens are synthesized by the sequence of glycoproteins. The genes encode glycosyltransferases, which carry out the sequence of glycoproteins. The erythrocyte surface glycoproteins have immunological properties which can induce allogeneic and heterogeneous immune responses. Different sequences of glycoprotein constitute the blood group system. According to the International Society of Blood Transfusion (ISBT), a total of 347 blood group systems have been identified, including the most common ABO blood group system and Rh blood group system. Described in this chapter are five blood group systems, ABO, Rh, Duffy, Kell, and MN systems.

X. Hu (✉) · Z. Zhang · S. Zeng
Department of Urology, Beijing Chao-Yang Hospital, Capital Medical University, Beijing, China
e-mail: huxp@ccmu.edu.cn; zzhang742@uwalumni.com; doctorzeng@mail.ccmu.edu.cn

Y. Wang (ed.), *ABO-incompatible Organ Transplantation*,
https://doi.org/10.1007/978-981-13-3399-6_2

1 ABO Blood Group System

- The ABO blood group system was the first human blood group system to be discovered. It was first reported by Landsteiner in 1901 [1], who found that A, B, and C could be recognized by mixing together erythrocytes and serum from different people. The following year von Decastello et al. [2] reported the fourth group (AB). Because the antibodies anti-A, anti-B, and anti-AB can be reactive at 37 °C in persons whose erythrocytes lack the corresponding antigens, so that if transfusions were to be given without regard to the ABO groups, lots of people would be incompatible. Therefore, the routine determination of ABO blood groups is the most important in transfusion practice. Moreover, because the regular presence of the immunological properties can induce immune responses, the ABO blood group system remains the most important aspect in organ transplantation immune response.

1.1 ABO System Phenotypes

The erythrocyte surface antigens are the primary basis to classify the ABO blood group system. The ABO blood group system can be categorized into four types, A, B, AB, and O, according to the species of agglutinogen (see Table 2.1). The group A only agglutinated the serum of group B, and the group B only agglutinated the serum of group A. In group AB, the serum neither agglutinate, and the erythrocytes are agglutinated by sera of all other groups. While in group O, the serum contains a mixture of two agglutinins capable to agglutinate A and B groups; the erythrocytes are not agglutinated by any serum. The ABO blood group system contains several subgroups, in which the subgroup of A group is the most common.

Table 2.1 Antibodies and antigens in the ABO system

Group	Subgroup	Antigens on red cells	Agglutinins in serum
O	–	None	Anti-A
			Anti-A_1
			Anti-B
			Anti-A, B
A	A_1	$A + A_1$	Anti-B
	A_2	A	
B	–	B	Anti-A
			Anti-A_1
AB	A_1B	$A + A_1 + B$	None
	A_2B	A + B	

1.1.1 Subgroups of A

A_1 and A_2

A group can be subdivided into A_1, A_2, and many other rare subgroups. About 80% of group A individuals belongs to subgroup A_1, almost all the rest being A_2. The most convenient method to distinguish them is to test erythrocytes with the lectin. The lectin agglutinates only subgroup A_1 in appropriate concentration.

It may be difficult to make a distinction between A_1 and A_2 in infants, because the erythrocyte of some infants can specifically present A_1, but they may not able to react with anti-A_1 regents when they are old. Test with anti-H lectin from *Laburnum alpinum* may be useful in such a situation: subgroup A_2 reacting much more strongly than subgroup A_1.

Differences Between Subgroups A_1 and A_2

As described in the following content, the number of A sites on subgroup A_1 is significantly higher than that on subgroup A_2. Due to the different cell population of individuals, the number of A sites per erythrocyte varies considerably for subgroup A_1 and A_2, but this difference is much greater for subgroup A_2 than for subgroup A_1 [3]. The difference in reactivity between subgroup A_1 and A_2 can be quantitative. It has been reported that a minimum of $2.5–4 \times 10^5$ A sites per erythrocyte were needed to agglutinate with anti-A_1 reagents [4]. Thus, the anti-A_1 can be considered as an antibody that reacts only with a certain minimum number of A sites.

Anti-A_1 was found in the serum of some subgroups A_2 and A_2B individuals. About 2–8% of subgroup A_2 individuals and 22–35% of subgroup A_2B individuals contained the anti-A. But the antibody is active at 37 °C only in rare individuals, so it can be ignored in blood transfusion and there is no need to distinguish A_1 from A_2 donors in routine practice. However, during blood collection, blood transfusion, and organ transplantation, a weak positive result or inconsistent test result of antigen and antibody may appear in consideration of the presence of A subgroups.

A_1- and A_2-specified transferases in serum differ quantitatively as well as qualitatively. Compared with subgroup A_1, the A_2-specified transferases had a base mutation of C to T at the 467 site, which caused the corresponding encoded protein mutation of proline to leucine at the 156 site. A base C deletion at the 1061 site led to the frame shift and more 21 amino acids. All these mutations weaken the activity of glycosyltransferase obviously, reduce the synthesize of A-antigen, and weaken the antigenicity.

In addition to qualitative differences, there are quantitative differences. Since the A_2-specified transferase has less activity than the A_1-specified transferase, the number of A sites on subgroup A_1 is significantly higher than that on subgroup A_2. The level of A-transferase in the serum of subgroup A_2 individuals is only about 10% of the level in subgroup A_1 individuals.

In addition, A_1 can convert type 3 H and type 4 H chains to type 3 A and type 4 A, while A_2 cannot. Thus, A_2 erythrocytes have more H and less A and lacked the type 4 A. It seems that anti-A_1 may recognize repetitive A structures, meanwhile anti-A may react with subgroup A_1 but not subgroup A_2 [5].

Other Weaker Forms of Subgroup A

The inheritance of rare alleles of subgroup A results in these phenotypes, and these subgroups cannot be recognized when the rare allele is paired with A_1 or A_2. These weaker forms of A have been described based on (1) the presence of reactions with anti-A, anti-A_1, anti-H, and anti-A, B, (2) the presence of anti-A_1 in serum, and (3) the presence of A and H substances in the saliva of ABH secretors.

1.1.2 Subgroups of B

Although no subgroup of B similar to subgroup A_2 existed, diverse types of B erythrocytes reacting weakly or not at all with anti-B have been described [6].

1.1.3 Cis AB

In the cis AB phenotype, the serum of most cis AB individuals contains anti-B, which means that the B in cis AB is different from normal B. The B antigen is usually very weak so that the phenotype cannot be confused with normal AB, while the A antigen is more strongly expressed than in A_2B but less strongly than in A_1B. This phenomenon happens occasionally in a family consisted with a group AB father, a group O mother, and an AB child.

1.2 Gene and Structure of the ABH, the Antigens

1.2.1 Gene of ABH Antigens

The gene of ABO is located at chromosome 9q34.1-34.2, including seven exons, with a total length of 18,000–20,000 base pairs. The base number of the largest exons, the seventh exon and sixth exon, accounts for 77% of the total coding sequence. The ABO gene has three major alleles: IA (A), IB (B), and I (O). The primary product of these allelic genes is glycosyltransferase. The IA allelic genes can bind the α-*N*-acetylgalactosamine to the β-D-galactose of the H antigen by encoding the α-1,3-*N*-acetylgalactosaminyltransferase and then form the A antigen. The IB allelic genes can bind the α-D-galactose to the β-D-galactose of the H antigen by encoding the α-1,3-D-galactosyltransferase and then form the B antigen. The lack of a nucleotide in the sixth exon of the I allelic gene can result in the abnormal expression of the corresponding encoded protein with the loss of enzyme activity. Thus, the O antigen is the original H antigen [7]. The major blood groups, including A, B, AB, and O, are formed by the three allelic genes. The H antigen was the precursor antigen of the blood group. The fucosyltransferase encoded by the H gene can transform the fucose to the oligosaccharide chains of glycoproteins or glycosphingolipids on the surface of the erythrocyte. This gene can express activity in all kinds of blood group of individuals. The glycosyltransferase encoded by the IA and IB allelic genes is comprised of transmembrane, C-catalytic domain, and N-terminal.

1.2.2 Structure of ABH Antigens

ABH antigens are carbohydrate structures. These oligosaccharide chains are usually conjugated with polypeptides to form glycoproteins or with ceramide to form glycosphingolipids. Each monosaccharide is catalyzed by a specific glycosyltransferase and then synthesizes the oligosaccharides step by step. Therefore the specificity of the antigens depends on the glycosyl of oligosaccharide chains. The antigenic determinant of A antigen is the *N*-acetylgalactosamine, while that of B antigen is D-galactose [8–10]. The structure of the oligosaccharide chain of the ABH antigens is presented in Fig. 2.1.

Glycoconjugates Expressing ABH Antigens

Glycosphingolipids consist of carbohydrate chains bound to ceramide. Two major carbohydrate chains on glycoproteins, N-glycans and O-glycans, express ABH antigens. Glycosphingolipid-borne ABH antigens are present predominantly on the lacto-series glycolipids, although ABH antigens can also be detected on other series glycolipids. The carbohydrate chains of most ABH-bearing glycoproteins and of

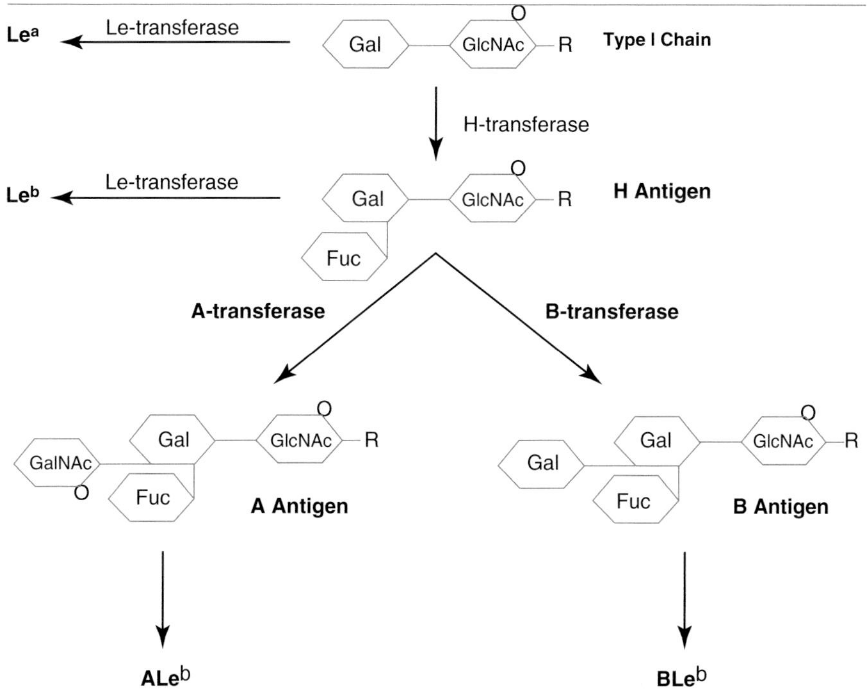

Fig. 2.1 Biosynthesis of ABH antigen in secretions. *Gal* D-galactose, *GlcNAc* *N*-acetyl-D-glucosamine, *Fuc* L-Fucose, *GalNAc* *N*-acetyl-D-galactosamine, *R* rest of molecule

lacto-series glycolipids are based on a poly-*N*-acetyllactosamine structure. Glycoproteins play a major role in erythrocyte ABH expression compared with glycolipids. All the study establishing the structures of the ABH determinants was carried out on body secretions [11]. ABH antigens in secretions are glycoproteins. In milk and urine, free oligosaccharides with ABH activity are also found [12, 13]. ABH determinants are present in plasma on glycosphingolipids, some of which may become compound of the erythrocyte.

1.3 Identification of ABO Blood Group

1.3.1 Principles of Identification of ABO Blood Group

In human serum, there contains natural agglutinins, antibodies, corresponding to the antigens mentioned above. For instance, in group A, the serum agglutinates only group B, and in group B, the serum agglutinates only group A. In group AB, the serum contains neither agglutinin, and the erythrocytes are agglutinated by sera of all other groups. While in group O, the serum contains a mixture of two agglutinins capable of agglutinating A and B groups, the erythrocytes are not agglutinated by any serum. If erythrocyte antigen in one of the four blood groups and its specific antibody exist at the same time, agglutinate action occurs. For example, when erythrocyte antigen in group A and anti-A antibody exist at the same time, the erythrocytes agglutinate together into clusters of irregular cells aggregation. Once the agglutination occurs, with the help of complement, erythrocytes are bound to lyse (hemolysis). Agglutination differs from blood coagulation. Agglutination is actually an antigen-antibody reaction, a kind of immune reaction, while the essence of blood coagulation is an enzymatic reaction in which fibrinogens in plasma change into insoluble fibrins, followed by multimeric fibrin interwoven into the net, which forms a lot of blood cells into blood clot.

Identification of ABO blood group is defined as a detection of ABH antigens. According to the presence or absence of the A antigen and (or) B antigen on the surface of erythrocytes, the blood group can be divided into four kinds: A, B, AB, and O. Red blood cell agglutination test can be used to identify ABO blood group accurately by positive and negative typing. The positive typing refers to use the standard anti-A and anti-B sera to determine whether the erythrocytes have the corresponding A antigen and B antigen. The reverse typing means to use the standard A and B groups to determine the presence or absence of anti-A and anti-B antibodies in the serum. The blood group should be confirmed only when the antigen identified on the examinee erythrocytes and the antibody identified in the serum are consistent with the results obtained. In addition, we should pay attention to the existence of A_2 and A_2B subgroups. Because of the weak antigenicity of A_2 antigen, the two subgroups can be easily mistaken for O group and B group, respectively.

1.3.2 Methods of Clinical ABO Blood Group Identification

A total of three major methods is used for identification: slide method, tube method, and microcolumn gel test (MGT).

1. Slide method: A and B are labeled at each end of the slide with a marker pen, and each drop is added with a drop of the corresponding standard serum. Disinfect the earlobe or fingertip with 75% alcohol cotton ball, puncture the skin with antiseptic needle, then stick to the glass slide A and B standard serum after blood sampling, and observe the agglutination phenomenon after 2–5 min. The method has the advantages of easy operation and material saving, but the weak agglutination reaction needs to be determined by microscope.
2. Tube method: Blood is collected with the same method mentioned above, and 1–2 drops of blood are mixed in a small tube containing 1 mL physiological saline to make erythrocyte suspension (concentration of about 5%). Then take two small tubes; mark "A" and "B," respectively. In each standard serum and each suspension of the erythrocyte, suspensions are divided into 1–2 drops, mixed and centrifuged at low speed for 1 min (1000 rpm). Flick the bottom of the tube lightly to make sure the sediment was bounced and then observe with light. The sediment group float indicates the occurrence of agglutination phenomenon; but if the sediment rises with smoke form, and serum back to the suspension state, it indicates no agglutination. Thus, the red cell suspension of O group cannot be agglutinated by any serum; in group A, the red cell suspension can be agglutinated by only the serum of group B, and in group B, the red cell suspension can be agglutinated by only the serum of group A. In group AB, the red cell suspension can be agglutinated by serum of all other groups. However, the decrease of the anti-A agglutinin titers can result to the A group mistaken for O group and the AB group mistaken for B group. Compared with the slide method, tube method has the advantage of reliability and accuracy as the method can reduce the concentration of non-specific antibody by diluting the examinee erythrocytes.
3. MGT: It is an immunological method of agglutination between erythrocyte antigen and corresponding antibody in gel microcolumn medium. The antibody of blood group belongs to monoclonal antibody. With reagents and specimens added to the blood serum, they can be directly observed with the naked eye or analyzed by a blood group instrument after centrifugation with a special centrifuge. This method is standardized and the results are accurate.

1.3.3 Reagent Requirement for ABO Blood Group Identification

Standard serum of anti-A and anti-B is collected from healthy individuals and should reach the following conditions:

1. Specificity: it can only agglutinate with the corresponding erythrocyte antigen without non-specific agglutination.
2. Titer: the titers of the anti-A and anti-B serum should be above 1: 128.
3. Affinity: the time of agglutination for the anti-A reacting with subgroup A_1, A_2, and A_2B is 15 s, 30 s, and 45 s, respectively; anti-B reacting with group is 15 s. The clot should be no less than 1 mm^2 when the agglutination strength is 3 min.
4. The titer of cold agglutinin should be below 1: 4.
5. Aseptic.
6. The complement should be inactivated.

1.3.4 Distribution of ABH Antigens in Human Body

There are three types of ABH antigens: (1) water-soluble glycoproteins, mainly found in human fluids, secretions, and tissues, but not in red blood cells and serum; (2) alcohol-soluble glycolipid, primarily found in red blood cells and other tissue cells, but not in brain tissue and body fluids; (3) and membrane glycoproteins, predominantly the ion exchange protein band 3 and the glucose transporter band 4.5. There are about one million band 3 proteins and 500 thousand band 4.5 protein monomers per adult erythrocyte.

The A and B antigens are primarily expressed in the form of glycoproteins and glycolipids on the erythrocyte. ABH antigens can also be found on leukocytes, platelets, and other tissue cells. In addition, tissue cells can synthesize and secrete soluble ABH antibiotics. Specific ABH substances can be found in all the secretion which is related to the inheritance of the ABH antigens, such as saliva, urine, tears, gastric juice, bile, amniotic fluid, and serum but not in the cerebrospinal fluid. These soluble antigens, also known as blood group substances, are classified as secretory and nonsecretory types in the presence or absence of it in the saliva. The dominant inheritance genes, Se genes that control the classification of the blood group substances, can synthesize soluble H precursors. The Se gene is not on the same chromosome as the ABO gene, and its inheritance is independent of the ABO and H genes. Approximately 80% of individuals have this gene, and all the rest are SeSe homozygous in which soluble H precursors cannot be synthesized. Thus, this group has no soluble A/B antigen, known as nonsecretory type.

In addition, as the water-soluble blood group substances can react with the corresponding antibody, they can be measured in a trace amount. The significance of blood type substance determination is as follows: (1) determination of blood group substances in saliva can help the identification of blood group; (2) neutralizing the natural antibody in the ABO blood group system can help examine in the level of immune antibody; (3) and check amniotic fluid, predict fetal ABO blood group, etc.

- ABO blood group antigens are also expressed in the gut, respiratory organs, and other organs, just as they do on the surface of erythrocyte. In the kidney, the A antigen and B antigen are found in the arteries, veins, glomeruli, capillaries, tubules, the basement membrane of some distal tubules, and the surface of the endothelial cells of the collecting duct.

2 The Rh System

2.1 Introduction

Rh is the most complex of the blood group systems, which include 54 antigens. In 1940, Landsteiner and Wiener [14, 15] made antibodies by injecting rhesus red cells into rabbits and guinea pigs. The antibodies, called anti-Rh, agglutinated rhesus monkey red cells but also agglutinated the red cells from 85% of white New Yorkers. Thus, this blood system was named as rhesus monkey system (Rh system). D antigen of Rh system is highly immunogenic that if a D-negative recipient was exposed to D antigen by blood transfusion, the anti-D antibody will be form in more than 90% of cases and thereafter cannot safely receive D-positive blood again. It was confirmed by Levine [16] that incompatibility of Rh blood type between mother and fetus may cause HDFN (hemolytic disease of the fetus and newborn), and more evidence supported that Rh system is associated with warm autoimmune hemolytic anemia; afterward Rh system has gradually gotten more attention.

2.2 Rh Antigens and Genes

2.2.1 Rh Genes

In 1943, RA Fisher proposed that there were three closely linked genes, *Cc*, *Dd*, and *Ee*, which determined corresponding antithetical antigens [17]. Application of the techniques of molecular biology has since shown that there are only two genes: *D*, which has no allele, and, a second gene, *CeEe* [18], which has many alleles. It is worth noting that it is convenient to use d to indicate the absence of *D*, rather than the real existence of allele gene d. The Rh antigens are encoded by two highly homologous genes on chromosome 1: *RHD* and *RHCE*. The first discovered and the most important antigen clinically is D (RH1), produced by *RHD* gene, which is often referred to as the Rh or rhesus antigen. D is present on red cells of about 85% of white people and is more common in Africans and Asians. In addition to the D antigen, C and c and E and e are two pairs of antigens controlled by the *RHCE* gene.

2.2.2 Common Rh Genotypes and Phenotypes

The Rh phenotype can be determined by the antisera. Theoretically, Rh antigens controlled by two pairs of alleles and a non-allele make the Rh blood group system have eight phenotypes (DCE, DCe, DcE, Dce, dCE, dCe, dcE, dce). In clinical practice, only D antigen can always be detected, thus D+, D- are used as the two clinical phenotypes of Rh system. Therefore, when D antigen on the surface of red blood cells exists, it is called Rh positive, marked as Rh (+); the lack of D antigen is Rh negative, marked as Rh (−). In all populations, the D-positive dominates the clear majority, accounting for about 83% of white people. Phenotype frequencies in most white people are similar, although in Basques have 20–40% D-negative. The D-negative in Burmese, Japanese, Maoris, Melanesians, American Indians, and Inuit is rarely less than 1%. In Chinese people, D-negative accounted for only 0.3–0.4%.

2.3 Structure of D Antigen

Rh polypeptides were first characterized biochemically as an approximate molecular weight of 30 kDa through 125I radiolabeled Rh proteins by sodium dodecyl sulfate-polyacrylamide gel electrophoresis of autoradiography [19, 20]. The complete D antigen has two polypeptides, one corresponding to the D

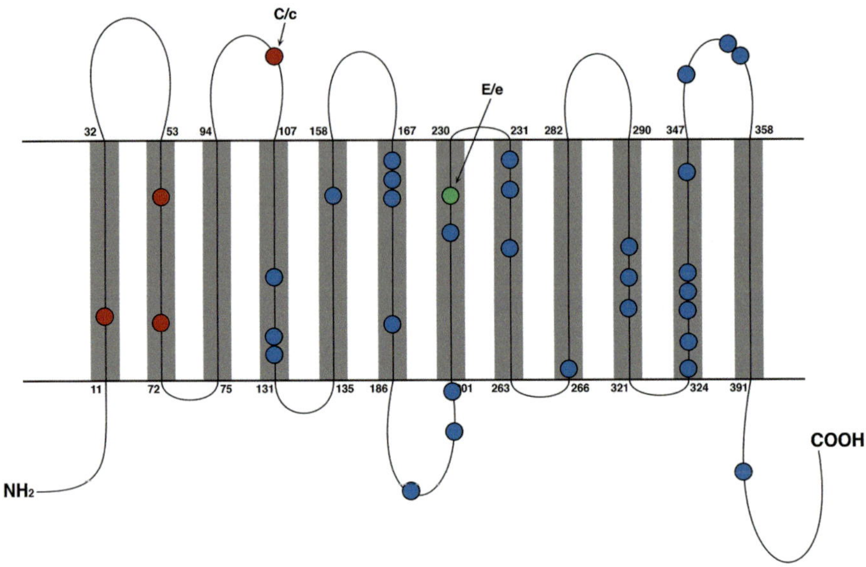

Fig. 2.2 Structure of D polypeptide

polypeptide and the other to the CE polypeptide. D polypeptide has 416 amino acids (417 amino acids including initial methionine) as shown in Fig. 2.2 [21]. C/E and D polypeptides are highly homologous, of which only 35/36 amino acid substitutions are different. C/c polymorphism mainly appears to depend on serine substitution by proline at position 103, while other amino acid substitutions also occur normally at positions 16, 60, and 68 [22]. E/e polymorphism is only determined by a single amino acid substitution which are proline and alanine at position 226 (Fig. 2.2) [23].

Unlike the *RHCE* gene, the *RHD* gene does not contain the corresponding recessive allele d, which represents that most of the D antigen-negative phenotypes are due to the deletion of the *RHD*. Chromosomal misalignment at meiosis and subsequent unequal crossing may result in a complete deletion of *RHD*, which is a common cause of D-negative in white people. While in the black Africans, in addition to the deletion of *RHD*, 67% of the D-negative always results from an inactive *RHD* by a nonsense mutation in exon 6 which creates a stop codon (Tyr269 to stop). Of the very rare D-negative in Asians, 32% of individuals are due to another variant of D antigen called weak D or Del [24].

Some variants of D antigen are very rare but known as partial D and weak D. The difference between them is mainly manifested in partial D antigen that lacks some of the D epitopes, while weak D expresses all epitopes of D antigen; both may have a lower site density than D. The variants result from the amino acid substitutions in D polypeptide, due to the missense mutations in *RHD*, or a gene conversion happened with *RHCE*.

2.4 Clinical Significance of Rh System

The clinical significance of the Rh blood group system is from the highly immunogenic of antigen D. If a D-negative recipient received D-positive blood from transfusion, the recipient forms anti-D antibodies in some 90% of cases and thereafter cannot safely receive D-positive red blood cells. Moreover, if a D-negative woman is pregnant with a D-positive fetus, the D-positive red blood cells from the fetus across the placenta may induce immune response of D antigen in about one sixth of cases. Part of the immune cells that recognize the D antigen can differentiate into memory cells. In a subsequent pregnancy, secondary immunization may lead to hemolytic disease in the infant due to the secreting of anti-D antibodies. In addition, Rh is also involved in some of the autoimmune hemolytic anemia, especially warm autoimmune hemolytic anemia.

In organ transplantation, when a D-negative recipient received an organ from a D-positive donor, it is defined as Rh blood group incompatible organ transplantation. Because Rh blood type antigens are mainly present on the surface of erythrocytes and less in solid organs or vascular endothelial cells, Rh-incompatible organ transplantation is generally possible without specific treatment and also has lower complications compared to ABO incompatible transplantation.

3 Other Blood Systems

In the remaining blood systems, the most clinically significant are Duffy, Kell, and MN.

3.1 Duffy (Fy) System

In 1950, Cutbush found a new red blood cell antibody (anti-FYa antibody) in the serum of a hemophilia patient with multiple transfusions and named the new blood group system as Duffy system [25]. The *Fy* gene is located in chromosome 1q21–q25, coding the codominant alleles *Fya*, *Fyb*, and a recessive gene Fy [26]. The only difference between the *Fya* and *Fyb* alleles is that the single base in the 44th codon is different, which represents aspartic acid in Fya antigen or glycine in Fyb antigen [27].

The codominant alleles *Fya*, *Fyb*, and recessive gene *Fy* that make the Duffy blood group system have four phenotypes (Fy a+b+, Fy a+b−, Fy a−b+, and Fy a−b−). More than 90% of Asians are Fya-positive, and about 80% of Caucasians are Fyb-positive. Fy (a−b−) (Duffy negative) are extremely rare in both Asians and Caucasians, but about 70% African Americans and close to 100% of West Africans are Duffy negative.

Common Duffy antibodies are anti-Fya and anti-Fyb. Anti-Fya is not infrequent and can be found in previously blood-transfused patients who have highly panel-reactive antibodies. Anti-Fyb is quite rare in clinical patients. Both may cause hemolytic transfusion reactions and HDFN but seldom severe, which is then usually slight to mild [28].

3.2 Kell (K) System

The original Kell antigen, K (KEL1), was found in the serum of a primigravida by Coombs test in 1946. KEL1 has about 9% of frequency in Caucasians but is rare in other ethnic groups. The allelic antigen, k (KEL2), is more common in all populations (about 95%) [29]. The remainder of Kell antigen includes 13 high-frequency and 3 low-frequency antigens. The polymorphism of KEL1/KEL2 is determined by methionine or threonine at position 193, which can be the important site to distinguish KEL1 from KEL2.

KEL1 and anti-K are the most important in clinical view and can cause hemolytic transfusion reactions and HDFN more frequently than any other blood systems beyond the ABO and Rh systems. Some of other Kell system antibodies were also known to cause delayed hemolytic transfusion reaction (DHTR).

3.3 MN System

MN system has a total of 48 antigens which is the second to Rh system in complexity. The antigens M and N were discovered by analysis of the specific antibodies in rabbit after injecting human blood in 1927 [30]. In the year of 1947, another antigen named S has been found as the linked antigen of M and N [31]. The MN antigens and S antigen are encoded by homologous genes, *GYPA* and *GYPB*, on chromosome 4, respectively. M and N antigens are differed by amino acids at positions 1 and 5. They are alleles that rise to three genotypes, MM, MN, and NN, with the frequencies of about 28%, 50%, and 22%. MN system also contains En, U, and other rare antigens and some other genotypes.

MN antigens are already present at the time of birth, and the complexity of the antigen is manifested in serology, genetics, and biology. This may be associated with hemolytic transfusion reactions and HDFN.

References

1. Landsteiner K. Über Agglutinationserscheinungen normalen menschlichen Blutes. Agglutination phenomena in normal human blood. Wien Klin Wochenschr. 1901;14:1132–4.
2. von Decastello A, Stürli A. Über die Isoagglutinie im Serum gesunder und kranker Menschen. München Med Wchnschr. 1902;26:1090–5.
3. Smalley CE, Tucker EM. Blood group A antigen site distribution and immunoglobulin binding in relation to red cell age. Br J Haematol. 1983;54:209–19.

4. Lopez M, Benali J, Cartron JP, et al. Some notes on the specificity of anti-A_1 reagents. Vox Sang. 1980;39:271–6.
5. Clausen H, Levery SB, Nudelman SS, et al. Repetitive A epitope (Type 3 chain A) defined by blood group A_1-specific antibody TH-1: chemical basis of qualitative A_1 and A_2 distinction. Proc Natl Acad Sci U S A. 1985;82:1119–203.
6. Doinel C, Ropars C, Salmon C. Quantitative and thermodynamic measurements on I and i antigens of human red blood cells. Immunology. 1976;30:289–97.
7. Mohiuddin MM, Ogawa H, Yin DP, et al. Antibody-mediated accommodation of heart grafts expressing an incompatible carbohydrate antigen. Transplantation. 2003;75:258–62.
8. Schenkel-Brunner H, Tuppy H. Enzymatic conversion of human blood-group-O erythrocytes into A_2 and A_1 cells by a α-N-acetyl-D-galactosaminyl transferases of blood-group-A individuals. Eur J Biochem. 1973;34:125–8.
9. Comenzo RL, Malachowski ME, Rohrer RJ, et al. Anomalous ABO phenotype in a child after an ABO-incompatible liver transplantation. N Engl J Med. 1992;326:867–70.
10. Wichmann MG, Haferlach T, Suttorp M, et al. Can blood group O red cells of donor origin acquire weak group A reactivity through serum A transferase of the recipient after bone marrow transplantation? Beitr Infusionsther Transfusionsmed. 1994;32:146–8.
11. Morgan WTJ, Van Heyningen R. The occurrence of A, B and O blood group substances in pseudo-mucinous ovarian cyst fluids. Br J Exp Pathol. 1944;25:5–15.
12. Kobata A. Isolation of oligosaccharides from human milk. Methods Enzymol. 1972;28:262–71.
13. Lundblad A. Oligosaccharides from human urine. Methods Enzymol. 1978;50:226–35.
14. Landsteiner K, Wiener AS. An agglutinable factor in human blood recognized by immune sera for Rhesus blood. Proc Soc Exp Biol N Y. 1940;43:223.
15. Landsteiner K, Wiener AS. Studies on an agglutinogen (Rh) in human blood reacting with anti-rhesus sera and with human isoantibodies. J Exp Med. 1941;74:309–20.
16. Levine P, Burnham L, Katzin EM, Vogel P. The role of iso-immunization in the pathogenesis of erythroblastosis fetalis. Am J Obstet Gynecol. 1941;42:925–37.
17. Race RR. An 'incomplete' antibody in human serum. Nature. 1944;153:771.
18. Colin Y, Chérif-Zahar B, Le van Kim C, et al. Genetic basis of the Rh-D positive and Rh-D negative blood group polymorphism as determined by Southern analysis. Blood. 1991;78:1–6.
19. Gahmberg CG. Molecular identification of the human Rho (D) antigen. FEBS Lett. 1982;140:93–7.
20. Moore S, Woodrow CF, McClelland BL, et al. Isolation of membrane components associated with human red cell antigens Rh(D), (c), (E) and Fy. Nature. 1982;295:529–31.
21. Le Van Kim C, Mouro I, Chérif-Zahar B, et al. Molecular cloning and primary structure of the human blood group RhD polypeptide. Proc Natl Acad Sci U S A. 1992;89:10925–9.
22. Anstee DJ, Mallinson G. The biochemistry of blood group antigens: some recent advances. Vox Sang. 1994;67(Suppl 3):1–6.
23. Mouro I, Colin Y, Chérif-Zahar B, et al. Molecular genetic basis of the human Rhesus blood group system. Nat Genet. 1993;5:62–5.
24. Touinssi M, Chapel-Fernandes S, Granier T, et al. Molecular analysis of inactive and active RHD alleles in native Congolese cohorts. Transfusion. 2009;49:1353–60.
25. Cutbush M, Mollison PL. A new human blood group. Nature. 1950;165:188.
26. Donahue RP, Bias W, Renwick JH, et al. Probable assignment of the Duffy blood group locus to chromosome 1 in man. Proc Natl Acad Sci U S A. 1968;61:949.
27. Meny GM1. The Duffy blood group system: a review. Immunohematology. 2010;26(2):51–6.
28. Goodrick MJ, Hadley AG, Poole G. Haemolytic disease of the fetus and newborn due to anti-Fy(a) and the potential value of Duffy genotyping in pregnancies at risk. Transfus Med. 1997;7:301–4.
29. Landsteiner K, Levine P. Further observations on individual differences of human blood. Proc Soc Exp Biol (NY). 1927;24:941.
30. Denomme GA, et al. Immunohematology. 2015;31(1):14–9.
31. Walsh RJ, Montgomery CM. A new human iso-agglutinin subdividing the MN blood groups. Nature. 1947;160:504–6.

ABO Blood Group Antibodies

3

Jiang Qiu and Changxi Wang

Abstract

In this chapter, the characteristics of an antibody, ABO blood group antibodies, and the detection of blood group antibodies are discussed. ABO blood group antibodies, the most important antibodies in the human body, have many common features with general antibodies in terms of basic functions and biological characteristics. Clearance of ABO blood group antibodies (mainly IgG and IgM) is the key to ABO-incompatible (ABOi) transplantation. Antibody removal technology includes plasma exchange technology, immuno-adsorption technology, and plasma double filtration technology.

Keywords

Antibody · ABO blood group antibody · Antibody removal technology

1 Introduction

The term "antibody" was first proposed in the conclusion of the paper "Experimental Studies on Immunity" published by Paul Ehrlich in October 1891, which states that "if two substances lead to the production of two different antibodies, the two substances must be different." In the early stages of immunological development, bacteria or their exotoxins were injected into animals. After a certain period of time, in vitro experiments proved that there is a component in serum which can specifically neutralize exotoxin, known as antitoxin, and a component that can specifically agglutinate bacteria, known as lectin. After that, this component with a specific

J. Qiu (✉) · C. Wang
Department of Organ Transplantation, The First Affiliated Hospital of Sun Yat-sen University, Guangzhou, Guangdong Province, China

Y. Wang (ed.), *ABO-incompatible Organ Transplantation*,
https://doi.org/10.1007/978-981-13-3399-6_3

response in serum was called an antibody (Ab), and the substance that can stimulate the body to produce antibody is called antigen (Ag), thus establishing the concept of antigen and antibody.

2 The Antibody and Its Characteristics

2.1 General Concept of the Antibody

The antibody, also known as immunoglobulin (Ig), is a type of Y-shaped protein that is produced by the proliferation and differentiation of B lymphocytes or memory B cells into plasma cells, which can specifically bind to the corresponding antigen, which is used by the immune system to identify and neutralize foreign substances such as bacteria and viruses. It is only found in body fluids, such as blood, of vertebrates, and on the B-cell membrane surface [1]. Antibody molecules have binding sites (binding clusters) that can bind to the corresponding antigenic determinants. After antibodies bind to different antigens, a different response is produced, so antibodies are often given different names, such as lectin, precipitin, antitoxin, hemolysin, and lysozyme. Antibodies are mainly distributed in the serum, as well as in tissue fluids and exocrine fluid.

At first, some researchers had proved via electrophoresis that antibody activity in the serum occurred in the γ-globulin. Therefore, the antibody was collectively referred to as γ-globulin. Later, it was found that not all antibodies were in the γ-area, and the globulin in the γ-area did not always have antibody activity. In 1964, in a special conference of the World Health Organization, globulin with antibody activity and antibody-related globulin were collectively referred to as *immunoglobulins*, such as abnormal Ig in the serum of patients with myeloma, macroglobulinemia, and cryoglobulinemia, and the natural Ig subunits in healthy people. Thus, Ig is a concept in structural chemistry, whereas the antibody is a concept of biological function. It can be said that all antibodies are Igs but not all Igs are antibodies.

2.2 Structure of the Antibody

An antibody is a globular blood protein macromolecule, weighing about 150 kDa. An antibody is also an Ig, because some amino acid residues contain sugar chains. The basic unit that can exert function is an Ig. The monomer of an antibody is a Y-shaped molecule with a symmetrical structure of four polypeptide chains, of which two chains are longer heavy chains (H chains) with a relatively high molecular weight, and two chains are shorter light chains (L chains) with a relatively low molecular weight. Interchain disulfide bonds and noncovalent bonds bind and form a monomer molecule composed of four polypeptide chains [2]. The whole antibody molecule can be divided into a constant region and a variable region. According to the composition of the constant region, there are two kinds of L chain (κ and λ), and five kinds of H chain (μ, δ, γ, ε, α). The variable region is located at the ends of both arms of the "Y." In the variable region, a small part of amino acid residues has a high degree of variability. The composition and sequence of these amino acid residues are more prone to variation, so it is known as the hypervariable region. The variable region outside the hypervariable region is called the framework region. Each H or L chain has three hypervariable regions and adjacent regions and four framework regions. The hypervariable region is located on the surface of molecular space structure, and the antibody space structure, determined by its amino acid sequence, is a part where the antibody specifically binds to the antibody, so it is also known as the complementary determining region. The hypervariable region consists of up to 17 amino acid residues, or only 2 or 3 residues. The two H (or L) chains on one antibody molecule are the same. When papain hydrolyzes the antibody, the N end (i.e., between the first and second constant regions) of its hinge region is cut, forming two identical antigen-binding fragments at the ends of both arms, known as the antigen-binding fragment (Fab). The "Y" handle is called the crystalline fragment (FC).

2.3 Function and Production Regularity Law of Antibodies

Activated B cells can differentiate into two kinds of cells with different functions: plasma cells, which produce soluble antibodies, and memory B cells, which are used to memorize the antigens contacted. The latter can exist in the body for many years, and when the body is reexposed to the antigen, it reacts more quickly. Antibodies in the fetus and newborn are provided by the mother, as a kind of passive immunity. Within 1 year after birth, newborns

can produce many different kinds of antibodies on their own. Because antibodies can be dissolved in the bloodstream, they are part of the humoral immune system. Antibodies in the circulation of body fluid are generated by B-cell descendants that respond to a particular antigen, such as a viral capsid. The main function of the antibody is to combine with antigens (both foreign and self) to effectively remove foreign bodies, such as microorganisms and parasites that are invading the body, and to neutralize the toxins released by these, or to remove some autoantigens, maintaining the normal balance of the body. However, sometimes an antibody also causes pathological damage to the body, such as anti-nuclear antibodies, anti-double-stranded DNA antibodies, or anti-thyroglobulin antibodies, leading to autoimmune diseases.

2.3.1 Biological Activity of Antibodies

Antibody function is closely related to biological activity, and the biological activity of an antibody is mainly manifested in the following aspects. (1) An antibody binds a specific antigen: the main difference of the antibody from other Ig molecules is that the antibody can bind to a specific antigen, causing physiological or pathological effects in the body; it produces various direct or indirect visible antigen–antibody binding reactions in vitro. Antibodies bind to the antigen by relying on the specific binding sites on the molecule. (2) Antibodies activate complement: after the antibody binds to the corresponding antigen, the complement system is activated by means of the exposed complement-binding sites, and the immunological action of complement bacteriolysis and cytolysis is also stimulated. (3) The antibody binds cells: different types of Ig can bind to different kinds of cells involved in immune response. (4) IgG can pass from the mother into the fetal blood through the placenta, forming a natural passive immunity for the fetus. IgA is a major factor in local mucosal immune response through the digestive tract and respiratory mucosa. (5) Antigenicity: the antibody molecule is a kind of protein and also has the ability to stimulate the body to produce an immune response. Different Ig molecules have different antigenicity. (6) Antibody resistance to physical and chemical factors is different from that of general globulin: it is not heat resistant and can be destroyed at 60°–70 °C. A variety of enzymes and substances that produce protein coagulation and degeneration can destroy the effects of antibodies. Also, antibodies can be precipitated by neutral salts. In production, ammonium sulfate or sodium sulfate can often be used to precipitate antibody-containing globulin from the immune serum, which is then purified via dialysis.

2.3.2 Antibody Function

The functions of antibodies are mainly manifested in the following aspects. (1) Antibodies can inhibit the growth and reproduction of pathogens; for example, antibacterial antibodies can agglutinate the invading bacteria and separate the bacteria from nutrients so that the bacteria cannot breed. (2) Antibodies can stop viruses or bacteria from getting close to human cells, so the invaders cannot reach or adhere to the cells; as a result, the invader cannot damage the cells or form an infection. Similar to plant seeds, they can only take root and germinate when they fall into the soil. Antibodies do not allow the virus to adhere to the cells, just like seeds floating in the air can never take root. (3) Antibodies can neutralize viruses, such as hepatitis B virus (HBV); there is a layer of protein structure on the surface that adheres to the surface of human liver cells, which is followed by access into the liver cells. However, it is very important for the antibody to meet with HBV before it binds to the surface, changing the protein on the surface of HBV and losing its ability to adhere to the hepatocytes, so that it cannot enter the hepatocytes, let alone replicate. The neutralizing effect of antibodies, such as "acid–base neutralization," causes HBV to be no longer infectious and it may soon be cleared by the body. (4) Antibodies can also identify the type of microorganisms. Each pathogenic microorganism that invades the human body automatically generates different antibodies according to different antigenic epitopes of microorganisms; for example, if a severe acute respiratory syndrome (SARS) virus invades the human body, that body will produce SARS antibodies; the human body will also produce a series of anti-hepatitis B antibodies in the case of HBV invasion.

2.3.3 Production Law of Natural Antibodies

Antibodies, as a special kind of immunoglobulins, exhibit a general law when exerting specific immune functions. Mastering the law of antibody production is of great significance in the prevention and diagnosis of disease. For example, the first vaccination should be carried out several weeks before the prevalence of disease, and people generally should be vaccinated more than two times; when a serological test is performed to diagnose infectious diseases, two samples of serum in the initial and late stages of the disease should be taken for comparative observation. If the serum antibody level at the second testing is more than four times higher than that at the first time, it indicates diagnostic significance.

1. Production of antibodies in primary response: When the antigen enters the body for the first time, it can produce antibodies after a certain incubation period, and not much antibody is produced; it is also maintained in vivo for a shorter time. Its main features are as follows: the latency of primary immune response is long, the concentration of antibody produced is low, and the antibody–antigen affinity is also low, mainly IgM.
2. Production of antibodies in secondary response: When the same antigen enters the body a second time, some of the original antibodies bind to the later antigen initially, so the original antibody amount is slightly reduced. Subsequently, as there is a rapid increase in antibody titer, it can be increased several times over the primary response, and its in vivo retention time is also longer. Its main features are as follows: the latency is usually as short as 1–3 days; antibodies will be produced in the blood, resulting in high antibody concentration; and the antibody–antigen affinity is high, mainly IgG.
3. Production of antibodies in anamnesis reaction: The antibodies produced by the antigens can gradually disappear after a certain period of time. At this point, if the antigen is contacted again, the antibody that had disappeared may be rapidly increased. If the antigen stimulating the body again is the same as that at the first time, it is known as the specific anamnesis reaction; if it is different from that in the primary response, it is known as a nonspecific anamnesis reaction. The increase of antibodies caused by a nonspecific anamnesis reaction is temporary and will decline rapidly in a short time.

2.4 Classification of Antibodies

2.4.1 Classification According to Action Objects

Antibodies can be classified as antitoxin, antibacterial, antivirus, and cytotropic (cell-binding immunoglobulin, such as IgE reagin antibodies in a type I allergic reaction, which can adhere to the target cell membrane).

1. Antitoxin that is produced in the early stage when the immunoglobulin is not clearly classified is a general term for a class of immunoglobulin. It is a specific antibody that can neutralize antibodies of toxin or serum containing this antibody. Also, it can neutralize the toxic effects of the corresponding exotoxin. Pathogens, such as diphtheria, tetanus, gas gangrene, and others that cause the body to produce exotoxin, can produce antitoxin. After formaldehyde treatment, the exotoxin can lose toxicity and maintain immunogenicity, becoming the toxoid. In medical practice, the application of toxoid in prophylactic vaccination

can make the body produce the corresponding antitoxin, preventing disease. In immunotherapy, the commonly used bacteria include exotoxin, toxins, or other poisons (such as snake venom); antitoxin can be produced in the horse after immune injection, and then the serum is drawn, purified, and concentrated into antitoxin, which not only can improve the potency but also reduces side effects. The animal-derived antitoxin serum has a dual effect on the human body: on the one hand, it provides patients with specific antitoxin antibodies to neutralize the corresponding exotoxin in the body, and has a role in prevention and treatment; on the other hand, it has the antigenic heterologous protein, which can stimulate the body to produce anti-horse serum protein antibodies, and hypersensitivity may occur later when receiving the horse immune serum. IgG molecules that have been hydrolyzed by pepsin retain F(ab)2 fragments with antibody activity, and the specific antigenic determinants are removed as much as possible, resulting in a dramatic increase in potency and a lesser chance of hypersensitivity.

2. Antibacterial antibodies and antivirus antibodies, a type of immunoglobulin produced by the body against infection and destruction of pathogens, such as bacteria and viruses, can maintain the function of physiological stability. After the virus breaks through the body's first line of defense, interferons and natural killer cells (NK cells) are important as the second line of defense. After the virus enters into the body, it can stimulate the body's macrophages, lymphocytes, and somatic cells to produce interferon. Interferon, which has a broad spectrum of antiviral effects, can induce antiviral albumin to block the emergence of new viruses, so it can block virus proliferation and proliferation. NK cells are lymphocytes, in addition to T cells and B cells, accounting for 5–10% of the total number of lymphocytes; they perform a "patrol" task in the blood circulation. When abnormal cells are found, the lymphocytes immediately release perforin to kill the abnormal cells. Host cells infected with the virus are abnormal cells and are therefore also within the attack range of NK cells. After the virus escapes from the second line of defense, it faces a third line of defense, namely, specific humoral and cellular immunity, with specific roles in fighting viral infections. Specific antibodies can neutralize viruses outside the host cell. After the antibody binds to the virus, the virus cannot enter the cell by binding to the corresponding receptor on the surface of the infected cell, so the virus is then phagocytosed and degraded by the phagocyte. Antibodies cannot enter an intracellular virus that has entered the infected cells, as in intracellular bacteria, and CD8 cytotoxic T lymphocyte (CTL) cells in cellular immunity are needed for clearing. CTL cells destroy the virus-infected cells. First, CTL cells and virus-infected cells make contact, and CTL cells then release biologically active substances such as perforin and granzyme. The CTL cells then leave and the virus finally infects the cells, leading to rupture and death. The virus that is released can be neutralized by specific antibodies. After the CD8 CTL cells leave, they can attack other infected cells repeatedly in the same manner.
3. A cytophilic antibody is a type of immunoglobulin that binds to cells, such as IgE reaginic antibody in type I allergic reactions, which can bind to mast cells and basophilic granulocytes. IgG can bind to macrophages and adhere to the

target cell membrane. The immunoglobulin that binds to the same type of cell is called a homocytotropic antibody, and immunoglobulin that binds to xenogeneic cells is called a heterocytotropic antibody. The Fc-terminus of a cytophilic antibody can be adsorbed on the immune cells of Fc receptors, including (1) IgE allergic antibodies ecotropic to mast cells and basophils; and (2) IgG antibody that can be adsorbed on killer cells (also known as K cell K). Only K cells with antibodies can effectively kill target cells with the corresponding antigens. (3) Antibodies adsorbed on macrophages can arm macrophages to enhance the ability of phagocytosis and killing target cells.

2.4.2 Classification According to Physical and Chemical Properties and Biological Functions

Antibodies can be divided into IgM, IgG, IgA, IgE, and IgD [3].

1. Immunoglobulin M (IgM) accounts for 5–10% of the total amount of serum immunoglobulin. It is the type of antibody that is present first on the cell membrane after rearrangement of the B-cell antibody gene (as follows), forming the B-cell receptor (BCR). Secretory IgM is a pentamer, and the J chain combines five IgM Fc segments, which is Ig with the highest molecular weight, namely, macroglobulin. Because of its high molecular weight, pentameric IgM usually does not pass through the blood vessel walls and is present mainly in the blood, containing ten F(ab) segments, and thus it has a higher antibacterial activity than IgG; moreover, it has five Fc segments, so it can activate more complement than IgG. The natural blood group antibody is IgM, and inconsistent blood transfusion can cause a serious hemolytic reaction. IgM is the first antibody to be synthesized and secreted during individual development, and the fetus synthesizes IgM at about the 20th week in the embryonic period. IgM in the body cannot pass the placenta, so if IgM appears in newborn blood, it indicates intrauterine infection; moreover, if IgM is increased in the umbilical cord blood, this indicates intrauterine fetal infection (such as rubella or cytomegalovirus infection). IgM, which is also the antibody appearing first in humoral immunity, acts as the "pioneer" of anti-infection, and is also the antibody secreted first in the immune response. After a period of time, the IgM antibody level gradually decreases and then disappears. IgM initiates the cascade of complement after binding to the antigen, and also connects the intruders and gathers them to be engulfed by macrophages. Therefore, the determination of IgM antibodies has clinical diagnostic value for some infectious diseases such as hepatitis. IgM detected in serum suggests a recent infection and can be used for early diagnosis. In children more than 1 year of age, serum IgM will reach the adult level. Many antimicrobial natural antibodies, such as cognate hemagglutinin (anti-type A and anti-type B blood), rheumatoid factor in rheumatoid diseases, and complement-binding antibodies in syphilis belong to IgM.
2. Immunoglobulin G (IgG) is an immunoglobulin component in serum, accounting for about 75% of the total serum immunoglobulin with a normal value of 9.5–12.5 mg/ml: 40–50% IgG is distributed in the serum and the remaining

resides in the tissues. With a molecular weight of about 150 kDa, IgG in human serum is mainly a monomer, and normal human IgG includes four subtypes: IgG1 (60–70%), IgG2 (15–20%), IgG3 (5–10%), and IgG4 (1–7%). These subtypes have different binding abilities in the classic pathway of complement activation. IgG, synthesized mainly by plasma cells in the spleen and lymph nodes, is the only antibody that can pass through the placenta, having an important role in preventing infections within a few weeks after birth. Its synthesis starts at the third month after birth, reaching the adult level at the age of 3–5 years, and gradually decreases after 40 years of age. IgG content varies widely among individuals and fluctuates in the same individual under different conditions. Most antibacterial, antivirus, and antitoxin antibodies produced by the body under antigen stimulation belong to IgG. Many autoantibodies, such as LE factor in systemic lupus erythematosus, and anti-thyroglobulin antibodies, also belong to IgG. IgG is the main anti-infective antibody in the body: it activates complement and neutralizes a variety of toxins. IgG persists for a long time and is the only antibody that protects the fetus across the placenta during gestation. Moreover, it is also secreted into the colostrum from the breast to protect the newborn. The functional role of IgG in body immunity is mainly protective. Antivirals, antitoxins, and most antibacterial antibodies belong to the IgG class. To handle the numbness of hepatitis A, for example, IgG can effectively prevent the corresponding infectious diseases. Therefore, IgG antibodies are important in the neutralization of toxins and antibacterial and antiviral activities. IgG is the only immunoglobulin that passes through the placenta. Thus, IgG from the maternal body is important in the prevention of diphtheria, measles, and poliomyelitis infections during the first few months of life. The maternal IgG delivered to the fetus has almost completely disappeared by 6 months after birth, whereas that produced by the baby itself is gradually increased from 3 months, so it is susceptible to infection after 6 months.

3. IgA content in normal human serum is second only to IgG, with serum immunoglobulin content of 10–20%. From the aspect of structure, IgA has monomer, dyad, trisomy, and polymer points. According to immune function, it is divided into two types of serotypes and secretions. Serum IgA is present in the serum, which accounts for about 85% of total IgA. Although serogroup IgA has certain functions of IgG and IgM, it does not show important immune function in the serum. Secretory IgA is composed of catenin and secretory components linked by a J chain, mainly in colostrum, saliva, lacrimal fluid, gastrointestinal fluid, bronchial secretions, and other exocrine fluids. It is the most important factor of mucosal local immunity. Secretory IgA, by binding to the corresponding pathogenic microorganisms (such as poliovirus), inhibits its adsorption onto susceptible cells; secreted IgA can also neutralize toxins such as those of *Vibrio cholerae* and *Escherichia coli*. Neonatal respiratory tract infection and gastrointestinal infections may be related to a lack of IgA synthesis. Chronic bronchitis attacks and secretory IgA reduction also have a certain relationship. IgA is also known as mucosal local antibodies. IgA cannot pass the placenta. Neonatal serum IgA antibodies can be maternal colostrum-secreted IgA passed to infants;

this is also an important natural passive immunization. Eosinophils, neutrophils, and macrophages express FcαR, and serotonergic IgA mediates phagocytosis and antibody-dependent cell-mediated cytotoxicity (ADCC). In addition, secreted IgA functions as an immune exclusion whereby secreted IgA binds to a large number of soluble antigens in the diet and the pyrogen released by normal intestinal microflora or pathogenic microorganisms, preventing them from entering the bloodstream.

IgA is mainly produced by mucosa-associated lymphoid tissues, most of which are synthesized by gastrointestinal lymphoid tissues; a small portion is synthesized by respiratory, salivary, and reproductive tract mucosal tissues. Maternal lactation gland tissue contains a large number of IgA-producing cells; these cells are mainly from the gastrointestinal tract. In humans, a small amount of IgA comes from the bone marrow. IgA is synthesized at 4 to 6 months after birth, and serum levels at 4 to 12 years of age reach the adult human level. Antibody enters the mucosal surfaces of the body, including the respiratory, digestive, reproductive, and other pipeline mucosa, as do infection factors. It is also possible to deliver this antibody, the most abundant and important class of antibodies, to the gut mucosa of the newborn through the colostrum of breast milk.

4. Immunoglobulin E (IgE) is mainly produced by plasma cells in the nasopharynx, tonsil, bronchial, gastrointestinal, and other mucosal lamina propria; molecular weight is 188 kDa, and in normal human serum this is the smallest amount of immunoglobulin, only 0.002% of the total Ig in serum. The secretion of IgE often occurs in response to allergen invasion and type I allergy. Serum IgE levels in patients with allergies and parasites are significantly higher than those in normal subjects. In 1966, the Swedish scholar Johansson and the Japanese scholar Ishizaka first isolated IgE from the serum of ragweed allergy sufferers and proved IgE to be a mediator of allergic reactions. IgE is a pro-type antibody. At the tail, basophils, such as mast cell membrane antibody- and antigen-binding basophils, and mast cells release histamine substances to promote the development of inflammation. This mode is also the path that triggers an immediate allergic reaction.

   The mechanism of IgE synthesis and regulation is not entirely clear. A variety of allergic diseases can be seen in the same patient, indicating the constitution of that allergic susceptibility, and in such patients, compared with normal serum, IgE is significantly increased, as is the number of mast cells, and more IgE receptors occur on the membrane. Studies have confirmed that the allergic constitution is autosomal dominant, but different members of the same family may suffer from different allergies; the nature of the antigen and the way it enters the body also affect the synthesis of IgE, although the antigens enter the body in the same way. Some antigens such as hairstyling products cause a strong allergic reaction, although others cannot, although the exact reason is not clear; but with the antigen itself, especially the characteristics of epitopes recognized by T cells, some drugs such as degraded penicillin, worm antigen, wormwood pollen, ragweed pollen, etc., can cause strong IgE-type allergic reactions. Antigens entering into the body and the frequency of antigen contact with the body produce antibodies having an impact; the mucosa easily produce the IgE response, and injection is caused by the production of IgG. The greater the number of allergens that are in contact with the body, the greater is the possibility of sensitization.

When the allergen is contacted again, binding to the IgE receptors on the cell membrane causes a series of biochemical reactions, which in turn release various bioactive mediators such as histamine and cause allergy and inflammation. Helper T cells and their contributing cytokines have a key regulatory role in the composition of IgE. Depending on the type of excreted cytokines, helper cells are categorized into two subsets, Th1 and Th2. The cytokines secreted by Th2 cells are mainly important in antibody constitution and allergic reaction. By cytokines and mutual regulation, under healthy conditions, Th1 and Th2 balance each other, and at the same time accept T helper cells in the control of helper T-cell deficiencies or contact with certain foreign proteins or more subtle molecules (such as dust mites, pollen, or seafood). Th2 overactivation results in Th2 cytokine excretion that is too high, prompting increased serum IgE concentration, thus triggering allergies. Supplementation with anti-hyperlipid probiotic strains has been shown to lower the level of serum IgE antibodies. Anti-allergic probiotics use a physiologically acceptable probiotic composition with enhanced anti-allergic properties that effectively alleviates the symptoms of allergy by regulating the secretion of interleukin 12 (IL-12) and interferon 7; this also regulates the Th1-type immune response and inhibits the immunoglobulin IgE Th2-type immune response to improve the phenomenon of excessive allergies. Anti-allergic probiotic bacteria and dendritic cells in the intestinal wall act on receptor binding; activation of intracellular translation of protein is moved to the nucleus and releases a large number of cytokines, a part of innate immunity. Polypeptide diabetes substances such as peptidoglycan, lipopolysaccharide, and polysaccharides in the innate immune system can indeed activate T-cell development.

5. Immunoglobulin D (IgD) is the most mysterious type of antibody known today. The specific role of IgD in the human is not known. IgD mainly appears on the surface of mature B lymphocytes, which may be related to cell recognition that responds to the corresponding pathogens for immune response, and may also be related to the differentiation of B cells. Its main cross-model exists in the B-cell surface, and the level of secretion to the serum is very low. IgD as found in human myeloma protein in 1995 has a molecular weight of 175 kDa and is mainly produced by plasma cells of the tonsils, spleen, etc. IgD concentration in human serum is 3–40 μg/ml, less than 1% of the total serum. The IgD hinge region is very long and sensitive to proteolytic hydrolysis, so IgD half-life is very short, only 2.8 days. The exact immune function of serum IgD is not clear. In differentiation to the mature B-cell stage, in addition to expressing SmIgD, the antigen appears to be immune tolerant after stimulation. SmIgD fades after activation of B cells, either upon activation or upon becoming memory B cells.

2.4.3 Classification According to the Presence of Visible Antigen-Binding Reaction

Antibodies can be divided into a medium reaction with the participation of the visible binding reaction of the complete antibody, the so-called antibody; or if no visible reaction occurs, they can suppress the antigen with its corresponding complete antibody binding to an incomplete antibody.

2.4.4 Classification According to the Origin of Antibodies

By origin, there are natural antibodies and immune antibodies.

1. Natural antibodies are also known as normal antibodies, that is, various antibodies that naturally occur in humans without significant infection by humans or animals or by artificial injection of antigens. Natural antibodies include not only antibodies against pathogenic microorganisms and their products, but antibodies against nonpathogenic substances, such as blood group antibodies. In addition to blood type, antibodies are mainly affected by genetic factors; the other natural antibodies may result from latent infection or common antigen stimulation. Because people or animals are constantly exposed to various antigens after birth, some observers think that natural antibodies are correct and are just customary. In a given region, the average level of natural antibodies for the diagnosis of disease has a certain reference value. The most important natural antibody is IgM.
2. An immune antibody occurs by the stimulation of antigen substances, by B-cell differentiation into plasma cells generated, with the corresponding antigen-specific binding reaction of immunoglobulin. Antibodies can be combined with antigens, both foreign and foreign, to effectively remove foreign bodies such as pathogenic microorganisms and parasites that invade the body, to neutralize the toxins they release, or to remove certain autoantigens to keep the body in good condition and balance. However, immune antibodies such as anti-nuclear antibodies, anti-double-stranded DNA antibodies, and anti-thyroglobulin antibodies can cause harm, sometimes pathological lesions, to the human body.

2.4.5 Classification According to Antibody Preparation Methods

The categories are polyclonal antibodies and monoclonal antibodies.

1. A polyclonal antibody (PcAb) (referred to as polyclonal), as its name implies, is a relatively "monoclonal" antibody in terms of antigen and is usually composed of multiple antigenic determinants that stimulate the body. An antibody produced by a B lymphocyte that receives the antigen is called a monoclonal antibody. By a variety of antigenic determinants to stimulate the body, corresponding to produce a variety of monoclonal antibodies, these monoclonal antibodies are mixed together as a polyclonal antibody; the body produces antibodies that are polyclonal antibodies in addition to antigenic determinants. Diversity is the same type of antigenic determinant but also stimulates the body to produce antibodies such as IgG, IgM, IgA, IgE, and IgD. The correct understanding of monoclonal

antibodies, in turn, allows further understanding of the significant role of polyclonal antibodies. Polyclonal antibodies from the body are from the outside of the heterologous antigen (macromolecular antigen, hapten, etc.) to stimulate the body's immune response; the body of plasma cells secrete a group of special immunoglobulin. Polyclonal antibodies are widely used in research and diagnosis because of their ability to recognize multiple epitopes, precipitating reactions, short preparation times, and low cost.

2. Monoclonal antibody (McAb) (referred to as monoclonal antibody, MAb) is known as the tumor "biological missile," resembling a drug that can be directly directed to the tumor; it is produced by a lymphocyte hybridoma, only for a single antigen molecule, with antigenic determinants of specific antibodies. A lymphocyte hybridoma is an artificial method to make myeloma cells (ascites tumor-like plasma cells of pure mice) fuse with lymphocytes that have been sensitized with antigens and can secrete certain antibodies (commonly used are sensitized animal spleen cells, which act as one of the B cells). After addition of HAT selection medium, unfused B cells die because they cannot survive for long periods of time, whereas myeloma cells cannot synthesize DNA through the DNA remediation synthesis pathway because of the lack of HGPRT enzyme and therefore also die. Survival of fusion cells, the final acquisition of monoclonal cells, compares the potency of antibodies between different monoclonal cells to select the appropriate monoclonal strain. The fusion cells not only have a large number of tumor cells, the characteristics of unlimited reproduction, but also the ability of B cells to synthesize and secrete specific antibodies. Antigens that can be used to produce monoclonal antibodies can be human or animal T cells, B cells, erythrocytes, tumor cells, or various microorganisms or proteins, nucleic acids, and other molecules.

   Because a B-cell clone produces antibodies to only one antigenic determinant, a single hybridoma cell from a B cell fused with a myeloma cell produces only a single antibody. The hybridoma cells are isolated by suitable means and subjected to a single cell culture to multiply in large quantities so that the cell clones that proliferate in the culture medium produce only perfectly uniform and monospecific antibodies, that is, monoclonal antibodies. Monoclonal antibodies of high purity, specificity, and high potency, and the use of different cells and microbial strains or strains, can be eliminated from serological cross-reaction, which greatly improves diagnostic specificity and sensitivity. In addition, these have a very important role in studying cell-surface markers, purifying soluble antigens, and further studying the structure and function of antibodies.

   In 1975, British scientists Kohler and Milstein fused antibody-producing lymphocytes and tumor cells and successfully established this monoclonal technology, winning the Nobel Prize in physiology or medicine in 1984. Since its advent in 1975, the monoclonal antibody has opened a new chapter in clinical immunology. It not only opens up a new path for the preparation of antisera, but also greatly improves the diagnosis and treatment of many clinical diseases.

Monoclonal antibody technology is an important tool in modern life science research, having an indispensable role in the study of the structure and function of genes and proteins. So far, monoclonal antibody technology is still irreplaceable in the immunological diagnosis of humans, animals, and plants. In recent years, monoclonal antibodies have been widely used in tissue and organ transplantation, which greatly improves the curative effect of transplantation and provides strong technical support for the rapid development of transplantation. Common clinical monoclonal antibodies include rituximab, cetuximab, and trastuzumab.

3. Single B-cell polymerase chain reaction (PCR) expression of antibodies in vitro is similar to the aforementioned polyclonal or monoclonal antibody; after immunizing a mouse or a rabbit with the antigen of interest, the animal's peripheral blood or spleen tissue is removed to prepare a cell suspension and incubated with the antigen of interest labeled with fluorescein. As the surface of the memory B cells that expresses specific IgG or IgM can express the desired antigen-specific antibody, it will bind to the antigen, which has been labeled with fluorescein; thus, memory B cells that bind the antigen will produce fluorescence under the laser-specific excitation of a flow cytometer. Cell sorting and lysis, single-cell messenger RNA reverse transcription into complementary DNA (complement DNA, cDNA), and the use of antibody variables and constant region primers for PCR increase the specific antibody sequence. It is then cloned into the antibody expression vector and transfected into common 293 cells to express the monoclonal antibody in vitro.

   The single-cell PCR method in vitro expression method rather than the traditional monoclonal antibody technology has certain advantages. (1) There is no hybridoma formation process, greatly saving time and cost. In addition, certain low abundance antibody information may be lost because of the relatively low efficiency of hybridoma technology. (2) Peripheral blood can also be used in this method for antibody expression. It is also possible to extract B cells from blood samples of infected individuals to obtain fully humanized monoclonal antibodies such as anti-SARS virus antibodies and AB blood group antibodies.

2.4.6 Classification According to the Antigen–Antibody Reaction in Various Manifestations

(1) Precipitin refers to the antigen and the precipitation reaction can occur with the antibody. (2) Lectin refers to the combination of particulate antigen aggregation antibody. (3) Lysin: with cell membrane antigen binding, the complement can make the cells appear as dissolved antibodies, such as lysozymes or hemolysin. (4) Complement fixation antibody refers to the combination of antigens that can activate complement antibody. (5) Opsonin refers to the role of conditioning with the combination of microorganisms that can promote swallowing by phagocyte antibodies. (6) When neutralizing antibodies are combined with the virus, the virus can lose the infectious antibodies.

2.5 Diversity of Antibodies and Its Production Mechanism

2.5.1 Diversity of Antibodies

The diversity of antibodies is the heterogeneity of antibodies. Antibody composition is extremely complex and consists of thousands and thousands of Ig molecules. These Ig molecules are both similar and different in shape, size, structure, and amino acid composition and arrangement. Their differences cause their electrophoretic activity to vary greatly. As the antibody has a binding site (antigen-binding cluster) corresponding to the antigenic determinant, the binding of the antibody to the antigen is specific. On the other hand, the antibody itself is a protein, with its own amino acid composition, arrangement, and three-dimensional structure; in the case of xeno animals, it is an antigen. Each Ig has an antigen specificity that is detectable by serological methods and shows different serological types. There are three specific Ig antigens. (1) In those isotype specific, all from the same species have common antigen specificity. Human Ig can be divided into five major categories (IgM, IgG, IgA, IgD, IgE), and two types (lambda and kappa), as well as several subclasses, subtypes, groups, and subgroups. However, the specificity of the binding of the antibody to the antigen is not related to the antibody class, subclass, type, etc. (2) In allotype specificity, the antigenic determinant is shared by some individuals of the same species (such as the human), which is determined by the genetic category, some of the heavy chain and light chain constant regions, and the replacement of individual amino acids to form Gm, Am, and Km, of each type. (3) Unique type specificity arises from a single B-cell clone of Ig molecules with unique antigenicity. This determinant is in the variable regions of the heavy and light chains, especially in the hypervariable regions of the variable regions. Because each individual antibody-forming cell is composed of polyclones, the idiosyncratic specificity is extremely large.

The diversity of antibodies is controlled by the B-cell system genes. The peptide chain is encoded by two different genes, respectively, of the variable or constant region; the constant region of the gene (C gene) is limited, although it can determine the type and subclass of Ig molecules, to cause Ig molecular diversity. However, the main reason for the diversity of immunoglobulin molecules lies in the heterogeneity of the variable region.

2.5.2 Antibody Diversity Mechanism

Antibody diversity has the following mechanisms [3].

1. VDJ gene fragment combination: The antibody forms a Y-structure from two identical heavy chains and two identical light chains. The specificity of the antibody for the antigen is determined by the variable region of the antibody. The heavy chain variable region of the human antibody consists of three VDJ gene segments located on chromosome 14: about 45 V gene segments, 23 D gene segments, and 6 J gene segments. During maturation of B cells to produce antibodies, the region of the antibody gene that contains the VDJ gene is rearranged; one for each of the VDJ fragments to form the variable region of the antibody, and

one of many constant region gene fragments is then taken to form the antibody heavy chain. As a result, 45 × 23 × 6 = 6210 kinds of antibodies are possible. The human light chain genes are k and λ, located on chromosomes 2 and 12, respectively. The light chain variable region consists of two VJ gene fragments: the number of Vk and Jk fragments is 40 and 5, and the number of Vλ and Jλ fragments is 30 and 4, respectively. Thus, possible k species are 40 × 5 = 200 and the possible k type is 30 × 4 = 120 species. The antibody consists of a heavy chain and a light chain such that there are 6210 × (200 + 120) = 1,198,700 species possibilities for the number of antibodies that result from the light and heavy chain V (D) J rearrangements.

2. Diversity of junctional connections among VDJ: Although the antibody diversity caused by the combination of VDJ gene fragments is about 2 × 106, the actual situation is far more than that, suggesting that there are other diversity mechanisms. The V (D) J gene fragment leaves the 3′-end of the sense strand and the 5′-end of the antisense strand before ligation, such as before the V and D gene fragments are ligated. Similarly, similar to the V gene fragment, the D gene fragment ends (the head end, the end to be linked to the V gene) are also dissociated by a recombinase to form a hairpin. When the V gene is linked to the D gene, the hairpin structures of the two gene segments are resected. However, the site of cleavage is not necessarily the original position, resulting in one strand in the double strand of the V (D) gene being longer than the other. The shorter one is filled to the blunt end and then to the D (V) gene fragment. Completed nucleotides are called P-nucleotides. The P-nucleotide is present between the DJ gene segments or the light chain VJ gene segments as the result of this mechanism. The presence of P-nucleotides greatly enriches the diversity of antibodies. In addition, after P-nucleotides are added, and also when terminal deoxynucleotidyl transferase (TdT) is active, the terminal transferase may add nucleotides after the P-nucleotide up to 20 nucleotides; these additions are called N-nucleotides. In addition to adding P- or N-nucleotides, deletions of nucleotides can also be made at the ends between the VDJ fragments of the antibody. The insertion and deletion of this nucleotide greatly enriches the diversity of antibodies.
3. Somatic high-frequency mutation of mature B cells in addition to the VDJ gene junction region and the precursor cells or other cells in the body is different; it was found that the VDJ gene is also different, suggesting a mature B-cell VDJ gene mutation, called somatic hypermutation. High-frequency somatic mutations have a crucial role in the diversity of antibodies, especially the specificity and affinity of antibodies. Through the combination of diversity and P-, N-, and other nucleotides, changes mostly produce low-affinity antibodies. Affinity maturation at this time has a function in the peripheral lymphoid organs (mainly lymph nodes) germinal center; in B cells with low-affinity binding antigen in the VDJ nucleotide, mutation occurs by mitosis, at a mutation frequency as great as one mutation per 1000 nucleotides. Mutated cells with more affinity to the antibody gain preponderance of growth, thereby greatly increasing the affinity of the antibody produced by the B cells.

3 ABO Blood Group Antibodies

3.1 Introduction

The ABO blood group antibody, which is one of the most important antibodies in the human body, has many features in common with general antibodies in terms of basic functions and biological characteristics. The relationship between ABO blood group antibodies and common antibodies is individuality and commonness. As the basic rules and characteristics of antibodies are mentioned earlier, this section focuses on the ABO blood group antibody personality characteristics.

3.2 Type of ABO Blood Group Antibodies

In the human ABO blood group system, there are blood group antigens on the erythrocyte membrane, the most important of which are the A antigen and the B antigen. The carbohydrate-linked glycoproteins or glycolipids of these two antigens are distributed on the surface of most tissues, including the vascular system of endothelial cells. Blood can be divided into four kinds of ABO blood groups according to the existence of A antigen and B antigen on the erythrocyte membrane: four blood types, namely, A, B, O, and AB. The surface of the human type A red blood cell contains A antigen (also known as agglutinogen), the serum contains anti-B antibody; the type B human erythrocyte surface contains B antigen, and the serum contains anti-A antibody. In the AB type of human red blood cells, the cell surface contains two antigens, A and B, but the serum has neither anti-A antibody nor anti-B antibody. The type O human erythrocyte cell surface has neither A antigen nor B antigen; the serum contains anti-A antibody and anti-B antibody. The ABO blood group system can be divided into several subtypes: for type A blood, there are at least two subtypes, A1 and A2, and in the A1 erythrocyte membrane two antigens, A and A1, in the A2 type erythrocyte membrane. Antigen B is only contained in the sera of type A sera, which contains only the A antigen. The serum of type A2 sera contains anti-B and anti-A1 antibodies. The A type is divided into A1 and A2 types, making AB type, which is also divided into A1B type and A2B type, or two subtypes. Among these blood types, the antigenicity of each blood group antigen is different according to the distribution of the antigen on the erythrocyte membrane of each blood group: the antigenicity of the AB blood group is strongest, the antigenicity of O-type blood is the weakest, and in the others, the blood group antigenicity is A1B > A > A2B > B > A2.

Inheritance of the human ABO blood group system is controlled by the alleles IA, IB, and i on chromosome 9. Only two of these three genes may appear on a pair of chromosomes, one for each offspring (except for the rare CisAB blood group). Three genes can be composed of six genotypes, because the A and B genes are genetically dominant. O-type genes are recessive, so in the blood type of expression of only four, the same blood type of their genetic type is not certain (Table 3.1). For example, in the phenotype of type A blood, the genetic type may be A1A1 or A1O;

Table 3.1 Genotype and phenotype, antigen and antibody, of ABO blood groups

Phenotype	Genotype	Erythrocyte antigen	Natural antibodies in serum
Al	Al Al	A1	Anti-B
	A1 O	A1 + H	
A2	A2 A2	A2	Anti-B (about 10% people have anti-A1)
	A2O	A2 + H	
B	BB	B	Anti-A
	BO	B + H	
A1B	AB	A1 + B	None
A2B	Al B	A2 + B	(About 25% people have anti-A1)
O	O	H	Anti-A + B

Note: All erythrocytes in the foregoing list generally have a certain H antigen on their surface and therefore do not produce anti-H antibodies (although some reports suggest that approximately 3% of A1B-type blood donors contain anti-H antibodies). To indicate that A2 antigen is weaker than A1, the H antigen is not marked in these blood types

in phenotype A2 type blood, the genetic type may be A2A2 or A2O; but for the red blood cells on the phenotype O, the gene type can only be OO. Because phenotypes A or B may originate from the AO and BO genotypes, respectively, it is entirely possible that parents of type A or B blood types will give birth to children whose phenotype is type O.

In the United States, about 20% of blood group A individuals showed A2, whereas most showed A1. In contrast, A2 is extremely rare in Japan [4]. However, although type A2 and A2B Han people in China accounted for a smaller proportion of type A and type AB, respectively, type A1 and type A2 A2B are agglutinated by type A1 erythrocytes, and the RBCs are less antigenic than A1 and A1B erythrocytes. Therefore, in view of this characteristic of blood type A2, in ABOi (ABO-incompatible) organ transplantation, studies have shown [4, 5] that the kidneys from the A2 blood group donors have corresponding preoperative and postoperative treatment. The extent to which antibody-mediated graft injury is undergone by technology is less severe than that of other blood donor donors. To some extent, this experimental result confirms the idea that the antigenicity of type A2 erythrocytes is weaker than that of A1 erythrocytes and has a role in future development of transplantation.

ABO blood group antibodies are divided into two categories of natural antibodies and immune antibodies; these blood group antibodies are mainly IgM and IgG class antibodies, with are a very small number of IgA antibodies. The origin of human blood group antibodies cannot be completely elucidated. It is generally considered to be caused by exposure to A and B blood group antigens or their analogues in the environment (bacteria, viruses, animals, plants, etc.). These antibodies can cause human blood group substance reactions, such as when type A individuals exposed to B antigens produce anti-B antibodies; this produces more antibodies to IgM. Pregnancy, blood transfusion, and transplantation have produced more blood group antibodies, which are IgG. In physiological circumstances, the newborn has not yet fully developed, so there is no blood ABO blood group antibody. At 2–8 months after birth the antibody begins to produce, with 18 months needed to reach a steady state, peaking at 8–10 years of age. Because of its molecular weight, the natural antibody, mostly IgM, cannot pass the placenta; therefore, in pregnant women with fetal blood group discrepancy, the natural antibodies in the body of the pregnant woman will not enter the fetus through the placenta, and will not cause fetal agglutination of red blood cells. An immune antibody in the body to accept their own does not exist in the stimulation of erythrocyte antigen produced. Immune antibodies are mostly IgG antibodies, so by their molecular weight they can enter the fetus through the placenta. Therefore, if the mother in the past has experienced exogenous A or B antigen in the body (such as in blood transfusion) and produces immune antibodies, fetal and ABO blood group incompatibility of pregnant women may be caused by entrance of maternal immune blood type antibodies into the fetus, causing fetal red blood cell damage, the occurrence of hemolytic disease of newborns.

3.3 Blood Group Antibody Removal Technology

Postoperative rejection is a major challenge for ABOi organ transplantation. Acute rejection has been the main factor impeding the long-term survival of ABOi organ transplantation. With the application and development of blood group antibody removal technology in organ transplantation, people have come to realize that this technology will become crucial for determining the success or failure of transplantation. Its significance lies in the ABO blood group antibodies (mainly IgG and IgM) in patients with clearance or reduced in vivo titers, so that ABOi transplant rejection is reduced to achieve effectiveness in enhancing graft survival or prolongation of the patient's life.

Blood group antibody removal technology includes plasma exchange technology, immuno-adsorption technology, and plasma double filtration technology.

1. Plasma exchange technology is a plasma separation device, the use of extracorporeal circulation of the patient's plasma separation and filtration, removal of abnormal plasma, and recovery of the blood to replace the physical components; some of the autoantibodies in plasma are removed in this method. In ABOi organ transplantation, the primary purpose of plasmapheresis is to remove anti-A and anti-B antibodies in patients and to reduce the incidence of postoperative acute rejection. Plasma exchange technology can effectively remove from the body small, medium, and large molecular substances, especially protein-binding substances, such as toxins and antibodies. The filtration effect of plasma exchange on various ABO blood group antibodies is shown in Fig. 3.1. Among the three

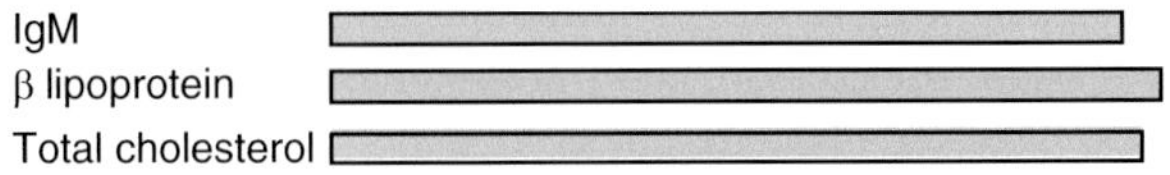

Fig. 3.1 Filtration composition and proportion of ABO blood group antibody in plasma exchange

blood group antibodies, the antibody IgG has the smallest molecular weight and IgM the highest molecular weight, and, therefore, the highest filtration rate is that of the IgG of the blood group antibody, and IgA is second, the lowest rate of IgM antibody filtration. We can see that among the three types of blood group antibodies, the blood group antibody IgM is most likely to be cleared in blood replacement. Plasma exchange technology is widely used in the United States and Japan, with anti-ABO blood group antibodies eliminated by one application reaching about 20%. The main advantage of plasmapheresis in the removal of ABO blood group antibodies is that, for example, freshly freeze-dried type AB plasmapheresis removes blood group antibodies and replenishes clotting factors; its major drawback is the risk of a viral infection. It is prone to allergic reactions, and the treatment is more costly. On the other hand, plasma exchange technology can be used alone to remove blood group antibodies and can also be used in combination with plasma double filtration.

2. Adsorption technology is a blood purification technology developed on the basis of plasma exchange in the past 15 years. The principle is that the separated plasma selectively removes related antibodies through an adsorber. In ABOi organ transplantation, immuno-adsorption occurs through the extracorporeal circulation, the highly specific antigen–antibody and adsorbent material of the adsorption column being selective for removal of antibodies in plasma, thereby reducing rejection after transplantation. Approximately 30% of anti-A and/or anti-B IgM antibodies are cleared by immunosorbent in a single treatment, and clearance of the anti-A and/or anti-B IgG antibody is approximately 20%, which will not cause other antibody changes [6]. In ABO-incompatible organ transplantation, the types and percentages of the immunosorbent-removed blood group antibodies are IgG1, -2, -3 (100%), IgG3 (30–80%), IgM (56%), and IgA (69%). Compared with plasmapheresis, immunosuppressive technology has obvious advantages in terms of curative effect and safety. For example, the adsorption of blood type antibody is specific; no albumin and other plasma component is lost, there is no need of replenishing fluid, and no risk of virus infection. However, immunosorbent technology also has its own shortcomings, such as the need to use specific adsorbers, which are more expensive.
3. Dual plasma filtration technology is the separation of the smaller plasma components through the membrane pores of the separator, and the clearance of the body of large molecular weight proteins, while leaving the small molecular weight albumin and other active ingredients, and adding the supplement liquid and returning it to the treatment. Plasma double filtration technology is a highly selective blood purification technology, which uses two different pore-size filters: one is a plasma separator, by centrifugation or filtration effect, and the other is the plasma filter. The pore size of the filter mainly allows no more than or less than the passage of albumin molecules, and substances greater in size than albumin will be cleared out. In the application of ABOi organ transplantation, because of the different pore size of the blood plasma filter membrane, the inhibition rate of the blood group antibody is also different. Therefore, plasma membrane filters with different pore sizes should be selected according to the molecular weight of

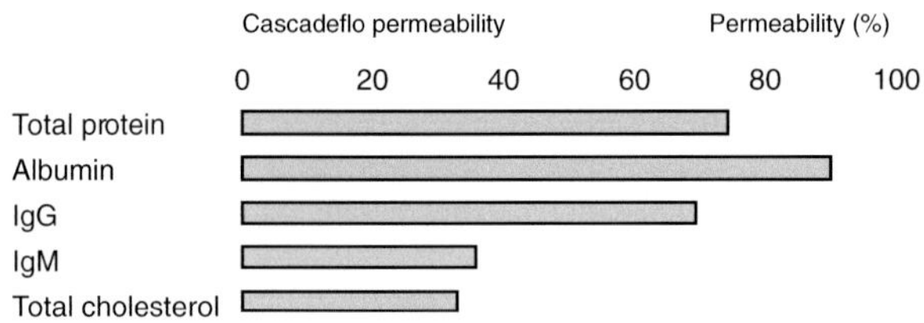

Fig. 3.2 Filtration composition and proportion of ABO blood group antibody in plasma double filtration

the pathogenic substance, to ensure not only the complete elimination of the corresponding antibodies, but also to minimize the loss of albumin. In ABOi organ transplantation, the double filtration technique of plasma filters with the filtration rate and the proportion of different components is shown in Fig. 3.2. Because of the large molecular weight of the blood group antibody IgM, it is difficult to be effectively removed through the blood plasma filter; blood group antibodies IgG have a relatively small molecular weight and pass through the plasma filter relatively more easily than IgM. The main advantage of the plasma double-pass technique in removing blood group antibodies is that the relatively selective elimination of ABO blood group antibodies and HLA antibodies reduces the loss of albumin and can generally be supplemented with albumin solution to effectively reduce the risk of infection, such as viruses, and allergic reactions. The main drawbacks are the large number of coagulation factors and macromolecular protein loss.

Filtration composition and proportion of ABO blood group antibody in plasma double filtration using a certain type of adsorption column are shown in Fig. 3.2.

The plasma exchange technique, immuno-adsorption technique, and plasma double filtration technique are important breakthroughs in the history of ABOi organ transplantation. These three techniques can effectively remove anti-A and anti-B antibodies from patients, when applied alone or in combination, to reduce the incidence of acute rejection after transplantation, and greatly improve the survival rate of graft and patients, thus having an important role in the development of ABOi organ transplantation.

4 Detection of Blood Type Antibody and Its Significance

4.1 Test Method for Blood Group Antibody

In the immune response, cellular immunity and humoral immunity are two closely related and mutually regulated physiological processes. There are many detection methods for both immune responses, but so far in clinical testing, the detection of specific antibodies is the most widely used. Antibody titer refers to the physical state of an antibody and its residence time in the body, and its immune response is expressed by how much it reacts with the antigen.

Both anti-A and anti-B antibodies include IgG and IgM. IgG can be detected by the indirect Coombs test, IgM antibody can be detected by the saline method; the bromelain method can be used to detect IgG and IgM, and has higher sensitivity than that of the other two methods. Micro-column gel Karl's method is a new method to display the reaction of erythrocyte antigen antibody in recent years. It has advantages such as simple operation, easy observation of results, and simultaneous detection of incomplete antibodies.

4.1.1 Saline Medium Agglutination Test

The antigen in the saline media agglutination test is a saline erythrocyte suspension. The antigenic determinant on the erythrocytes binds to the antigen-binding site on the corresponding antibody molecule and crosslinks to form a macroscopic agglutination mass. The saline media agglutination test is used to detect, identify, and cross-match blood tests with IgM antibodies as well as to blood group systems identified by saline antibodies such as ABO, MN, P, or S. In the saline medium agglutination test in the determination of blood type and cross-matching blood, results of the observation are available immediately after centrifugation, with the advantages of easy operation, saving time, and low consumption. However, because the distance between erythrocytes in saline solution is about 25 nm, the shortest distance between the two most adjacent Fab ends of IgM antibody molecules is more than 35 nm, and the distance between two Fab ends of IgG antibody molecules is generally less than 25 nm, IgG antibodies do not agglutinate with the red blood cells of the corresponding antibodies in the saline medium, whereas IgM antibodies do agglutinate. However, low detection sensitivity and low sensitivity to incomplete antibodies can lead to serious consequences as well as disadvantages such as unstable results and poor interpretation, and such methods have therefore been either eliminated or used only for preliminary tests of blood compatibility testing.

4.1.2 Colloidal Media Agglutination Test

Agglutination of IgG antibodies usually does not occur in saline media. However, if an erythrocyte suspension is prepared in colloidal medium, the antibodies on erythrocytes agglutinate with the corresponding IgG antibodies in serum, and the colloidal medium affects the second phase of the agglutination reaction. The erythrocyte surface is rich in sialic acid; red blood cells in a neutral environment are negatively charged and because of the same charge repel each other in a suspended state. Electrostatic theory holds that the higher the cell-surface charge, the dielectric constant of the smaller media, the greater the potential, the greater the power between the red blood cells, and the greater the distance between cells; on the other hand, the distance between the red blood cells is small. The main role of colloidal media is to maintain the dielectric constant and shorten the distance between the red blood cells, the IgG antibodies sensitized erythrocytes agglutination phenomenon. The substances used to form the colloidal medium include bovine serum albumin (BSA), human albumin, AB type serum, and gum acacia. It is most convenient to take AB type serum, and the best is bovine albumin, which is also used more often. Colloidal media agglutination tests increase the sensitivity of the reaction, especially for IgG class antibodies. However, the operation of such methods is complicated and the test requirements are also high; there is also a problem of subjective interpretation. At present, only a few laboratories in the United States use certain BSA-boosting antibody-enhancing solutions: 18% use 22% BSA, and only 3% use 30% BSA. Other methods neutralize the negative charges on the surface of red blood cells by using low ionic strength solution (LISS) or polyethylene glycol (PEG) added with molecular substances, and shorten the distance between the red blood cells to enhance the direct agglutination reaction.

4.1.3 Enzyme-Treated Erythrocyte Agglutination Test

The erythrocyte surface is rich in sialic acid, making it negatively charged in the neutral environment, which is why red blood cells exclude each other. Proteolytic enzymes digest and destroy this sialic acid, reducing the negative charge on the surface of red blood cells, thereby promoting agglutination. Common enzymes are bromelain and papain. The enzyme method can be divided into one-step and two-step methods; the one-step method is not as sensitive as the two-step method, but is easy to operate, and more convenient for cross-matching blood, and the two-step method is generally used for antibody screening and antibody identification if the positive result is too much. The enzyme method can significantly enhance the antigen–antibody reaction of the Rh and Kidd systems. However, proteases can destroy M, N, S, s, Fya, and Fyb antigens and cannot be treated with enzymes for such antigens. Although the enzymatic method is more sensitive, the application of such methods has been limited for some of these reasons. The use criteria recommended by the Swiss Red Cross Blood Transfusion Service (BTSSRC) suggest that one-step enzymatic methods are not sensitive enough to be eliminated, but enhanced two-step enzyme assays are necessary for pregnant women. Gerbr believes that the enzymatic assay is not suitable for routine work; too many positive results are caused by unrelated clinical factors. In Finland, enzymatic methods have been phased out since the 1980s to avoid interfering with meaningless antibodies. In the UK, a survey of 50,776 pregnant women who had "records" showed that the positive rate was 6.6% for initial screening tests, 4.7% was still positive again, and only 1.4% (731 cases) contained identifiable potentially clinically relevant erythrocyte alloantibodies, of which 117 cases were detectable only enzymatically; 54 of 117 patients had antibodies with potential clinical significance to the fetus. Results of these 54 follow-up studies showed that only 3 patients were detected by PEG-IAT at later stages of pregnancy (anti-D 0.9 IU/ml; anti-D 1:32; anti-C 1:1), with only one infant showing signs of hemolytic disease of the newborn (HDN). It can be inferred that the results of the enzyme test are not effective for the detection of the morbidity and mortality of the fetus or the newborn and a role in the prenatal examination. The abolition of the enzymatic test and the introduction of the automatic processing program and data acquisition will probably compress the huge workload. Similarly, the use of enzymatic crossover tests is also not recommended in the UK. The results of the UK National Objective Quality Assessment Program (NEQAS) showed that although the IAT assay is sensitive to detect weak RH antibodies by enzymatic assays, the IAT is weakly detectable in the most sensitive anti-D method, which is based on experimental evidence.

4.1.4 Antiglobulin Test and Its Improved Method

The antiglobulin test, established in 1945 by Coombs et al., is also known as the Coombs test. The establishment of an antiglobulin test is very important for blood group serology. The erythrocyte surface is coated with IgG antibody molecules or complement molecule C3, C4 fragments, but cannot produce agglutination. IgG antibodies and complement are human globulin, and with these human immunoglobulin immunization animals or hybridoma technology can be made of anti-human globulin The specificity of such antibodies against the Fc fragment of IgG molecules or complement C3, C4 fragments can be coated on the red blood cells and antibody complement molecules, agglutination of red blood cells. Anti-human globulin molecules take part in bridging. The antiglobulin test is divided into the direct anti-human globulin test (DAT) and indirect anti-human globulin test (IAT). The traditional method is saltwater as a medium, test tubes by centrifugation, widely used in cross-matching blood, blood type identification, and antibody screening. In the UK, only 82% of the test-anti-D programs in 1985 adopted the indirect anti-human globulin test (IAT), but reaching 98% in 1992 and 100% in 1994 [7]. A survey of 59 hospitals in Ontario conducted by the Toronto Red Cross Society Toronto Center in 1993 showed that two thirds of hospitals used IAT for antibody screening experiments. Although tube centrifugation of anti-human globulin assays is considered an acceptable technique for detecting antibodies to erythrocytes, data suggest that the reaction between 1+ and 2+ is easy because of improper interpretation in standard IAT tube centrifuge assays, being wrong especially more often than 20% on a large scale. Because many clinically significant erythrocytic antibodies are IgG, many improvements have been made to increase the sensitivity of anti-human globulin assays: the medium is changed to low ionic strength solution (LISS), polyethylene glycol (PEG), and the like. These improved tests are sensitive in tubes or microplates. As can be seen from the data provided by NEQAS, almost all laboratories in the UK and Scotland have adopted enhanced anti-human globulin methods, usually using low ionic strength media plus two-step enzymatic methods. These methods are recommended because they improve sensitivity and show good performance in detecting clinically relevant antibodies and also have excellent records in NEQAS experiments in Scotland. Molds believes that in the hands of a skilled serologist, LISS—antiglobulin test (AGT) and PEGAGT—have like sensitivity, but the latter will produce less ambiguous results. LISS-AGT or PEG-AGT experiments are all available if only antiglobulin-reactive antibodies are tested, but both are flawed in the detection of mixed antibodies. From a report from the Netherlands, Overbeeke said that their choice of the PEG-IAT method was based on a comparative study of a large sample of plasma containing known antibodies and a large sample of unknown patients. They found that the PEG-IAT method was more sensitive than the standard centrifuge tube IAT assay using albumin. Several clinically significant antibodies are detected by the PEG-IAT method but not by the albumin IAT method, such as Jka antibodies, Jkb, antibodies and E antibody. The only problem with this technique is that IgM hemolysins (such as anti-Vel antibodies and anti-P antibodies) are detectable using the multispecific antiglobulin reagent IAT but not with PEG-IAT. The main problem with anti-human globulin is the interpretation of the results. When the anti-human globulin method is used in a large number of sample experiments, and results are negative, it is very difficult to maintain accurate interpretation. In addition, there are some problems such as cumbersome operation, heavy workload, and being time-consuming, which restrict their application.

4.1.5 Low-Ion Polybrene Test

In 1980, Lalezari and Jiang first applied polybrene technology to blood bank operations. Polybrene is a high-priced cationic quaternary ammonium salt polymer that can produce much positive charge when dissolved to redirect the surface of the negative charge, so that the distance between the red blood cells can be reduced; the normal erythrocyte can cause reversible nonspecific agglutination. If the antibody-sensitized erythrocytes are agglutinated by agglutinants, the agglutination is irreversible. In the polybrene test that detects the activity of antibodies, erythrocytes and serum are first incubated in a low-ionic medium to promote the binding of antibodies to erythrocytes, followed by the addition of polybrene to agglutinate the cells. After centrifugation, the agglutinated cells are no longer suspended, added to the resuspension, agglutination of polybrene can be neutralized by addition of sodium citrate, the agglutination of normal erythrocytes dissolved, and antibody-induced agglutination still exists. Chen Heping et al. improved the technique of agglomerating amines. The modified polybrene technique is characterized as fast, simple, and sensitive. Especially for Rh system antibodies, its sensitivity is higher than that of the anti-human globulin method; for example, the detection of anti-D is possible to 1 ng/ml, much higher than the antiglobulin method of about 10 ng/ml. This feature provides a powerful tool for the detection of weak Rh system antibodies. In 1983, Fisher used the saltwater method, papaya enzyme method, low ionic saline anti-human globulin method, the polybrene method, and other four different methods to detect the ability of alloantibodies and found that the polybrene method detected alloantibodies with higher sensitivity than other methods. Since then, European and American blood bank laboratories have adopted this method. However, the coagulation amine method still cannot detect all the incomplete antibodies, such as anti-k antibody, so its application has been limited.

4.1.6 Microtube Gel Test

The micropipette gel detection method has gradually emerged in recent years as a new immunoassay method. First invented by Dr. Yves Lapierre in France in 1986, it combines a gel column with an anti-human globulin method, etc., and is a product of the combination of biochemical gel filtration and immunological antigens. The gel is the key to microtubule gel detection technology; the concentration of gel controls the size of the gel gap so that the gap can only allow the passage of free red blood cells. So, free red blood cells and red blood cells gather to distinguish the reaction. If by centrifugation, erythrocyte sedimentation in the bottom of the test tube indicates that no agglutination of erythrocytes is a negative reaction; if the red blood cells are in the upper part of the gel band, it indicates agglutination of red blood cells, a positive reaction. In addition, the gel has been added to anti-human globulin and various types of blood group antibodies, thus simplifying the operation; just add the sample. This type of technology in blood type identification, cross-matching of blood, and antibody screening and identification has a wide range of applications. Gel detection technology is a new technology, currently in the stage of improvement and promotion, that is also gradually being taken seriously. Some hospitals in Canada use gel detection technology to experiment as they think this technology is simple and the results easy to determine. Gel detection technology has also drawn considerable attention in the United States. Garratty stated that the study of alloantibodies produced the detection of very good results. He believes (and hopes) to automate all compatibility experiments quickly. ABO and D blood group identification and antibody screening by blood recipients and blood donors in the United States will be automated and electronic: that is, computerized cross-matching will be used, and gel cards can easily achieve this goal. In 1994 NEQAS received feedback from 380 hospital blood banks which showed that approximately 65% of the cross-match blood tests were performed with gel technology using low-ion-concentration solution centrifugation (BTSSRC) in antibody studies based on 6-month results of the comparative experiment and the subsequent operational experience. Several smaller studies of other technologies have also consolidated their choices. In addition to high sensitivity and high specificity, gel experiments also seem to have high reproducibility, relying on experimental staff: small, long-term preservation of experimental results can be reviewed at any time, which may have so far unknown advantages. Two different techniques were also chosen, traditional centrifugation tube antiglobulin and gel technology, based on the pathological changes of plasma in some patients, such as plasma protein disorders and strong cold or thermal antibodies. Specimens, known as HLTA antibodies, are more easily detectable by the tube method than the gel method. As a reference laboratory, problematic samples are very common: more than 50% of cross-matched blood shows unpredictable responses in different blood types. Approximately one-third of Finnish hospital laboratories, including three-fifths of the university hospitals, chose the condensate method. The data obtained from KUOPIO University Hospital show that screening with the gel method has important clinical implications for increasing the percentage of antibodies identified. Many published data show that this gel anti-human globulin approach meets or exceeds conventional anti-human globulin approaches when examining weak antibodies. Voak and Ouvehand have developed rapid validation techniques for evaluating new methods and using the LISSIA method correctly. This work, as well as many articles covering the new IAT method, shows that the effects of the new antiglobulin method, that is, gel technique and the polyethylene glycol (PEG) centrifuge antiglobulin method, are at least equivalent to the LISS tube centrifugation globulin method. Therefore, with the correct use of high-quality screening cells, they can meet the antibody screening experiments. In addition, data from the NEQAS in the UK demonstrated this, with 38 of the 188 subjects using the IVTG assay for 1 weak anti-antibody missing, whereas only 1 of 53 using the microtubule method missed the check. Many advantages of gel detection techniques are increasingly being applied because of their sensitivity, ease of operation, and long timeframe for interpreting results. As the key to gel technology is control of the quality of the gel, variations in gel cards have also drawn the same attention. Data from two Finnish Red Cross Blood Centers at university hospitals using DiaMed-ID gel cards indicate that the number of positive anti-human globulin experiments in cross-matched blood tests is unbelievably high (1:400), whereas that from the third laboratory using the traditional method was low (1:3000), and they concluded that at least some batches of DiaMed experiments are overly sensitive to very weak IgGs on the erythrocyte surface. Gel card variations and ABO compatibility (i.e., B plasma and A2B cells compatible) may cause gel cards to miss-check; this was first discovered in sophisticated experiments in the UK and has been confirmed by Cummuns and Downham. They believe that the application of gel microcolumn technology in cross-matching experiments remains to be further studied. Under Spain's recently enacted law, the saline method and the traditional anti-human globulin method will be eliminated to detect ABO and other incompatibilities when cross-matching blood. Because of the advantages and automation of gel cards, their use will be greatly increased. This result suggests that the widespread use of gel technology in other countries to detect red blood cell antibodies will become a trend.

4.2 Significance of Blood Group Antibody Test

4.2.1 Significance in Blood Transfusion

Because each person has his or her own blood type and corresponding antibody, when blood transfusions are needed clinically for surgery, it is necessary to first identify the blood type of recipients and donors, and then cross-match the blood type. When a different type of blood is infused, it can cause severe hemolysis that can endanger the recipient's life. Because O-type blood has neither A nor B antigens, many people think that O-type blood is a universal donor, and this idea is not desirable. Because type O blood plasma contains antibodies A and B, in a small amount of blood transfusion the antibody may be diluted in the recipient blood and the secretion of blood type substances and will not have a significant impact, and when a large number of infusions take place, antibodies in the plasma can react with hematopoietic cells of the recipients to cause hemolysis. In addition, studies have shown that some O-containing anti-A or anti-B antibodies that cannot be neutralized by blood group substances can cause a hemolytic reaction. Similarly, that AB is a universal recipient of blood is not correct, in addition to the need to be careful as to A1 and A2 subtypes. Therefore, only the same group of blood is infused, and a different group is used as a last resort.

4.2.2 Significance in Organ Transplantation

The ABO blood group is a strong antigen and therefore needs to be considered for donor ABO blood grouping in organ transplants or hematopoietic stem cell transplants, which otherwise cause hyperacute rejection, especially skin grafts. With the development of science and technology, it has been possible to overcome the ABO blood group disorder. For removal of AB antibodies (such as removal of donor erythrocytes by centrifugation during hematopoietic stem cell transplantation) by immunosorbent, plasmapheresis, or similar methods preceding transplantation, and successful transplantation of T (B) cells using immunosuppressive agents after ABO blood incompatible transplantation, see the following chapter.

4.2.3 Significance in Neonatal Hemolysis

In humans, about half a year after babies are born, because of contact with the nature of the A or B antigens the AB antibody begins to appear in the blood, mainly including IgM and IgG. Neonatal hemolysis occurs in the mother when the blood type is O, and the most common fetal blood group is A or B, and caused by heavier jaundice; others such as the mother's blood group A, fetal blood group B or AB; mother's blood group B, fetal blood group A or AB are less common, and cause less jaundice. Because of the presence of A/B antigens in nature, ABO hemolysis can occur in the first child. Although Rh-negative mothers develop only when the second fetus is Rh-positive and the first fetus is also Rh-positive, although the first child, a history of blood transfusions could cause the mother to produce Rh antibodies.

4.2.4 Other Significance

The ABO blood groups can also be used for kinship identification and forensic identification. Second, the ABO blood group is also associated with disease. The study found that in type A, B, and AB individuals, the probability of squamous cell carcinoma is lower than in the individual with O-type blood. The probability of individual type O blood pancreatic cancer is lower than in other blood types. In terms of coagulation, individuals with type O blood and individuals with level VI and vWF are lower than those with other blood types and tend to have bleeding. Accordingly, studies have shown that A1 and B increase the risk of venous thrombosis, whereas A2 and O decrease the risk.

References

1. Litman GW, Rast JP, Shamblott MJ, et al. Phylogenetic diversification of immunoglobulin genes and the antibody repertoire. Mol Biol Evol. 1993;10:60–72.
2. Woof JM, Burton DR. Human antibody-fc receptor interactions illuminated by crystal structures. Nat Rev Immunol. 2004;4:89–99.
3. Market EA, Papavasiliou FN. V(d)j recombination and the evolution of the adaptive immune system. PLoS Biol. 2003;1:E16.
4. Warner PR, Nester TA. ABO-incompatible solid-organ transplantation. Am J Clin Pathol. 2006;125(Suppl):S87–94.
5. Rydberg L. ABO-incompatibility in solid organ transplantation. Transfus Med. 2001;11:325–42.
6. Valli PV, Puga Yung G, Fehr T, et al. Changes of circulating antibody levels induced by ABO antibody adsorption for ABO-incompatible kidney transplantation. Am J Transplant. 2009;9:1072–80.
7. Crew RJ, Ratner LE. ABO-incompatible kidney transplantation: current practice and the decade ahead. Curr Opin Organ Transplant. 2010;15:526–30.

Tissue Matching of ABO-Incompatible Organ Transplantation

4

Jiqiu Wen

Abstract

The principle of tissue matching of ABO-incompatible organ transplantation was similar to ABO-compatible organ transplantation. The objective of histocompatibility testing is predicting humoral rejection potential in transplant recipients, which depends upon accurate donor typing and sensitive and specific testing for antibodies to human leukocyte antigen. This chapter will describe the basic idea of major histocompatibility complex (MHC), human leukocyte antigen (HLA), and panel-reactive antibody (PRA) and then introduce the evolution techniques of HLA typing, antibody screening, and crossmatching. Depending on the help of these current widespread practices, the clinician can evaluate the immunologic risk assessment of the solid organ transplant recipient and can benefit the allograft/receipt survival.

Keywords

Histocompatibility · Major histocompatibility complex · Human leukocyte antigen · Panel-reactive antibody (PRA) · Crossmatch · Donor-specific antibody

1 Introduction

The fundamental objective of histocompatibility testing was to evaluate humoral immunologic risk of a transplant recipient in the context of their potential donor(s). The advances in techniques for human leukocyte antigen (HLA) typing and the new

J. Wen (✉)
Kidney Transplant Center, National Clinical Research Center of Kidney Diseases, Jinling Hospital, Nanjing University School of Medicine, Nanjing, China

Nanjing General Hospital, PLA, Nanjing, China
e-mail: wjqdoctor@163.com

Y. Wang (ed.), *ABO-incompatible Organ Transplantation*,
https://doi.org/10.1007/978-981-13-3399-6_4

techniques of detection methods for antibodies to HLA antigens and non-HLA allo-immune targets can help transplant physician to improve the recognition of tissue match. This testing evaluates the risk that the recipient immune system will accept a potential allograft as foreign to self and thereby initiate rejection resulting in allograft damage.

HLA laboratory testing was considered as the immunologic component of the pretransplant risk assessment, and antibody analysis was also studied posttransplant, as noninvasive predictors of acute and chronic rejection. It is important for the clinician to understand the complex and interactive nature of these available histocompatibility testing methods in order to fully identify the immunologic risk status of a potential recipient or transplant patient.

This chapter will discuss the basic concepts and the detecting methods of major histocompatibility complex, HLA typing testing, antibody screening, and cross-matching, which provide a practical reference of histocompatibility for the clinician.

2 Basic Concepts of MHC, HLA, PRA, and DSA

2.1 MHC

The major histocompatibility complex (MHC) was first found in inbred mice strains by Clarence Cook Little, who found that there was a rejection between the different mice in the tumor tissue transplantation experiment. George Snell named the antigen which caused the rejection histocompatibility antigen and pointed out that the H-2 complex is the main histocompatibility complex of mice, and this is the earliest discovery of MHC locus [1]. For his contribution, Snell received the 1980 Nobel Prize in Physiology or Medicine.

The major histocompatibility complex (MHC), also known as the major histocompatibility complex gene, is a gene family that exists in most of the vertebrate genome. MHC is widely present in the body of various tissue cell surfaces, and the genes that control the antigens are inherited according to Mendelian law. The location of the gene in the chromosome is called the tissue compatibility site. The major histocompatibility gene of the human body is located on chromosome 6 and is linked by several sites, called the major histocompatibility complex. A group of antigen systems produced by MHC is called the major histocompatibility system (MHS). The MHC glycoprotein of human is also called human leukocyte antigen (HLA) [2]. The cell surface antigens encoded by some genes are a "characteristic" of each human cell and are also the basis for the immune system to distinguish self from nonself.

2.2 HLA

In 1958, Dausset discovered the first human leukocyte antigen and opened the prelude to the HLA [2]. Human MHC locus, also known as HLA, located on the short arm of chromosome 6, is about 4000 kb and composed of 3.6 million base pairs. HLA has the highest genetic density and is the most abundant polymorphic region as far as is known, hence called "chemical fingerprints of human beings."

Over the past three decades, the development of HLA is closely related to the development of organ transplantation. Histocompatibility antigens can be divided into three categories according to their immune performance: Human class I genes encode the transplanted antigen HLA-A, HLA-B, and HLA-CR. The transplantation antigen is responsible for the exclusion of foreign tissue. It exists in the killer T leukocyte and is necessary for cell-mediated immune responses. The second class is involved in the information transmission of immune response process between the cells. The human class II, called HLA-D, can be divided into four subregions, arranged in order DR, DQ, DZ/DO, and DP [3]; complement protein provides the third class of MHC which is located in the S region [4, 5]. The encoded protein is the composition of the serum and is responsible for antigen-antibody complex to cause cell lysis.

HLA-I region has three loci: A, B, and C; each locus has dozens to more than 200 alleles. There are F, G, H, J and other locus in HLA-I region, known as class I-like genes. There are DQ, DR, and DP loci in HLA-II region, and several alleles per locus are more than 100 alleles [6]. HLA-III class has complements C2, C4, Bf, and other loci. HLA locus is closely linked and located on the same chromosome and constitutes a haplotype. As HLA genotypes have a lot of alleles and there are numerous combinations, unless the genetic factors are identical twins, the probability that different individuals have the same HLA haplotype is minimal. Human leukocyte antigen (HLA) has the strongest antigenicity, and it has human specificity. HLA is the most concentrated on the surface of leukocytes. Therefore, it is convenient for clinical examination and is considered to be the main histocompatibility antigen of the human body. It is known that human HLA antigen systems have five adjacent sites, known as HLA-A, HLA-B, HLA-C, HLA-D, and HLA-DR.

2.3 PRA and DSA

Sensitization to HLA antigens occurs with previous exposure to nonself HLA during pregnancy or after blood transfusion or prior transplant. Panel-reactive antibody (PRA) is currently the method to evaluate the anti-HLA level, and it represents the anti-HLA levels of blood circulation. PRA $\geq$ 10% is positive, PRA < 50% is low sensitized, and PRA $\geq$ 50% is high sensitized. Some of these antibodies are directed against the transplanted kidney, which is called donor-specific antibody (DSA). DSA refers to the specificity of the donor tissue antigen produced by the recipient after organ or tissue transplantation, including HLA-I, class II antibodies [7], and some non-HLA class antibodies (such as anti-endothelial cell antibodies [8], anti-vimentin antibodies [9], anti-MICA antibodies, anti-MICB antibodies [10], etc.). These DSAs will cause damage to the transplanted kidney, leading to chronic humoral rejection. DSA is an important indicator of allergic recipients before and after organ transplantation and is closely related to transplant rejection and graft survival. If the patient has been exposed to HLA (human leukocyte antigen) in previous transfusion or organ transplantation, it will produce strong resistance and is not conducive to organ transplantation [11]. In the kidney transplant, the group of PRA-positive recipients are called sensitized recipients. These recipients often have DSA, and they are high-risk populations for transplantation. If there is a large number of DSA before transplantation, hyperacute rejection will immediately occur after transplantation and directly lead to renal failure. Even a small amount of DSA (especially HLA-II) can lead to acute humoral rejection in the short term, affecting the survival rate of the transplanted kidney [12, 13]. Most patients with failed grafts have anti-HLA antibodies. Through the detection of population-reactive antibody, the level of anti-HLA antibody in recipients before and after transplantation can be assessed and can avoid hyperacute rejection to a certain extent. However, some recipients and anti-HLA antibodies coexist in peace.

3 Detection Methods of HLA and DSA

At present, the most frequently detected antibodies in clinical practice are HLA-type donor-specific antibody. The reasons for this are as follows:

1. HLA gene is highly polymorphic and highly associated with rejection in organ transplantations.
2. It is agreed in the academic community that HLA antibodies are involved in hyperacute rejection, and it is necessary to perform CDC test before transplantation. With newer detecting methods such as anti-globulin CDC and FCXM, the sensitivity and specificity for HLA antibody detection have greatly improved.
3. HLA antibody-mediated rejection is intimately associated with acute and chronic injuries of the allograft.
4. The clinical significance of HLA antibody has already been widely recognized, and its detection method has already been standardized.

Clinically, HLA antibody detection method has evolved from CDC or FCXM that based on live cells to ELISA and Luminex that based on HLA antigen-coated solid-phase absorption. LSA is at present the most widely recognized DSA detection method that has both high sensitivity and specificity.

3.1 CDC

CDC has been the gold standard for detecting HLA antibodies since its first reported application in 1969 [14]. This method operates on the principle that antibodies in the recipient that activate corresponding antigens on the donor lymphocytes will lyse lymphocytes and increase cell permeability, all of which can be quantified by calculating the percentage of destructed cells using dye. It is generally conceived that CDC < 10% is suitable for kidney transplantation, while CDC > 10% is unsuitable. The main disadvantage for CDC is that this method is insensitive and is prone to false-negative results. Although still performed in many centers, this method is low yield and cannot be used for patient DSA screening.

3.2 Flow Cytometry Crossmatching

This method was used for HLA antibody screening due to its high sensitivity. Nonetheless, it was quickly replaced by FlowPRA™ beads due to the low specificity and reproducibility of FCX. To perform FlowPRA™ beads, recipient serum is incubated with purified HLA antigen-coated beads [15]. A fluorescent-conjugated anti-human IgG is added, which binds to and detects HLA antibody on its antigen target that can be analyzed by flow cytometer. This method is similar with CDC in the sense that all these two methods were based on live cells. Nevertheless, FlowPRA™ beads test is much more rapid than CDC since no lymphocyte separation is necessary. False-positive results have been reported for FlowPRA™ beads test, possibly due to its high sensitivity.

3.3 ELISA

ELISA was developed as a rapid and sensitive detection method for detecting HLA antibody in the 1990s. Purified HLA antigens were solubilized, then affixed to a solid matrix in ELISA, and analyzed by flow cytometry [16]. No live cells were used in this method and its sensitivity is also satisfying. Abundant transplant labs use ELISA as a routine technique for detecting PRA. ELISA, although sensitive, is only limited to serological typing of HLA antibodies. Another limitation for ELISA is that this method is tedious and cross-contamination often results in false-positive results.

3.4 Luminex Single Antigen (LSA) Microbead

The introduction of fluorescently labeled beads changed the landscape of HLA antibody testing during the middle of 1990s. Commercially available kit which consists of beads impregnated with differing ratios of two fluorochromes (red and green, respectively, for species and intensity) resulting in a unique signal for each bead and which have one or several types of HLA molecules attached [17]. With this new technique, important studies that revealed the role antibody played in rejection enhanced our understanding significantly.

The introduction of LSA revolutionized patient DSA monitoring and management post-kidney transplantation. To date, LSA is considered to be the most sensitive method for detecting DSA in highly immunized patients. The most frequently used kit in China is Luminex100 and Luminex200.

The main parameter for LSA characterization of DSA is mean fluorescence intensity (MFI). The cutoff point for DSA positivity varies from labs to labs, with some labs define MFI > 1000 as DSA-positive, while some consider MFI > 2000 to be clinically significant DSA-positive. In a study by Malheiro et al. [18], the authors found in 462 patients that only when HLA-DSA MFI > 3000 in preoperative serums did HLA-DSA associated with antibody-mediated rejection. This association rose to 0.857 when HLA-DSA MFI > 4900. In a word, the cutoff point for HLA-DSA MFI is arbitrary. It is recommended that organ transplant centers establish MFI criteria based on individual clinical data.

3.4.1 The Advantages of Luminex Method for Detecting Donor-Specific Antibody [17]

High Accuracy

HLA is highly polymorphic complexes consisting of a series of tightly linked loci. To date, there are 4585 HLA antigens, including 3348 HLA class I antigens and 1237 HLA class II antigens. Currently, medium-resolution typing of anti-HLA antibodies (DRB1*04:01/DRB1*07:01) can be detected by LSA method, while only low-resolution typing (DR4/DR7) can be discerned by previously used ELISA. LSA is able to accurately determine whether anti-HLA antibodies are DSA, so it can facilitate screening of transplanted donors, effectively shorten the highly sensitized patients' waiting time, and avoid donor waste. Meanwhile, it is a powerful technology for the diagnosis and treatment of AMR. Therefore, LSA can better meet the clinical needs of kidney transplantation.

High Sensitivity

For using microbeads coated by highly purified single HLA antigen, LSA has higher sensitivity. It is reported that the sensitivity of LSA is much higher than that of ELISA, which is the representative technology for testing anti-HLA antibody in recipient. Wang Qinghua et al. conducted a comparative study of the two methods in 34 recipients with living related transplant. Using Luminex method, 18 cases were antibody positive. Fourteen cases among them were anti-HLA class I antibody positive; the positive rate was 41.2%. Thirteen cases among them were anti-HLA class II antibody positive; the positive rate was 38.2%. However, using ELISA, only one case was anti-HLA class I antibody positive, the positive rate was 2.9%, and three cases were anti-HLA class II antibody positive, the positive rate was 8.8%. The positive rate of anti-HLA antibody with Luminex in renal transplant recipients was significantly higher than that of ELISA. Studies reveal that anti-DQ antibody of HLA class II is the common antibody involved in rejection, which is significantly related to transplant glomerulopathy. Anti-HLA-DQ antibody is a direct risk factor for the prognosis of renal allograft and a critical indicator of early intervention and removal of immune risk factors. In recent years, studies have shown that donor-specific anti-HLA-DP antibodies can mediate acute and chronic graft rejection. Detection of anti-HLA-DQ/anti-HLA-DP antibodies by ELISA is often a miss. LSA owns more monoclonal antigen-coating locus than ELISA; hence, this method can increase the width of anti-HLA antibody detection.

High Automation

LSA is a semiautomatic anti-HLA antibody detection system. Assisted by Luminex 200 Analyzer and related analyzing software, it is able to detect the type and percentage of DSA. Ninety-six samples can be tested simultaneously one time in only 2–3 h. Using software to read and analyze date automatically, this method increases the accuracy of the results by reducing the error of subjective judgment. Compared with the previously used ELISA for the detection of anti-HLA antibodies, only a smaller amount of recipient serum (5 μL) is needed. The instrument with a vacuum-washing device is easily operated and can avoid pollution by repeatedly washing plate manually.

3.4.2 The Disadvantages of Luminex Method for Detecting Donor-Specific Antibody

As a highly sensitive method for detecting anti-HLA antibodies, LSA is able to detect very low concentrations of antibodies, but it is prone to false-positive results and cannot distinguish complement-fixing antibody from non-complement-fixing antibody. To solve this problem, intensive studies were performed and showed that the membrane attack complexes against target cells caused by activating complement are a critical pathway for antibody-induced renal damage.

Clq is a subunit of component C1, which is the initiating factor of the classical pathway of complement activation. Loupy et al. [19] found that in 1064 cases of renal transplant, a 5-year survival rate of DSA and C1q double-positive patients is 54%, DSA-negative patients is 93%, and DSA-positive and C1q-negative patients is 94%. Consequently, the joint detection of DSA and C1q can enhance a positive rate. Single antigen-coating microbeads fail to cover the differences in HLA and alleles across the population. For example, the African Indian population carry a large number of novel alleles and unique HLA haplotypes. Hence, such rare HLA antibodies cannot be found.

3.4.3 The Significance of Luminex Single Antigen Microbead Method for Detecting Donor-Specific Antibodies

At present, LSA is the most sensitive way to assess hyperacute rejection. Among previously used methods for detecting anti-HLA antibodies, the sensitivity of CDC is low, FCXM is easier to cause false positive, and ELISA has lower resolution. What's more, both CDC and FCXM require live lymphocytes. In terms of sensitivity, LSA > ELISA/FCXM > CDC. There is no conclusive evidence that ELISA is more sensitive than FCXM. It is certain that in order to improve the specificity of detecting DSA, LSA will gradually replace ELISA. Although the sensitivity of DSA detection has improved, LSA still cannot completely substitute CDC, which is the gold standard of anti-HLA antibody test. CDC positive is still the contraindication of kidney transplantation.

Detecting DSA by LSA before renal transplantation can determine whether unacceptable donor antigens are present. The risk of postoperative AMR emerging can be reduced, especially for highly allergenic recipients. Avoiding receiving unaccepted antigens from donors and starting desensitization therapy timely may increase the surgical opportunity of these recipients and shorten preoperative waiting time. Monitoring the production of DSA after transplantation and determining the type of postoperative graft rejection can help clinicians to develop appropriate treatment programs without delaying of the illness. If DSA is found before transplantation, desensitization therapy, such as plasma exchange, immune-absorption, and intravenous infusion of immunoglobulin, can be used to reduce the level of DSA to safe transplantation. However, the effect was not satisfactory. It is reported that bortezomib, a proteasome inhibitor, can inhibit plasma cell-secreting antibodies so as to reduce the DSA titer, promote the reversal of transplant rejection, and improve the function of the transplanted kidney. However, bortezomib is mainly used to prevent DSA forming in clinical because of lacking uniform, standard, and optimized treatment procedure. LSA for detecting DSA has been widely recognized in the field of transplant. It deepens our understanding of AMR occurrence, development, diagnosis, and treatment. Using LSA to screen DSA has its advantages along with disadvantages as well, such as lacking of internationally standardized operating procedures and a unified cutoff value. The main causes of these disadvantages are that the kits are produced by different manufacturers and that the amount of beads coated by antigen and the production lot number are different. Standardization of cutoff values facilitates the comparison of multicenter antibody detection data, provides more accurate information for the clinic, and enables physicians to better assess the risk stratification so as to develop appropriate individualized treatment programs timely. Of course, in view of clinical status after transplantation, several affecting factors should be put into consideration. The effect of DSA and complement activation on long-term survival of transplanted kidney needs further study. For highly allergic patients, try not selecting donors with specific antigens to reduce the risk of dnDSA and early AMR occurrence after transplantation [20].

4 Clinical Significance of Crossmatch

For organ transplantation with ABO incompatibility, HLA match is as important as transplantation between patients with compatible ABO blood type. The antigens in different loci function differently. It is well-known that HLA-DR and HLA-D antigens are the most important, while HLA-B and HLA-A are less important than the former ones. Allograft rejection is related with the existence of HLA in the donor that was lacking in the recipient [21]. The survival rate of patients with transplantation from a living related donor is closely related with match of HLA-A and HLA-B. Due to the inherited linkage, the similarity between HLA-A and HLA-B means that HLA-D is possibly alike to HLA-B. Therefore, the survival rate is significantly higher in recipient whose HLA-A and HLA-B match to the living related donor than those patients whose HLA-A and HLA-B don't match to that of the donors. Among transplantations from deceased cardiac donors, some studies reported that the survival rate was obviously higher in receivers with HLA-A and HLA-B match to the donors than those without. However, the significance of HLA-D has been confirmed not only in renal transplantation but also in allogeneic skin and bone marrow transplant. Studies also demonstrated that the match level of HLA-DR was also associated with the prognosis.

The successful HLA match can successfully improve the survival rate of the transplant. The survival rate of graft with complete match of HLA-A, HLA-B, and HLA-DR between recipient and donor is significantly higher than that without HLA-A, HLA-B, and HLA-DR match [22]. In transplantation from deceased cardiac donor, the HLA-DR match is more important than the match of HLA-A and HLA-B. The effectiveness of HLA-DR match can be summarized as follows: (1) in kidney transplantation, the more HLA-DR mutually possessed by donor and recipient, or the less mismatch detected in HLA-DR, the survival rate will be higher; (2) in patients with pretransplantation transfusion, the DR match can improve the survival rate; and (3) in the case of immunization in recipients, transfusion is not suggested before bone marrow transplantation. In addition, because the donated kidney has to be pretreated with radiation and agents, the HLA match will be more critical than ABO blood type between recipients and donors.

Some research indicated that in patients with uremia, the panel-reactive antibody (PRA)-positive rate was significantly higher in female than male patients. Similarly, the difference was also observed among patients with different ages, which was lower in patients with junior age and higher in patients in middle age. The frequency of antibodies produced is different according to different alleles. The number of antibody types detected by ELISA about HLA-A, HLA-B, HLA-CW, HLA-DR, and HLA-DQ alleles is 20, 27, 5, 13, and 7, respectively. Alleles that have frequently occurring antibodies include A2, A25, A23, A24, and A66; B7, B13, B57, B44, and B60; CW4, CW6, CW10, CW7, and CW8; DR11, DR1, DR7, DR9, and DR12; and DQ6, DQ5, DQ7, DQ8, and DQ2. But their frequencies are not all consistent with that in Chinese population.

The new method is very sensitive to detect PRA, which can judge whether the graft has the risk to occur chronic humoral rejection by detecting the quantity of the serum antibodies and existence of antibodies targeted to the recipient. If the antibodies to the donated kidney has been detected, patients should be cared in an active way to prevent humoral rejection reaction, even without elevated creatinine.

Therefore, regular detection of PRA is necessary for patients after kidney transplantation. If the PRA is elevated, treatment agents should be adjusted in time, or extra management should be added to lower the PRA levels in case of further injuries. If patients are accompanied with increasing creatinine, biopsy of the transplanted kidney is needed to clarify whether there is chronic humoral rejection and patients should be treated actively [11]. For patients with stable creatinine and negative PRA in the first time, it is suggested to have a follow-up 6 months and 1 year after the surgery and one time a year after that.

For patients who are detected to have positive PRA in the first time, further examinations should be taken to clarify the specific subtype of the antibodies, such as type I, type II, and MICA antibodies. The aim of further examination is to define the type and concentration of the antibodies and whether these antibodies target the transplant kidney (donor-specific antibody, DSA). If recipients have DSA, they need to be treated actively. If those antibodies are not transplant kidney targeted, patients need to be observed regularly. If positive antibodies are found, patients are suggested to have a follow-up every half year to evaluate the changes of the antibodies and decide treatment measures. Methods to lower antibodies included the following three aspects: (1) to eliminate the antibodies in a physical way, plasma exchange, immunosorption, double plasma filtration etc.; (2) to eliminate the drugs that induce antibodies, anti-CD20 monoclonal antibody, bortezomib, etc.; and (3) drugs targeting complement.

Transplantation with ABO blood type incompatibility is similar with those with ABO compatibility. The high level of PRA in recipients is detrimental to the transplant kidney, which leads rejection to the graft. In patients with positive crossmatch, the immunized humoral HLA is the main reason, presenting higher ratio of positive PRA. Based on the PRA results, it is possible to distinguish the recipients with potential risk for severe rejection to happen and those without immunized state, which can be considered as an immune sign to choose appropriate recipients. Dynamic evaluation of the PRA can provide the best opportunity for surgery, and CDC can assess the choice of the immune agents, the usage time, the dosage, and the prediction of rejection level. Even if patients accept transplantation after the PRA decrease to the normal range, the possibility of rejection is still higher than other populations. Thus, usage of effective postoperation immunosuppressive drug is also very critical.

In fact, in whatever way, none of them can avoid hyperacute rejection and acute humoral rejection completely. Ideal match is an important way to reduce rejection, especially for hypersensitive recipients, for whom strict match to choose an ideal donor is important to reduce superacute rejection.

As a process of complicated immune reaction-related inflammatory injury, organ transplantation rejection is composed of cellular and humoral immune reactions. The cellular immune reaction is more important in transplantation immune. In the transplantation rejection reaction, in addition to direct contact of MHC I antigen with precursor Tc cells and B cells, the process of antigen-presenting cells (rich of MHC II antigen) handling the antigens as the first signal and presenting them to Th/Td cells is more significant. During this process, APC-derived IL-1 activates Th/Td cells as the second signal. IL-2, IL-4, IL-5, IL-6, and IFN-γ are released after Th/Td cell activation, participating Tc and B cells' differentiation into effective Tc and functional plasma cells, which leads to graft injury.

Sensitized T cells are mainly cytotoxic cells and $CD8^+$ cells which can induce delayed allergic reaction. In addition to that special cellular immune reaction, nonspecific Nk also participates in cellular reaction after IL-2 and IFN-γ ECT stimulation. Because most of the current transplantation belongs to allogeneic transplantation between recipients and donors without kinship and there are differences about HLA compatibility between them, it is possible for rejection to occur in different stages after operation, injuring the graft function and leading to the failure of transplantation and death of the recipients. As the knowledge of the preoperation tissue matches popularization, the technology and the surgical skill progress, the usage of the immunosuppressive agents, and combination of the multiple detection methods, the rejection reaction has been moderately estimated and controlled to some extent. Overall, the rejection is still one of the main factors that affect the graft's normal function and the recipient's long-term survival.

As a special immune reaction, the rejection has its typical immune pathological mechanism. According to different pathogenesis mechanisms, there will be corresponding onset time and specific histological changes. On the one hand, this pathomorphological change is the basis of the graft lost; on the other hand, in the initial of the pathological changes, multiple pathological biopsy methods can be applied to diagnose and guide clinical treatment effectively via observing the histomorphology changes, which is also key to ensure the success of the transplantation.

After the transplantation of the homologous organs, two types of rejections can happen based on the different immune directions. One of them is host versus graft reaction, which is the usually called rejection reaction. The other one is graft versus host disease, which means the immune directs to the host, resulting in graft versus graft disease. The rejection reaction can be divided into hyperacute reaction, accelerated rejection, acute reaction, and chronic reaction according to different pathogenesis mechanisms, onset time, clinical presentations, and pathomorphological changes.

Organ transplantation with ABO blood type incompatibility is same to the organ transplantation with ABO blood type compatibility. The difference between recipients' and donor's antigen is the immune basis of the rejective reaction. The survival quality is closely related with the antigen compatibility between recipients and donors. When the ABO incompatibility recipients' desensitization reaches the requirements, the more compatible the HLA is, the less the rejection happens, and the higher survival quality the graft will have. Otherwise, the worse the match is, more frequently the rejection occurs, which is detrimental to the survival of the graft and can lead to loss of allograft function.

References

1. Klein J. George snell's first foray into the unexplored territory of the major histocompatibility complex. Genetics. 2001;159:435–9.
2. Ono SJ, et al. Chemokines: roles in leukocyte development, trafficking, and effector function. J Allergy Clin Immunol. 2003;111(6):1185–99; quiz 1200
3. Schreuder GM, et al. HLA dictionary 2004: summary of HLA-A, -B, -C, -DRB1/3/4/5, -DQB1 alleles and their association with serologically defined HLA-A, -B, -C, -DR, and -DQ antigens. Hum Immunol. 2005;66(2):170–210.3.
4. Prodinger WM, et al. Complement. In: Paul WE, editor. Fundamentals in immunology. Philadelphia: Lippincott Williams & Wilkins; 2003. p. 1077–103.
5. Gammie JS, Pham SM, Colson YL, et al. Influence of panel-reactive antibody on survival and rejection after lung transplantation. J Heart Lung Transplant. 1997;16:408–15.
6. Marsh SG. Nomenclature for factors of the HLA system monthly updates 2006–2008. 2008. http://www.anthonynolan.com/HIG/nomen/updates/updates.html. Accessed 14 June 2010.
7. Gebel HM, Bray RA. Sensitization and sensitivity: defining the unsensitized patient. Transplantation. 2000;69(7):1370–4.

8. Regele H. Non-HLA antibodies in kidney allograft rejection: convincing concept in need of further evidence. Kidney Int. 2011;79(6):583–6.
9. Rose ML. Role of anti-vimentin antibodies in allograft rejection. Hum Immunol. 2013;74(11):1459–62.
10. Zou Y, Stastny P, Süsal C, Döhler B, Opelz G. Antibodies against MICA antigens and kidney-transplant rejection. N Engl J Med. 2007;357(13):1293–300.
11. Lachmann N, Terasaki PI, Budde K, et al. Anti-human leukocyte antigen and donor-specific antibodies detected by luminex posttransplant serve as biomarkers for chronic rejection of renal allografts. Transplantation. 2009;87:1505–13.
12. Arnold ML, et al. Anti-HLA class II antibodies in kidney retransplant patients. Tissue Antigens. 2005;65(4):370–8.
13. Gupta A, et al. Pretransplant donor-specific antibodies in cytotoxic negative crossmatch kidney transplants: are they relevant? Transplantation. 2008;85(8):1200–4.
14. Patel R, Terasaki PI. Significance of the positive crossmatch test in kidney transplantation. N Engl J Med. 1969;280(14):735–9.
15. Saw CL, Bray RA, Gebel HM. Cytotoxicity and antibody binding by flow cytometry: a single assay to simultaneously assess two parameters. Cytometry B Clin Cytom. 2008;74:287–94.
16. Zachary AA, et al. Characterization of HLA class I specific antibodies by ELISA using solubilized antigen targets: II. Clinical relevance. Hum Immunol. 2001;62(3):236–46.
17. Pei R, et al. Single human leukocyte antigen flow cytometry beads for accurate identification of human leukocyte antigen antibody specificities. Transplantation. 2003;75(1):43–9.
18. Malheiro J, Tafulo S, Dias L, Martins LS, Fonseca I, Beirão I, Castro-Henriques A, Cabrita A. Analysis of preformed donor-specific anti-HLA antibodies characteristics for prediction of antibody-mediated rejection in kidney transplantation. Transpl Immunol. 2015;32(2):66–71.
19. Loupy A, Lefaucheur C, Vernerey D, Prugger C, Duong van Huyen JP. Mooney N, et al. Complement-binding anti-HLA antibodies and kidney-allograft survival. N Engl J Med. 2013;369(13):1215–26.
20. Gebel HM, Bray RA, Nickerson P. Pre-transplant assessment of donor-reactive, HLA-specific antibodies in renal transplantation: contraindication vs. risk. Am J Transplant. 2003;3(12):1488–500.
21. Bray RA, Gebel HM. Allele specific HLA alloantibodies. Implication for organ allocation. Am J Transplant. 2005;5(s11):488.
22. Wissing KM, et al. HLA mismatches remain risk factors for acute kidney allograft rejection in patients receiving quadruple immunosuppression with anti-interleukin-2 receptor antibodies. Transplantation. 2008;85(3):411–6.

Indications for ABO-Incompatible Organ Transplantation

5

Chunbai Mo and Jinpeng Tu

Abstract

The time that ABO-incompatible (ABOi) organ transplantation has been used successfully in clinical is not long; however, important organ transplantation including heart, liver, lung, and kidney has their own different development histories. Early ABOi heart transplantation was conducted with infants of lower blood group antibody titer and underage children as main recipients. ABOi lung transplantation, however, has started from using the adult donor lung for underage children. Early ABOi liver transplantation, as a lifesaving measure, was applied mainly for liver function failure and severe liver disease patients failing in the conventional therapy, in order to help them go through the anhepatic phase. ABOi kidney transplantation has come from constant attempts and medical errors to learn lessons, sum up experience, and continuously improve preparative regimens. Meanwhile, the primary diseases and complications of a variety of organs are different. Hence, ABOi transplantation for a variety of organs has also various indications.

Keywords

ABO-incompatible · Organ transplantation · Indication · Contraindication

---

C. Mo (✉) · J. Tu
Department of Organ Transplantation, Tianjin First Center Hospital, Tianjin, China

Tianjin Clinical Research Center for Organ Transplantation, Tianjin, China
e-mail: cbmo@medmail.com.cn; tjpgold@126.com.cn

Y. Wang (ed.), *ABO-incompatible Organ Transplantation*,
https://doi.org/10.1007/978-981-13-3399-6_5

1 Selection of Donors and Recipients

At the selection of organ transplantation recipients and donors, many factors are needed to be estimated with caution and seriousness, such as primary disease category, age, general state of health, and complications of recipients and donors; on the other hand, in order to ensure that organs are first assigned for patients who need them the most, improve transplantation effects, and resolve the problem of shortage of organs at a certain degree, laws, regulations, and relevant policies of various countries, relevant ethical standards, and procedures of donor protection, informed consent, and donation acquisition are needed to conduct with the principles of justice, equity, and publicity.

1.1 Selection of Recipients of ABOi Organ Transplantation

1.1.1 Indications

Organ transplantation is the most effective treatment for end-stage organ failure and the only effective treatment option for important organs without effective replacement therapies, such as the heart, lung, and liver. Although there are hemodialysis, peritoneal dialysis, and renal transplantation for end-stage renal disease patients, transplantation is still the best choice. Because of the lack of donors and reasons of laws, regulations, and ethics, ABOi organ transplantation sometimes has to be carried out.

Similar with ABO-compatible (ABOc) organ transplantation, the selection of ABOi organ transplant patients also involves transplantation indications, contraindications, surgical timing, preoperative preparation and evaluation, etc., but ABOi organ transplantation has unique characters, due to the emergence of new immunosuppressive drugs and blood purification technology changing with each passing day. General indications for several important ABOi organ transplantations are described below.

Heart Transplantation

Being a visceral organ transplantation surgery, heart transplantation, on the premise of the consent of donor himself and relatives, generally will take the complete human heart from persons who are diagnosed as brain dead and match with organs. Heart transplantation is not a routine treatment for heart disease, but a treatment of saving the life of patients with end-stage heart disease and improving their quality of life. As the nonconventional treatment for advanced congestive heart failure, the expense of heart transplantation is very expensive, both on ABOc heart transplantation and ABOi heart transplantation. Heart transplantation, hence, is a surgical transplantation mainly for patients with advanced congestive heart failure and severe coronary artery disease and neonates with severe congenital heart disease, who require heart transplantation.

In general, indications for ABOi heart transplantation are applicable to advanced heart disease patients with NYHA Class IV who fail in various treatments. Indications for ABOi heart transplantation include mainly:

1. A variety of severe cardiomyopathy
2. A large area of myocardial infarction, heart failure patients without opportunity of coronary artery bypass surgery
3. Cureless complex congenital heart disease
4. Rheumatic heart disease combined with valvulopathy patients with extensive cardiomyopathy
5. Neonates with severe congenital heart disease
6. Obstinate, refractory, malignant arrhythmia patients failing in treatments [1] of internal and surgical medicine
7. Above patients who urgently need to undergo heart transplantation but without compatible blood type donors

Liver Transplantation

A part of the liver from the healthy liver donors is resected to be transplanted in patients, as is called living liver transplantation; if there is blood relationship between liver donors and liver recipients, it is called living related liver transplantation. Living liver transplantation is important to resolve the shortage of liver supply in the world. Early living liver transplantation is mainly to alleviate the shortage of donors, especially in children undergoing liver transplantation. In Europe, 15–20% of children with liver disease die each year during waiting for liver transplantation, and the presence of living liver transplantation has greatly eased the tension between supply and demand [2].

With the continuous development of living liver transplantation, indications for liver transplantation are increasing; patients with all kinds of acute or chronic liver diseases failing in other treatments of internal and surgical medicine who are expected to die unavoidably during a short term (6–12 months) is an indication for liver transplantation [3]. At first, liver transplantation is only a lifesaving process, and now with the continuous development of surgical techniques, the use of new immunosuppressive agents and clinical experience accumulation, liver transplantation peri-surgical complications and mortality rate decreasing significantly, and post-surgical survival rate and survival time increasing, the symptoms caused by liver diseases result in a serious decline in their quality of life, as has become one of the primary indications for liver transplantation.

The disease category treated by orthotopic liver transplantation is increasing in recent years; thus far, according to incomplete statistics, liver transplantation has been successfully applied to over 60 kinds of liver diseases, generally including end-stage cirrhosis disease, malignant liver disease, congenital metabolic disease, and acute or subacute liver function failure based on the nature of diseases. The contraindication of transplantation has been continuously reducing with the accumulation of experience in liver transplantation. Many previously considered absolute contraindications now become relatively contraindications, and many previously relative contraindications now become indications.

Generally, all diseases that can conduct conventional liver transplantation can perform ABOi liver transplantation [4]

1. Liver parenchymal diseases caused by nonpathogenic microorganisms: such as alcoholic cirrhosis; acute and chronic liver function failure caused by drugs, chemical poisons, etc.; congenital hepatic fibrosis; cystic fibrosis liver disease; huge liver cysts; Budd-Chiari syndrome; severe refractory trauma; autoimmune hepatitis; etc.
2. Liver function failure and portal hypertension caused by various types of hepatitis and cirrhosis induced by various pathogenic microorganisms: including severe acute and chronic hepatitis, cirrhosis, schistosomiasis, hepatic echinococcosis, etc. caused by hepatitis B virus (HBV) and hepatitis C virus (HCV), in which HBV infection-related severe acute and chronic hepatitis, cirrhosis, and liver function failure are commonest indications in China, almost accounting for 80–90% of all cases.
3. Congenital dysbolism diseases: such as hepatolenticular degeneration (Wilson's disease), Pompe's syndrome, hyperammonemia, antitrypsin deficiency, familial nonhemolytic jaundice, tyrosinemia, etc. Because of the abnormal metabolism of certain substances, such diseases may cause children premature death or abnormal development, as are more common indications in pediatric liver transplantation.
4. Cholestatic diseases: such as congenital biliary atresia, primary biliary cirrhosis (PBC), primary sclerosing cholangitis (PSC), secondary biliary cirrhosis, Calori's disease, intrahepatic biliary atresia (Byler disease), etc. Patients with such diseases are characterized with jaundice in clinical; such patients may have severe jaundice but can keep normality in liver synthesis function for a long time. There are risks of relapses for PBC and PSC after transplantation.
5. Liver tumor: Malignant liver tumor without extrahepatic metastasis and invasion of large vessels can also be used as the indication for liver transplantation. When the 2000 World Congress was held in Milan, Italy, "Milan standards" were recommended for liver transplantation for liver cancer by the Congress, i.e., single tumor diameter ≤5 cm, multiple tumors of no more than three, a maximum of no more than 3 cm, and no major vascular invasion. According to this standard, liver transplantation for liver cancer is up to 80% in the disease-free survival rate for 5 years, as is obviously superior to the traditional treatment. Through nearly 20 years of research, a "Hangzhou standard" for liver transplantation for liver cancer breaking through international conventions has been acquired by the hepatobiliary and pancreatic surgery department, which has been led by Academician Zheng Shusen, a director of the First Affiliated Hospital of Medical School of Zhejiang University in China. The standard suggests that liver cancer patients with the cumulative tumor diameter ≤8 cm can undergo liver transplantation; patients with the cumulative tumor diameter >8 cm can also receive transplanta-

tion, if there is serum AFP of ≤400 ng/mL with high or middle differentiation in the tumor histological grade. It is understood that liver cancer patients in China have accounted for more than 40% of the total worldwide patients. The "Hangzhou standard" enables more liver cancer patients to have new lives through liver transplantation.

6. Cirrhosis after a variety of hepatitis: (1) cirrhosis after alcoholic hepatitis, (2) cirrhosis after HBV hepatitis, (3) cirrhosis following autoimmune hepatitis, (4) and severe acute hepatitis.
7. Of other severe liver diseases with unknown causes, it is generally believed that the lesion of degree should accord with the following conditions: (1) ascites difficult to reverse, (2) the form of portal hypertension with hemorrhage of digestive tract, (3) severe liver function damage (child class C), (4) the emergence of hepatorenal syndrome, (5) the presence of progressively aggravated hepatic encephalopathy, (6) and liver cirrhosis complicated with liver cancer. Patients can undergo liver transplantation immediately when above two to three signs are noted.

Renal Transplantation

Successful renal transplantation can make patients complete recovery of health, live for ages, and return to work; hence, renal transplantation is the optimal alternative therapy for uremia. In general, all patients with chronic renal failure in the end stage failing in generally conservative treatment are suitable for renal transplantation [8]. Like the ABOc renal transplantation, the general requirements of the selection of patients for ABOi renal transplantation include:

1. Patients with the age range better from 4 to 65 years old
2. Patients with irreversible renal failure caused by end stage of chronic nephritis or other renal diseases
3. After hemodialysis or peritoneal dialysis, patients with favorable general conditions, no latent infectious foci in vivo, and the tolerance of renal transplantation
4. Patients without histories of active ulcer, tumor, hepatitis, and tuberculosis or histories of mental and neurological diseases

In recent years, the selection of primary diseases and age range of patients has been increasing relatively; however, of the selection of primary diseases, glomerular nephritis is still the first choice, followed by chronic pyelonephritis and interstitial nephritis, and thirdly polycystic kidney. In addition, the number of transplantation for diabetic nephropathy is also increasing; especially, the development of simultaneous pancreas-kidney transplantation provides a new approach for diabetic nephropathy and renal failure. Simultaneous pancreas-kidney transplantation is a more reasonable treatment for patients with advanced diabetes complicated with renal failure, if single kidney transplantation or hemodialysis is not a fundamental solution.

All end-stage renal diseases develop into chronic renal failure, with urea nitrogen being continuously over 35.7 mmol/L, serum creatinine being over 707–884 μmol/L, and creatinine clearance rate being below 5–10 mL/min in the uremia stage; renal transplantation can be considered to conduct at the time of receiving no obvious effects from general internal medicine. The common primary diseases are chronic glomerulonephritis, chronic pyelonephritis, polycystic kidney, diabetic glomerulosclerosis, the absence of single kidney or double kidneys caused by trauma or diseases, and other rare diseases. Generally, the age is required no more than 60 years old. If the patient's age is more than 65 years old, transplantation [5] could also be considered to perform for those with normal heart, lung, and liver functions, stable hypertension, and a satisfactory mental state.

But because of the lack of donor kidney sources, ABOc kidney transplantation has been unable to achieve when acute renal failure patients urgently need kidney transplantation. At this time, breaking through blood type disorder, ABOi kidney transplantation [6] cannot only resolve the problem of insufficient kidney sources at present in the world but also reduce the time of patients waiting for donor kidneys and save lives of patients as well.

Lung Transplantation

It refers to resecting unilateral or bilateral lungs with serious diseases and transplanting healthy lungs from brain dead donors, in order to make recipients recover health and even return to normal life and work, as is the only effective method for advanced pulmonary parenchymal diseases and advanced pulmonary vascular diseases. Lung diseases requiring lung transplantation mainly include tracheal lesions (emphysema, bronchiectasis, cystic fibrosis, and chronic bronchitis), pulmonary hypertension (primary pulmonary hypertension (unknown causes) and secondary hypertension (secondary to another heart or lung lesion)), and interstitial lung diseases (pulmonary fibrosis, sarcoidosis, silicosis, pneumoconiosis, scleroderma, calcinosis cutis, Raynaud's phenomenon, esophageal dyssynergia syndrome, telangiectasia, eosinophilic granuloma, idiopathic pulmonary fibrosis, hemosiderosis, pulmonary-renal syndrome).

In addition, lung transplantation can be divided into single lung transplantation and double lung transplantation, with different indications.

Small Intestine Transplantation

It has become the optimal standard treatment for patients with intestinal failure. The intestinal epidermis for absorption is damaged in such patients due to intra-abdominal diseases, such as volvulus, toxic enterocolitis, and trauma. Small intestine transplantation, at present, should be only for patients who are unable to tolerate chronic parenteral nutrition with no other choice for survival. It is reported for the first time that grafts survive for over 1 year and show complete small intestine functions, after small intestine transplantation. The question that needs to be asked is a suitable length of small intestine segments for transplantation, systemic vascular drainage or portal venous drainage used for grafts, the continuous suitability of grafts in the gastrointestinal tract of recipients, and the effect of lifestyle of related allogeneic intestinal donors. Due to the presence of gut-associated lymphoid tissues, graft versus host disease (GVHD) is a problem in small bowel transplantation, significantly larger than other allotransplantations with vascular organs. This is an interesting experimental study: cells causing GVHD are removed before transplanting the small intestine, which may reduce the immunogenicity of organs. Indications for small bowel transplantation mainly involve:

1. Short bowel syndrome following massive resection of small intestine resulted from a variety of reasons, including congenital atresia of small intestine, extensive necrosis of small intestine caused by intestinal twist, necrotizing enterocolitis, trauma, thrombosis or ischemia of mesenteric vessels or portal system, and extensive resection of small intestine caused by repeated surgeries for Crohn's disease
2. Disorders of motility of digestive tract, chronic intestinal pseudo-obstruction, visceral neuropathy, and absence of ganglion cells in the digestive tract (Hirschsprung's disease)
3. Severe malabsorption caused by congenital intestinal mucosal lesion such as microvillus inclusion disease and villous enteropathy
4. Radiation damage
5. Uncontrollable secretory diarrhea
6. Autoimmune enteritis
7. Congenital malformation of digestive tract such as gastroschisis and congenital atresia of small intestine
8. Localized desmoid tumor
9. Multiple polyposis, such as Gardner's syndrome

1.1.2 Contraindications

With the continuous improvement and perfection of the transplantation technology, contraindications for organ transplantation will gradually reduce, especially for absolute contraindications. The common contraindications faced by transplantation recipients include the following.

Peptic Ulcer Diseases

The treatment principle involves H2 receptor antagonists [7] that are administrated for patients with peptic ulcer and hemorrhea history, who show active stage of ulcer by endoscopy before transplantation; surgery could be conducted for stubborn ones. Transplantation is not absolutely forbidden for patients without active bleeding stage or severe gastric mucosal erosion; however, the dosage of hormone should be small after surgery, antacid drugs ought to be administrated at the same time, and endoscopy should be rechecked regularly.

Infections

Systemic and active infections are contraindications for transplantation.

Hepatitis of HBV and HBC

Such patients are not generally encouraged to perform transplantation; especially in cases that donor organ sources are in short supply, non-hepatitis B patients are given priority. In view of China's national conditions, transplantation centers in China, in fact, do not strictly refuse the positive HBV patients.

Other Diseases

Patients with the following conditions are not encouraged to perform transplantation, such as abnormal coagulation functions, diabetes, positive serum HIV (taxonomic diagnosis), severe vasculopathy, malignant tumors, psychosis, acute drug addiction, etc.

1.2 Selection of Donors of ABO-Incompatible Organ Transplantation

Studies on long-term transplantation survival have great achievements in recent years; however, the rejection after transplantation cannot be controlled completely. The occurrence of rejection is one of major causes to result in failure of organ transplantation. Hence, the selection of donors and recipients, reasonable tissue matching, and preoperative preparation are significant to improve long-term survival of recipients or organs. Of ABO-incompatible organ transplantation, it is crucial to select reasonable, lawful, and suitable donors; factors of donors influence effects after transplantation; meanwhile, the selection of donors is significant for the organ transplantation success. Hence, it is necessary to strictly select and treat donors for ABO-incompatible organ transplantation. However, standards that we select cannot be all the same because a variety of donors for organ transplantation are different.

1.2.1 Classification of Donors of ABO-Incompatible Organ Transplantation

In accordance with donors' life state, they can be divided into deceased donors and living donors.

Deceased Donors

They can also be divided into donors after brain death (DBD), called heart-beating dead donors in the past, and non-heart-beating donors (NHBD), now named as donors after cardiac death (DCD) [7], based on death state. Once donors of brain death are determined, a series of treatments including circulatory and respiratory functions should be maintained; transplanted organ injury from donors ought to be minimized as far as possible until organs are allowed to be removed. In general, of donors after heart death, warm ischemia time for donor organs cannot exceed a certain time; for instance, warm ischemia time should not exceed 30 min for donor kidneys, 15 min for donor livers, 10 min for donor small intestines, etc. [8].

Living Donors

They can be divided into living relative donors and living nonrelative donors according to their relatives. Living relative donors include spouses and relatives with blood relationship. Living nonrelative donors include friends, anonymous donors, and donors who cross donations.

The new concept of living donors has relieved the problem of organ shortage to a certain extent and injected a trend of thought into the development of organ transplantation. However, donating living organs is a new medical project in China. In this regard, we must give it sufficient respect and protection and must not impede its development due to improper use.

Living donors must accord with five basic conditions: (1) donors are legal adult; (2) patients must have a right of informed consent at organ donation, with completely free will, free of charge, and free from pressure, coercion, or inducements; (3) donors completely have civil capability; (4) donors must completely understand potential risks and dangerousness after organ donation; (5) and donors must meet selection standards of medicine.

1.2.2 Contraindications of Donors of ABO-Incompatible Organ Transplantation

Contraindications (Table 5.1) of donors of ABO-incompatible organ transplantation

With the rapid development of relevant organ transplantation technology, such as the development of transplantation surgery technology, the development and utilization of new immunosuppressive drugs, improvement of treating postoperative patients and postoperative rejection, indications of organ transplantation, and the requisite number of donor organs are increasing continuously. Although ABOi organ transplantation solves the difficulty of organ shortage to a great extent, it is a long way to go for completely resolving the difficulty of organ shortage in a certain period, due to the limitation of personal feeling, cultural customs, religious belief, and ethics problems.

On the one hand, we continuously promote organ transplantation technology for increasing the success rate of transplantation, meanwhile, and positively advocate the use of a variety of measures expanding donor sources. For instance: (1) encourage individuals and families to donate organs, (2) further improve donation procedures, (3) enhance educations of public and medical staff, (4) and revise relevant regulations for donor use.

Table 5.1 Contraindications of donors of ABO-incompatible organ transplantation [1]

Absolute contraindications	Relative contraindications
Transplanted organ-related chronic diseases (such as kidney, liver, heart, and lung diseases) Age more than 70 years Malignant tumors Severe hypertension patients Uncured bacterial septicemia Positive HIV antibody Active stage of syphilis Warm ischemia time for too long	Age more than 60 years or less than 5 years Positive HBV or HCV in serology Cured infectious diseases Donors suffering from internal diseases (such as diabetes, systemic lupus erythematosus, etc.) Enteric perforation with overflow of intestinal contents Intravenous drug users

2 Preoperative Evaluation and Inspection

The following examinations are to determine whether patients are suitable for transplantation, whether the timing of transplantation is reached, and whether there are contraindications of surgery or not. Transplantation can cause patients severe physiological changes, especially the use of extracorporeal circulation. Now used immunosuppressive agents all have toxic side effects and may cause some organs severe damage; hence, recipients must perform detailed examinations before surgery, in order to determine whether functions of organs free from lesions are normal or not, whether lesions can be corrected or not, etc. Hence, it is necessary to timely understand and find patients' conditions such as heart failure, infection, etc. before surgery; relevant treatments are conducted.

2.1 Evaluation of Preoperative Donors

Before a donor organ is obtained, it is essential to understand histories of donors in an all-round way and perform necessary physical and laboratory examinations. For example, if donors have septicemia, chronic liver disease, AIDS, viral hepatitis, viral encephalitis, recent drug poisoning, active tuberculosis, malignant tumor outside the central nervous system or severe liver trauma, etc., they should not be suitable for donors of liver transplantation.

2.2 Evaluation of Preoperative Recipients

It is essential to thoroughly estimate recipients before surgery, including systemic and nutritional status; functions of the heart, lung, liver, kidney, and other important organs; infectious diseases; the state of social psychology and economy, etc.

2.2.1 Assessment of Systemic and Nutritional Status

Most patients receiving organ transplantation have different levels of nutritional deficiency, because of suffering from long-term exhaustion of diseases before surgery. Studies have demonstrated that patients with malnutrition are slow to recover after transplantation and susceptible to infection, their mortality increasing significantly. Although there are meticulous and careful clinical practices, nursing, and drug and laboratory tests, postoperative complications and prognosis of patients with malnutrition have not still been predicted. Therefore, it is necessary to fully conduct history collection and relevant examinations before surgery, in order to understand the nutritional status of organ transplantation patients and predict risks of postoperative complications; relevant support and symptomatic treatment are given to improve the postoperative survival rate.

Consultation of Detailed Histories

It involves preoperative general state of health, nutrition (food intake, food variety, frequency, and body weight change), constitution, with or without other chronic diseases, and with or without fever and latent infection.

Physical Examinations and Laboratory Examinations

The nutritional status of patients are estimated; the main evaluation indexes and the practical value are shown in Table 5.2.

2.2.2 Evaluation of Important Organs Such as the Heart, Lung, Liver, and Kidney

Doctors need to understand functional status of the patients' heart, lung, liver, kidney, and other important organs in detail by a variety of medical imaging data during the period of waiting for organ transplantation, as follows.

Evaluation of Lung Function

Chest X-ray and CT, arterial blood gas analysis, and lung function tests are conducted; MRI, pulmonary angiography, etc. are performed if necessary.

Evaluation of Heart Function

General ECG, 24-h dynamic ECG, UCG, and treadmill exercise test are performed; cardiac radioisotopic examination and coronary angiography are conducted if necessary.

Table 5.2 Anthropometric relevant indexes as the main contents for evaluation in clinical

	Evaluation indexes	Evaluation and estimation
Anthropometry	The percentage of body weight and ideal body weight	Completely evaluate the nutritional status
	The thickness of triceps skinfold	The index is relatively objective, because of no water-sodium retention in the upper arm
	Arm circumference	The index is relatively objective, because of no water-sodium retention in the upper arm
Serum monitoring indexes	Albumin	The index is objective, due to reflecting the level of protein synthesis of the liver
	Transferring	Better reflect the ability of protein synthesis of the liver
Immunological indexes	Blood lymphocyte count	$<1000/\mu L$ indicates immune function reducing
	Skin delayed hypersensitivity	Be more accurate to estimate the immune status of patients
Nitrogen balance index	The ratio of creatinine and height	Reflect balance status of bodies

Evaluation of Renal Function

Urine analysis, urine protein quantification, blood urea nitrogen, creatinine test, glomerular filtration rate, creatinine clearance rate, and ultrasound examination for the kidney are conducted; renal biopsy is performed when necessary.

Evaluation of Liver Function

Five markers of HBV and HCV, full indexes of biochemical test, coagulation function, etc. are carried out.

2.2.3 Evaluation of Infectious Diseases

Systemic latent infection is a contraindication for transplantation; meanwhile, surgical trauma and the application of immunosuppressive drugs and hormone drugs reduce patients' immunity, as is easy to cause systemic infectious diffusion, resulting in septicemia, bacteremia, increased mortality, etc. During the period of waiting for transplantation, comprehensive examinations are carried out to determine whether patients have pathogenic microorganism infection or not; the immunity of patients to these microorganisms are estimated, as are significant to predict infectious risks of patients after surgery. Hence, infectious diseases of patients are detected and estimated; treatment regimens and preventive measures are designed based on estimated results; preventive use of antibiotics is performed before and during surgery, to improve survival rate for transplantation.

Assessment of Viral Infection

It mainly detects whether there are the following viral infections: *Cytomegalovirus*, *Epstein-Barr virus* (EBV), HBV, HCV, and HIV.

Estimation of Bacterial Infection

It is mainly to understand whether there are histories of bacteremia and tuberculosis infection or not.

Estimation of the Infection Status of Fungi and Parasites

In accordance with the pathogen epidemic status of living regions of patients, we should understand whether patients have fungal infection of skin, oral cavity, lung, etc. or not.

Evaluation of the Vaccination Status

Patients receive long-term immunosuppressive treatment after transplantation, which may cause them some infectious diseases. Thus, previous vaccination situation of patients is understood, and the corresponding immunity is evaluated.

2.2.4 Comprehensive Evaluation of Social Psychology and Economic Status, etc.

In order to understand whether patients can undergo surgery, well cooperate with treatments, perfectly well afford to support transplantation, receive immunosuppressive treatment for a long time after surgery, and other things, social psychology status, economic conditions, etc. of patients are estimated before transplantation. Patients do not insist on appropriate immunosuppressive therapy, the family does not attach importance to routine health maintenance of patients, and so forth, as are commonest causes of graft rejection and infection at the end stage of transplantation. Hence, it is very significant to conduct psychological comprehensive evaluation before transplantation. The evaluated contents include past mental and psychological diseases, current status of social psychology and coping mechanisms, the status of family and social support system, drug abuse history, history of mental disease, psychological disease and drug abuse of family, mental status examination, neurological examination, identification and grasping of general knowledge, trust to medical staff of transplantation, etc.

References

1. Shi C. Implantology. Beijing: People's Medical Publishing House; 2011.
2. Toso C, Al-Qahtani M, Alsaif FA, et al. ABO-incompatible liver transplantation for critically ill adult patients. Transpl Int. 2007;20:675–81.
3. Egawa H, Oike F, Buhler L, et al. Impact of recipient age on outcome of ABO-incompatible living-donor liver transplantation. Transplantation. 2004;77:403–11.
4. Gordon RD, Iwatsuki S, Esquivel CO, et al. Experience with primary liver transplantation across ABO blood groups. Transplant Proc. 1987;19:4575–9.
5. Montgomery JR, Berger JC, Warren DS, et al. Outcomes of ABO-incompatible kidney transplantation in the united states. Transplantation. 2012;93:603–9.
6. Tanabe T, Ishida H, Horita S, et al. Decrease of blood type antigenicity over the long-term after ABO-incompatible kidney transplantation. Transpl Immunol. 2011;25:1–6.
7. Merion RM, Ashby VB, Wolfe RA, et al. Deceased-donor characteristics and the survival benefit of kidney transplantation. JAMA. 2005;294:2726–33.
8. Chinese Medical Association. Clinical technical operation specification: organ transplantation. Beijing: People's Military Medical Press; 2010.

Pathophysiology of ABO-Incompatible Organ Transplantation

6

Zhiqiang Liu

Abstract

Plasma pretreatment is one of the most important procedures before ABO-incompatible organ transplantation compared to the ABO-compatible organ transplantations, with the purpose of eliminating the recipient's antibody titer in vivo. However, three most common methods, the plasmapheresis, the double filtration plasmapheresis (DFPP), and the immunosorption, will inevitably affect pathophysiological progress in recipients at different extents, such as hypoproteinemia, coagulation disorder, tissue hypoperfusion, or disorders of fluid, electrolyte, and acid-base balance. Hence, comprehensive understanding of these pathophysiological processes and correct treatment for these negative factors before operation are critical for successful implementation of the transplantation. In this chapter, we will introduce the pathophysiological alternations of ABO-incompatible organ transplantation, as well as the process of pathophysiology in acute and chronic graft dysfunction using ABO-incompatible kidney transplantation as the example.

Keywords

ABO-incompatible organ transplantation · Pathophysiology · Acute and chronic graft dysfunction · Chronic graft nephropathy

Z. Liu (✉)
Department of Physiology and Pathophysiology, School of Basic Medical Science, Tianjin Medical University, Tianjin, China
e-mail: zhiqiangliu@tmu.edu.cn

Y. Wang (ed.), *ABO-incompatible Organ Transplantation*,
https://doi.org/10.1007/978-981-13-3399-6_6

Abbreviations

AGD	Acute graft dysfunction
AKI	Acute kidney injury
AM	Adhesion molecules
AP	Potential action
ATP	Adenosine triphosphate
BMP-7	Bone morphogenetic protein-7
CAD	Chronic allograft dysfunction
CAN	Chronic allograft nephropathy
CGD	Chronic graft dysfunction
CMV	Cytomegalovirus
CNI	Calcineurin inhibitor
DFPP	Double filtration plasmapheresis
DGF	Delayed graft function
EMT	Epithelial-mesenchymal transition
FGF23	Fibroblast growth factor 23
FUS	First-use syndrome
GF	Growth factors
HBO	Hyperbaric oxygen
HIV	Human immunodeficiency virus
ICAM1	Intercellular adhesion molecule 1
IFN-γ	Interferon gamma
IFTA	Interstitial fibrosis and tubular atrophy
IL-1	Interleukin 1
IL-2R	Interleukin-2R
IL-6	Interleukin 6
MAR	Maximum platelet aggregation rate
MMF	Mycophenolate mofetil
NGAL	Neutrophil gelatinase-associated lipid
PAI	Plasminogen activator inhibitor
PTH	Parathyroid hormone
RAS	Renin-angiotensin system
ROS	Reactive oxygen species
TA-TMA	Transplantation-associated thrombotic microangiopathy
TEM	Transmission electron microscope
TGF-β	Transforming growth factor beta
TNF-α	Tumor necrosis factor alpha
t-PA	Tissue plasminogen activator
VCAM1	Vascular cell adhesion molecule 1
VLA-4	Very late antigen-4

1 Pathophysiological Alternations After ABO-Incompatible Organ Transplantation

1.1 Summary

Since the middle of the twentieth century, the transplantation immunology has been gradually established and completed, the transplantation techniques have been greatly improved, new immunosuppressive drugs have been developed and applied to clinic, and the organ transplantations crossing blood types, including kidney, liver, heart, lung, bone marrow transplantation, have been successfully carried out that significantly improved the survival rate and life quality of patients receiving organ transplantation. In the meantime, immune and pathophysiological mechanisms of organ transplantation and a variety of organ rejections have been understood comprehensively, leading to the emerging of a new subject, *transplantation pathology*, which is an inter-discipline combining the pathology and transplantation [1].

Transplantation pathology describes pathological basic knowledge and methods to organ transplantation implementation and basic research [2]. It mainly focuses on observing and studying the related alternations, mechanisms, and pathological histology features during transplantation and helps doctors to accurately diagnose and differentiate posttransplant complications based on these theories as well as clinical observations and examinations, thus guiding doctors to establish therapeutic regimens and carry out relevant basic researches. For example, after the ABO-incompatible organ transplantation, recipients may have multiple complications, such as graft ischemia-reperfusion injury, various types of rejection, immunosuppressive drug toxicity injury, coagulation disorders, microthrombopathy, infection, and original disease relapse. The best way to identify and diagnose these complications is pathological diagnosis for graft biopsy, which is the intension of the new subject transplantation pathology.

However, different organ transplantations have different immunopathophysiological responses; herein, we take kidney transplantation as an example to briefly introduce the ABO-incompatible organ rejection mechanisms after transplantation. It has been reported that the acute rejection incidence is 9–12% after renal transplantation based on renal biopsy, and subclinical acute rejection can be seen in nearly one third of the transplanted kidneys with stable function via biopsy examination. Grimm et al. compared the invasive cell phenotypes in the acute and the subclinical kidney rejection and found that $CD8^+$ and $CD68^+$ cells in the acute clinical kidney rejection were slightly more than the subclinical acute kidney rejection, despite two rejection types had the same Banff scores in immunohistochemistry and image analysis [3]. Moreover, although the lymphocyte activity products, including CD25, perforin, and TNF-α, had no significant difference between two rejections, the activated macrophages had significant difference, revealing that macrophages may act a pivotal role in the transplantation rejection-induced organ injury [4].

In addition, an important alternation in kidney transplantation is the elevated expressions of the adhesion molecules (AM) in vascular endothelial cells and epithelial cells of the renal tubule. For example, Lin et al. found that VCAM-1 was up-modulated in the renal epithelial cells after renal rejection, which can functionally bind with VLA-4; therefore the adhesion of potentially graft-damaging lymphoid cells was enhanced [5]. Schwarz et al. reported that adhesion molecule, expressed in donor biopsies, could be regarded as a postischemic acute renal allograft failure development marker rather than an early allograft rejection predictor [6].

1.2 Pathophysiological Alternations After Plasmapheresis

In order to remove abundant antibodies in the recipient's body, it is necessary for recipients to have preoperative blood purification before ABO-incompatible organ transplantation. Currently common methods include plasmapheresis, double filtration plasmapheresis (DFPP), and immunosorption, but all these methods can lead to a certain extent of pathophysiological alternations of organ transplantation recipients in vivo.

1.2.1 Pathophysiological Changes After Plasmapheresis

Due to multiple infusions of substantive plasma products, the following responses may occur:

1. Virus infection. Fresh frozen plasma may potentially contaminate hepatitis virus or human immunodeficiency virus (HIV), and since replacement of 1 unit plasma requires about 10–15 units of fresh frozen plasma, therefore virus infection can't be ignored. Currently, there has no effective measures to prevent virus infection; therefore detections of fresh frozen plasma must be particularly counted on before the application.
2. Anaphylaxis. Syndromes often occur during the fresh frozen plasma infusion; major symptoms include chills, skin rash, fever, and hypotension, but laryngeal edema and cardiopulmonary failure are very rare. Application of anti-allergic medicines such as corticosteroids, promethazine, adrenaline, etc. before plasmapheresis can reduce the severity and incidence of these allergic reactions. Some separate case also reported recipient allergies to membrane separator disinfector in membrane plasma separation.
3. Alkalemia. Albumin solution does not contain potassium ions, and the recipient's serum potassium concentration will reduce about 25% after every unit of plasma replacement; therefore, patients with hypokalemia should be paid more attention. Moreover, hypokalemia tends to cause metabolic alkaline, which easily leads to alkalosis inverse.
4. Cardiac insufficiency. Large amounts of plasma infusion also increase cardiac load and cause cardiac insufficiency with pathophysiological alternations such as pulmonary edema.

1.2.2 Pathophysiological Changes After Double Filtration Plasmapheresis

When removing a large number of antibodies in vivo before ABO-incompatible organ transplantation, it is inevitable to cause loss of other important components, such as coagulation factors, serum proteins etc.; therefore it may cause complications including coagulation disorders, hypoproteinemia, and massive hemorrhage.

1.2.3 Pathophysiological Changes After the Immunosorption

A few cases of first-use syndrome (FUS) have been reported after the first immunosorption dialysis because the cellulose of dialysis membrane contains low biocompatible fibers. Clinical manifestations of the FUS include hemolysis, bleeding, coagulation dysfunction, hypotension, hypocalcemia, and arrhythmia. In addition, contamination and even hypersensitivity may occur when patient's blood contacts with plasma separation membrane or is adsorbent during the adsorption process.

1.3 Coagulation Disorder

Coagulation disorders are common complications after ABO-incompatible organ transplantation. Generally, the following factors are main causes for coagulation disorders:

1. Blood purification before ABO-incompatible organ transplantation in patients can result in the loss of some coagulation factors.
2. During the surgery, donor organs or the adjacent tissues and organs will undergo stretch and compression, which will result in ischemia in these organs and tissues; therefore they are easily to produce abundant metabolic waste, and the latter will affect the body coagulation function when absorbed into the blood.
3. Defiber effect from the blood vessel endothelium around vascular anastomosis area can also result in coagulation functional disorder.

ABO-incompatible renal transplantation perioperative period patients may have different degrees of coagulation abnormalities, and main characteristics include:

1. APTT is significantly prolonged during a 3-day period after the operation and distinctly shortened after 1 week; the fibrinogen level is slightly decreased during a 3-day period after the operation compared to the level before operation, the D-dimer level increases immediately after operation and becomes significant at the third day after operation, and the antiprothrombin activity is significantly decreased during a 3-day period after the operation.
2. From pre-operation to the third day after operation, the platelet count is lower than the normal level or in a low normal level, and the maximum platelet aggregation rate (MAR) is also lower than the control group.
3. The activity of tissue plasminogen activator (t-PA) is obviously higher during a 3-day period after the operation, whereas PAI starts to increase 3 days after the operation.

These characteristics indicate that the number of platelets decreases, aggregation function of platelet is weakened, and parts of the platelets are activated in the early stage after ABO-incompatible renal transplantation due to uremia, blood purification, or surgical trauma; that blood coagulation will decrease because of blood dilution and blood coagulation factor consumption at the early stage after operation, and then the blood tends to be hypercoagulability 1 week later; and that hyperfibrinolysis at the beginning (the obviously increasing t-PA activity) and gradually suppressed t-PA (PAI dominant) are one of the possible mechanisms causing hemorrhage in the early stage and hypercoagulability later.

1.4 Transplantation-Associated Thrombotic Microangiopathy (TA-TMA)

The transplantation-associated thrombotic microangiopathy (TA-TMA) has been reported after ABO-incompatible organ transplantation about 20 years ago [7]. Since the last decade, the incidence of TA-TMA has increased with the rapid development of various types of organ transplantation, especially the establishment of the ABO-incompatible organ transplantation [8, 9]. We will take the ABO-incompatible kidney transplantation as an example to introduce the pathophysiological alternations of the TA-TMA.

Pathological changes of the TA-TMA are generally the same with the classical TMA, i.e., microvascular endothelial cell damage and activation of local coagulation system leading to micro-thrombosis formation and fibrin deposition. Immunopathological examination shows that both immunoglobulin and complement are negative. There are two types of renal pathological changes by light microscope examination:

1. Glomerular type: capillary cavity is obstructed due to glomerular capillary endothelial cell hyperplasia and swelling, the basement membrane incrassates, and subendothelial space broadens with the double track sign; occasionally, segmental fibrinoid necrosis of the glomerular capillary and microthrombus intracapillary can be observed.
2. Renal vascular type: arteriole and interlobular arterial endothelial cell hyperplasia and swelling, the basilar membrane tectorium broadens, and the lumen are stenosis; occasionally micro-thrombosis and fibrinoid necrosis of arterial wall can be seen, and finally endarterium hyperplasia can result in concentric circle onionskin changes in the later stage of disease.

Some cases mainly present only either one of the above two types [10].

Transmission electron microscope (TEM) exanimation shows that besides glomerular capillary endothelial cell proliferation and swelling, basement membrane tectorium widening and no electron dense deposition are also its characteristic changes [10].

The clinical presentations of the TA-TMA include multiple organ injuries caused by intravascular hemolytic anemia, thrombocytopenia, and thrombosis in microcirculation. It has been reported that the prognosis of TMA with glomerular lesions was much better. However, Bren et al. found that the glomerular-vascular mixed-type TMA was more serious than the glomerular-type TMA in the early stage, and renal function improved 1 year after gradual reduction treatment of ciclosporin, but the glomerular filtration rate (GFR) had no significant difference between two types with 1-year follow-up [11].

1.5 Graft Ischemia-Reperfusion Injury

Graft ischemia-reperfusion injury is the main reason for primary graft dysfunction or delayed graft function after ABO-incompatible organ transplantation. The donor organs undergo a series of procedures including excision, lavage, preservation, transportation, and blood circulation reconstruction for donors and recipients via vascular anastomosis during the whole process, and organs are in an ischemic situation at all the time before vascular anastomosis reopens. Moreover, after organs are separated from the donor's body and in cold preservation process, due to excessive ATP consumption in cells and sodium pump disorder on cytomembrane, sodium and calcium ions as well as water can come into cells and organelles, and endoplasmic reticulum vacuolization, mitochondrial swelling, and irreversible changes of membrane structure will occur. In addition, although cell metabolism can be decreased in low temperature for preservation, the low-temperature condition can also damage the cells and reduce the cell membrane sodium pump activity as well as the membrane potential action (AP), which aggravates cellular edema in return. After the vascular circulation reconstruction completed and reperfusion happens, oxygen free radical deriving from intra-organ can cause significant ischemia and ischemia-reperfusion injury to the organ.

It has been reported that injuries by warm ischemia within 10 min could be recovered quickly, whereas injuries by warm ischemia over 30 min required 1 week or longer to recover [12], which was consistent with the result observed by Booster and Shoskes [13, 14]. Troppmann et al. reported that although the kidneys had good tolerance to cold ischemia for 24–72 h, the possibility of delayed graft function incidence could be 23% [15]. As to the ABO-incompatible renal transplantation, the direct result of ischemia-reperfusion is the acute tubular necrosis of transplant kidney. Pathophysiological events of ischemia-reperfusion injury are the result of reactive oxygen species (ROS) production, microvascular vasoconstriction, and ultimately endothelial cell-neutrophil adhesion with subsequent neutrophil infiltration of the affected tissue. Initially thought to increase the amount of free radical oxygen in the system, hyperbaric oxygen (HBO) has demonstrated a protective effect on tissues by influencing the same mechanisms responsible for ischemia-reperfusion injury [16]. Recent studies have also found apoptosis and the emergency of inflammatory factors in ischemia-reperfusion play important roles in transplant organ injury [17]. In addition, ischemia-reperfusion injury is also closely related to graft rejection. In the pathophysiology of renal allograft rejection, the complement system which is made up of soluble and cell membrane-bound components of the innate immune system has unequivocal roles. Remarkably, the inevitable ischemia-reperfusion injury inherent to transplantation is regulated by means of the terminal complement activation products C5a and C5b-9. Moreover, antigen presentation and T-cell priming can be modulated by biologically active fragments C3a and C5a produced during complement activation, ultimately resulting in allograft rejection. The C3 synthesized in renal tubule cells rather than in hepar acts as the primary source of C3 driving these effects, which has been identified by earlier work [18].

2 Process of Pathophysiology in Acute and Chronic Graft Dysfunction

2.1 Acute Graft Dysfunction

Acute graft dysfunction (AGD), also named acute graft functional disorders, is caused mainly by immune and nonimmune reasons. These reasons can cause tissue and organ ischemic or immune injuries in short or long terms and ultimately result in serious consequences.

After organ transplantation, histocompatibility antigens from donor and recipient tissues will combine together, and antibodies in recipient's body will activate the complement system and damage target cells directly or induce vascular hyperpermeability and neutrophil infiltration via active fragments produced by complement activation; these processes can result in capillary and minute vessel endothelial cell injury, fibrin deposition, large number of platelet aggregation, and consequently thrombosis formation. Ultimately, graft will suffer irreversible ischemia, degeneration, and necrosis. This is the fundamental pathophysiological process for immunological mechanism [19].

Besides immunological mechanism, other factors such as poor perfusion or long-time ischemia of donor organs can also lead to hyperacute graft rejection, which results in acute graft dysfunction.

The serum creatinine concentration is the traditional diagnostic criteria for the acute graft dysfunction. However, increasing serum creatinine is regarded as a sign of delayed kidney injury but not a predictive marker, because serum creatinine only increases when kidney has been damaged. Fortunately, with the development of new technology like functional genomics and proteomics, some new biomarkers aiming at acute kidney injury (AKI) have been found and considered, such as neutrophil gelatinase-associated lipocalin (NGAL) transport protein, cystatin C, kidney injury molecule-1 (KIM-1), IL-18, urinary NGAL, etc. These biomarkers are recognized only in the graft transplantation AKI but not in the non-transplant AKI, thus indicating them promising in clinical perspective [20].

2.2 Chronic Graft Dysfunction

Chronic graft dysfunction (CGD), caused by a variety of immune and nonimmune factors after organ transplantation, is the description of the loss of function in allografts [21], for example, occlusive arterial disease caused by immune factors and ischemia-reperfusion injury caused by nonimmune factors. The short-term outcome of kidney transplantation has significantly improved over the past two decades; however, the progress of how to improve the longer-term survival of the allografts moves in a slow pace. A second-time organ transplant operation is generally demanded in patients with CGD. Here, we will take kidney transplantation as an example to introduce CGD. Allograft dysfunction after a kidney transplant is often clinically asymptomatic with increasing serum creatinine level corresponding with decline of the glomerular filtration rate [22].

Immune factors leading to chronic graft dysfunction include (1) poor HLA match; (2) relative insufficiency of immunosuppression; (3) short-term and frequent occurrence of acute rejection; (4) allograft nephropathy; (5) loss of Klotho, an antiaging protein hindering pro-fibrotic effects of TGF-β1; and (6) cytokines like TNF-α, TGF-β, IFN-γ, IL-1, and IL-6. Nonimmune factors include (1) donor source properties, such as the kidney derived from male, too old donors, or too young donors; (2) ischemia-reperfusion injury; (3) delayed allograft kidney function; (4) bacterial and viral infections, especially cytomegalovirus (CMV) infection; (5) long-time cold ischemia; (6) mismatch of organic size between donor and recipient; (7) hypertension and hyperlipidemia; (8) nephrotoxicity of immunosuppressive drugs; (9) elevated body mass; and (10) genetic, epigenetic, and environmental factors [23].

Renal graft dysfunction, one of the most common reasons to end-stage transplantation renal failure, leads to a secondary kidney transplantation which is required by more than 20% kidney transplant patients in the United States. On the grounds of this theory, it is generally accepted that chronic rejection is the main reason for graft dysfunction within 1 year after renal transplantation.

The concept of chronic allograft nephropathy (CAN) was firstly put forward in the 1990s, elucidating characteristics of chronic tubular atrophy and interstitial fibrosis within the renal allograft 3–6 months after transplantation. CAN, the leading cause of renal allograft loss in renal transplant recipients, results from immunological and nonimmunological mechanisms, including acute rejection episodes, calcineurin toxicity, hypoperfusion, ischemia-reperfusion, infection, calcineurin inhibitor (CNI), induced renal toxicity [24], and so on. The development of CAN is often insidious and may be prior to subclinical rejection in a well-working allograft, and classic histological findings include tubular atrophy, interstitial fibrosis, fibro-intimal hyperplasia and arteriolar hyalinosis, glomerulosclerosis, and the typical clinical manifestations including aggressive elevated serum creatinine, hypertension, and albuminuria. Amelioration of immunosuppression has given rise to greater 1-year graft survival rates, chronic graft loss remains relatively unaltered, and opportunistic infectious complication is still a hard nut to crack.

As to the treatment, reducing CNI or using alternative immunosuppressive reagents except CNI may decrease the risk of renal toxicity and increase transplant kidney will lengthen. Current clinical experience indicates that new immunosuppressive medicines without nephrotoxicity, such as mycophenolate mofetil (MMF), could improve renal function and survival time of graft, while CNI can be reduced or even abandoned in the early stage on the premise of no increased risk of rejection [25]. New immunosuppression regimens, tighter supervision of the renal allograft, and management of subclinical rejection may reduce immune injury leading to CAN but must be balanced with the risk of increased calcineurin inhibitor nephrotoxicity and immunosuppression. Some of such kinds of new reagents have been evaluated in clinic, including sirolimus, everolimus, and FTY720, as well as protocols that use immune-depleting antibodies such as Campath or anti-interleukin-2R (IL-2R) antibodies in a high dosage of immunosuppression at the early stage of transplantation to decrease long-term immunosuppression either by discontinuing CNIs or by discontinuing steroids [26]. Belatacept, another new CTLA4-Ig antibody, also has been implied triumphantly in adult kidney transplantation to replace CNI [27]. Aiming at preventing renal fibrosis, such as bone morphogenetic protein-7 (BMP-7) that can limit nonimmune renal injury and extending the survival of renal transplants, many original agents are under exploration.

In summary, CAN is a main causation of allograft functional loss, with results from a combination of both nonimmune and immune injuries occurring cumulatively from both donor and recipient causes as time goes by. New immunosuppression regimens may potentially retard CAN progression but must be equilibrated with more universal hazards of immunosuppression.

References

1. Solez K, Axelsen RA, Benediktsson H, Burdick JF, Cohen AH, Colvin RB, Croker BP, Droz D, Dunnill MS, Halloran PF, et al. International standardization of criteria for the histologic diagnosis of renal allograft rejection: the Banff working classification of kidney transplant pathology. Kidney Int. 1993;44:411–22.
2. Chen S, Guo H. Pathophysiology. Beijing: People's Health Publishing House; 2009.
3. Grimm PC, McKenna R, Nickerson P, Russell ME, Gough J, Gospodarek E, Liu B, Jeffery J, Rush DN. Clinical rejection is distinguished from subclinical rejection by increased infiltration by a population of activated macrophages. J Am Soc Nephrol. 1999;10:1582–9.
4. Rush D, Nickerson P, Gough J, McKenna R, Grimm P, Cheang M, Trpkov K, Solez K, Jeffery J. Beneficial effects of treatment of early subclinical rejection: a randomized study. J Am Soc Nephrol. 1998;9:2129–34.
5. Lin Y, Kirby JA, Browell DA, Morley AR, Shenton BK, Proud G, Taylor RM. Renal allograft rejection: expression and function of VCAM-1 on tubular epithelial cells. Clin Exp Immunol. 1993;92(1):145–51.
6. Schwarz C, Regele H, Steininger R, Hansmann C, Mayer G, Oberbauer R. The contribution of adhesion molecule expression in donor kidney biopsies to early allograft dysfunction. Transplantation. 2001;71(11):1666–70.
7. Rizza V, Coletti G, Mazzotta C, Clemente K, Di Cocco P, Del Reno F, Margiotta G, Famulari A, Pisani F. A rare case of colic thrombotic microangiopathy in renal transplantation. Transplant Proc. 2010;42(4):1362–4.

8. Ikeda T, Okumi M, Unagami K, Kanzawa T, Sawada A, Kawanishi K, Omoto K, Ishida H, Tanabe K. Two cases of kidney transplantation-associated thrombotic microangiopathy successfully treated with eculizumab. Nephrology (Carlton). 2016;21(Suppl 1):35–40.
9. Daly AS, Xenocostas A, Lipton JH. Transplantation-associated thrombotic microangiopathy: twenty-two years later. Bone Marrow Transplant. 2002;30(11):709–15.
10. Lu M, Zou WZ, Zhang Y, Wang SL, Wang W. Kidney injury in transplantation-associated thrombotic microangiopathy. Beijing Da Xue Xue Bao Yi Xue Ban. 2008;40(4):392–4.
11. Bren A, Pajek J, Grego K, Buturovic J, Ponikvar R, Lindic J, Knap B, Vizjak A, Ferluga D, Kandus A. Follow-up of kidney graft recipients with cyclosporine-associated hemolytic-uremic syndrome and thrombotic microangiopathy. Transplant Proc. 2005;37:1889–91.
12. Florack G, Sutherland DE, Squifflet JP, Cavallini M, Heidecke C. Effect of warm and cold ischemia on functional survival of canine pancreatic grafts. Life Support Syst. 1985;3(Suppl 1):696–700.
13. Booster MH, Wijnen RM, Vroemen JP, van Hooff JP, Kootstra G. In situ preservation of kidneys from non-heart-beating donors—a proposal for a standardized protocol. Transplantation. 1993;56(3):613–7.
14. Canes D, Berger A, Aron M, Brandina R, Goldfarb DA, Shoskes D, Desai MM, Gill IS. Laparo-endoscopic single site (LESS) versus standard laparoscopic left donor nephrectomy: matched-pair comparison. Eur Urol. 2010;57(1):95–101.
15. Troppmann C, Wiesmann K, McVicar JP, Wolfe BM, Perez RV. Increased transplantation of kidneys with multiple renal arteries in the laparoscopic live donor nephrectomy era: surgical technique and surgical and nonsurgical donor and recipient outcomes. Arch Surg. 2001;136(8):897–907.
16. Francis A, Baynosa R. Ischaemia-reperfusion injury and hyperbaric oxygen pathways: a review of cellular mechanisms. Diving Hyperb Med. 2017;47(2):110–7.
17. Rovcanin B, Medic B, Kocic G, Cebovic T, Ristic M, Prostran M. Molecular dissection of renal ischemia-reperfusion: oxidative stress and cellular events. Curr Med Chem. 2016;23(19):1965–80.
18. Nauser CL, Farrar CA, Sacks SH. Complement recognition pathways in renal transplantation. J Am Soc Nephrol. 2017;28(9):2571–8.
19. Zhang Q, Liang LW, Gjertson DW, Lassman C, Wilkinson AH, Kendrick E, Pham PT, Danovitch GM, Gritsch HA, Reed EF. Development of posttransplant antidonor HLA antibodies is associated with acute humoral rejection and early graft dysfunction. Transplantation. 2005;79:591–8.
20. Halawa A. The early diagnosis of acute renal graft dysfunction: a challenge we face. The role of novel biomarkers. Ann Transplant. 2011;16:90–8.
21. Knoop C, Estenne M. Chronic allograft dysfunction. Clin Chest Med. 2011;32(2):311–26.
22. Goldberg RJ, Weng FL, Kandula P. Acute and chronic allograft dysfunction in kidney transplant recipients. Med Clin North Am. 2016;100(3):487–503.
23. Zununi Vahed S, Samadi N, Mostafidi E, Ardalan MR, Omidi Y. Genetics and epigenetics of chronic allograft dysfunction in kidney transplants. Iran J Kidney Dis. 2016;10(1):1–9.
24. Naesens M, Kuypers DR, Sarwal M. Calcineurin inhibitor nephrotoxicity. Clin J Am Soc Nephrol. 2009;4(2):481–508.
25. Wang P, Que W, Li H, Yan L, Fu Z, Ye Q, Chen G, Dou K, Lu S, Yang Z, Zhu Z, Peng Z, Zhong L. Efficacy and safety of a reduced calcineurin inhibitor dose combined with mycophenolate mofetil in liver transplant patients with chronic renal dysfunction. Oncotarget. 2017;8(34):57505–15.
26. Harmon W, Meyers K, Ingelfinger JR, McDonald R, McIntosh MJ, Ho M, Spaneas LD, Palmer JA, Hawk M, Geehan C, Tinckam K, Hancock WW, Sayegh MH. Safety and efficacy of a calcineurin inhibitor avoidance regimen in pediatric renal transplantation. J Am Soc Nephrol. 2006;17:1735–45.
27. Riella LV, Gabardi S, Azzi J. Belatacept and long-term outcomes in kidney transplantation. N Engl J Med. 2016;374(26):2599–600.

Pathology of ABO-Incompatible Organ Transplantation

7

Jiqiu Wen

Abstract

Organ transplant pathology occupies a very important position in organ transplantation medicine. Although the super-acute rejection seen in ABO-incompatible organ transplantation compared with ABO-compatible organ transplantation is no different on the basis of pathological diagnosis, comparison shows that transplantation with ABO incompatibility is more prone to vascular thrombosis, C4d deposition, and other problems, as stated in the content of this chapter.

Keywords

Pathology · Vascular thrombosis · C4d deposition

Organ transplantation technology has become an effective means of treating various end-stage organ diseases. Since the middle of the twentieth century, the immunological theory of organ transplantation has been gradually established and improved. Surgical techniques of organ transplantation and perioperative treatment have been continuously advanced. New immunosuppressive drugs are emerging and have been successfully applied in clinics. These advances have not only prolonged the survival of patients with organ transplants but also improved their quality of life. These improvements also rendered ABO blood type-incompatible organ transplantation a reality. With the rapid development of organ transplantation, it also faces various new opportunities and challenges, such as immune pathological and physiological adaptation, immune tolerance, and the mechanisms of various rejection reactions of organ transplantation, which warrant further investigations.

J. Wen (✉)
Kidney Transplant Center, National Clinical Research Center of Kidney Diseases, Jinling Hospital, Nanjing University School of Medicine, Nanjing, China
e-mail: wjqdoctor@163.com

Y. Wang (ed.), *ABO-incompatible Organ Transplantation*,
https://doi.org/10.1007/978-981-13-3399-6_7

The pathological manifestation of immune rejection is an emerging subdiscipline that combines pathology with transplantation.

Transplantation pathology is the interdisciplinary study of the basic knowledge and methods of pathology applied to the medical procedures of organ transplantation. This research mainly observes and studies the related pathological changes, their mechanisms of occurrence, and histopathological features. Combined with clinical observation, clinical biochemistry, and imaging examination, the diagnosis and differential diagnosis of postoperative complications can be accurately and reasonably used to guide the clinical development of treatment plans and related basic research.

1 Special Staining Methods in Transplantation

1.1 Periodic Acid–Schiff Stain

Periodic acid oxidizes ethylene glycol on the polysaccharide to glyoxal, and glyoxal interacts with the colorless magenta in the Schiff reagent to form a purple-red product. Periodic acid–Schiff (PAS) is mainly used to dye polysaccharides such as glycogen, glycoproteins, and glycolipids. In renal pathology, PAS is capable of staining the glomerular capillary basement membrane (GBM), mesangial matrix, tubular basement membrane, renal capsule (or Bowman's capsule), and peritubular capillary basement membrane. In membranous glomerulonephritis, diffuse glomerular basement membrane thickening is present from deposition of immune complexes, and PAS is the most suitable stain. The display of subendothelial nodule-like hyaline deposits (hyalinization) caused by calcineurin-inhibitor toxicity is also a highlight of PAS staining.

1.2 Periodic Acid–Schiff Methenamine Silver Stain

Periodic acid–Schiff Methenamine Silver (PASM) staining (also known as Jones staining and silver staining) is similar to PAS staining for displaying the basement membrane. The principles of these two methods are similar. The tissue is oxidized by iodic acid to expose the polysaccharide in the basement membrane to the dialdehyde group, and the hexamine silver is reduced to black metallic silver. Gold chloride replaces silver and becomes a more stable metal gold. The PASM staining is black, the contrast is higher, the background is clearer, and it is particularly effective for displaying the fine structure of the glomerular basement membrane; it can replace some functions of the electron microscope in places where medical conditions are limited. It is often used to observe pathological changes in the glomerular basement membrane such as spur formation, rupture, hyperplasia, folding, and double-track signs. However, PASM does not completely replace PAS staining. The hyaline changes described here may be negative in PASM staining.

Table 7.1 Special stains frequently used in kidney biopsy pathology

	PAS	PASM	Masson
Basement membrane	Red	Black	Deep blue
Mesangial matrix	Red	Black	Deep blue
Collagen	Negative	Negative	Light blue
Cytoplasm	Negative	Negative	Red
Nucleus	Violaceous	Varies	Violaceous
Immune complex	Negative	Negative	Red
Fibrous tissue	Light red	Negative	Red
Cast	Red	Black	Light blue

Modified from [1]
PAS periodic-acid Schiff; *PASM* periodic acid-silver metheramine

1.3 Masson's Trichrome Stain

Masson trichrome stain colors collagen and cartilage into blue or green (glomerular basement membrane, tubular basement membrane, mesangial matrix, renal interstitial) according to the size of anionic dye molecules and tissue permeability. It is red and the nucleus is blue-violet or brown. Masson staining is particularly effective in staining fibrous connective tissue, identifying renal interstitial edema (in pale) and fibrosis (in green), and early or mild fibrosis with edema may be difficult to detect. Staining characteristics of kidney specimens by the three special stains commonly used are summarized in Table 7.1.

1.4 Other Special Staining Techniques

In the case of amyloidosis, Congo red staining is usually used, and under the observation of polarized light, apple green is refraction. Elastic fiber staining is mainly used to show vascular lesions. Immunohistochemical staining, especially for C4d staining, has an important role in renal antibody-mediated rejection.

2 Biopsy of Kidney Transplantation

2.1 Zero-Time Biopsy

Zero-time biopsy refers to a needle biopsy of the donor kidney before transplantation, and the underlying lesions of the donor kidney are observed by pathology, to rationally distribute the transplanted organs and predict organ function after transplantation. The concept of zero-time biopsy was first introduced by Gaber et al. [2]. Following Gaber's report that zero-time biopsy glomerular sclerosis was positively correlated with renal failure after marginal donor transplantation, performance of zero-time biopsy began at transplant centers around the world.

Biopsy techniques of zero-time biopsy differ widely among transplant centers. Most transplant centers take a wedge biopsy, which is a wedge-shaped tissue about 1 cm in length and 0.5 cm in depth, harvested with a scalpel before transplantation. There are also transplant centers that use a fine needle of 16 G or 18 G to puncture different parts of the kidney with two needles. Studies have shown that wedge biopsy may be too superficial whereas fine-needle biopsy reflects renal vascular disease to greater advantage [3].

Most research centers usually perform punctures just before the transplant, and whether the kidneys are available at the last moment, and how the pathological changes are determined. The pathological features at the two time points do not differ much. However, the latter has undergone low-temperature transport (mechanical perfusion), and its molecular expression profile may have changed, which has great influence on predicting delayed renal function recovery and renal failure from the molecular level. There are also a small number of transplant centers that perform biopsies after the transplanted renal vessels are connected. At this time, the kidney undergoes ischemia-reperfusion and the damage can be immediately observed, and the host-mediated rejection may be observed shortly after the blood vessel is connected. Koo and Hass et al. observed that the pathology of the donor after reperfusion has been observed in the host neutrophil infiltration, but the renal pathology of the living donor has not [4, 5]. Takahashi performed renal pathology 1 h after ABO-incompatible kidney transplantation (ABOi-KT), and found that 16.1% of patients had positive C4d staining of perivascular capillaries, suggesting that low levels of ABO blood group antibodies were deposited in transplanted kidneys [6]. Kanetsuna et al. reported that this ratio is even as high as 57% [7].

The application of zero-time biopsy is mainly to evaluate the donor kidney, to determine whether the donor kidney is suitable for transplantation, determine the kidney allocation, and evaluate the prognosis and guide the treatment. In the United States, zero-time biopsy-detected glomerular sclerosis is the most common reason for kidney discard. In Europe and other countries, organ allocation is less likely to be based on zero-time biopsy. To expand the kidney source, the Italian "Double Kidney Transplant Team" performed a double-kidney zero-time biopsy for kidneys more than 60 years old, with a medical history of diabetes, high blood pressure, and mild proteinuria, for quantitative scoring of pathological changes of glomeruli, renal tubules, and vessels, based on which the decision to perform double kidney transplantation was determined. Double kidney transplantation allows some of the kidneys that may have been discarded to be utilized, expanding renal utilization. They found, during follow-up, that in kidneys assigned according to the pathological score, the incidence of postoperative delayed graft function (DGF), survival rate, and patient survival rate were not related to age [8–10].

Although a few studies have found that zero-time biopsy may be associated with postoperative DGF, most studies have found that glomerular sclerosis and interstitial fibrosis tubular atrophy found in zero-time biopsy were not so associated. The correlation between zero-time biopsy pathology and postoperative renal failure is also controversial. Correlation between zero-time biopsy and postoperative renal function has been confirmed by abundant reports, but correlation between specific pathological changes and renal function is inconsistent [11–13]. It has been reported in the literature that the degree of glomerular sclerosis is directly related to postoperative estimated glomerular filtration rate (eGFR). It has also been reported that renal arteriosclerosis and arterial hyalinosis are the main factors. It can be confirmed that interstitial fibrosis/tubular atrophy (IF/TA) should not be the main influencing factors [13–15].

2.2 Protocol Biopsy

Protocol biopsy refers to biopsy and pathological examination of transplanted kidneys at a fixed time, regardless of renal function. There is currently no uniform date for protocol biopsy. Acute rejection without significant tissue damage can present with normal creatinine levels, which is termed subclinical rejection. However, at this time the damage has already begun, and early intervention can achieve better results. Protocol biopsy can explore subclinical rejection (and other subclinical lesions) to support early intervention.

The safety of protocol biopsy often leads to suspicion that biopsy can cause complications such as bleeding. However, with the maturity of the technology, the risk when using ultrasound-guided puncture is relatively small. Second, because the transplanted kidney is usually located in the iliac fossa and is more superficial than the physiological kidney, the risk is even smaller. Peter et al. evaluated 2127 puncture events, finding that in the first 4 h after transplantation, 3 cases of bleeding required intervention, 3 cases required blood transfusion, and 3 cases of peritonitis occurred. Graft failure occurred in 1 case. Overall, the incidence of complications is relatively low [16].

Early protocol biopsy studies found that subclinical rejection could appear as early as 1 week after transplantation, and the biopsy rejection rate after 3 months was as high as 30% [17]. However, as tacrolimus gradually replaced cyclosporine as an immunosuppressive agent, the probability of rejection was reduced, and the significance of protocol biopsy was controversial. Rush et al. [18] randomized 121 patients who underwent triple immunosuppression of tacrolimus, mycophenolate mofetil, and hormones into two groups. One group had a biopsy at 0, 1, 2, 3, and 6 months after transplantation, and one group was at 0 and 6 months. Frequent biopsy does not seem to benefit patients. Moulin et al. reviewed data from several centers in France and found that patients who underwent programmed biopsy 12 months after transplantation had no difference in immunosuppressive use and renal function compared with those not biopsied [19]. Christina also found no correlation between renal fibrosis at 6-week biopsy and pathology at 1 year post-biopsy [20]. However, some studies have indicated that subclinical rejection found at 2 weeks after surgery has a 10-year survival rate of 30% lower after surgery [21].

Therefore, on one hand, protocol biopsy can detect subclinical lesions, on the other hand, the risk and cost of complications and patient compliance should also be considered. We should determine different protocols for different patients when deciding whether to perform protocol biopsy. It is generally believed that protocol biopsy in patients with a high risk of rejection can detect subclinical lesions early and obtain a better prognosis. Therefore, we believe that protocol biopsy is indicated for patients who meet one of the following criteria. (1) Patients receiving marginal donors or donors with DGF have an increased risk of rejection and a poor prognosis. (2) The underlying disease is focal segmental glomerulonephritis, membranous nephropathy, and lupus nephritis, and the risk of recurrence is high. (3) The risk of rejection in transplanted patients with high sensitization is higher than that in those not sensitive. (4) Predisone or tacrolimus was discontinued in their postoperative immunosuppressive regimen. (5) There has been evidence of rejection or previous biopsy-found rejection, and the risk of re-rejection increased. Studies have shown that in ABO blood group-incompatible transplantation the probability of subclinical rejection after surgery increased to 28% in 1 year after surgery [22].

2.3 Biopsy Indication

Renal biopsy acts as a pivotal point in the diagnosis and treatment of postoperative renal failure. Specifically, renal biopsy can be diagnostic in the following cases: (1) DGF lasts for 2–3 weeks; (2) transplanted kidney function is unexpectedly low; (3) serum creatinine increased rapidly or continuously increased; (4) proteinuria was >1 g every 24 h; (5) urine sediment changes could rule out urinary tract causes; or (6) to determine the underlying changes before immunosuppressive therapy [23].

DGF is a risk factor for rejection. The study reported that when a kidney biopsy was performed every 7–10 days during DGF, rejection was detected on the second or third biopsy. During DGF, because of the need for dialysis maintenance, it is impossible to indicate whether rejection occurs through changes in renal function. Therefore, regular biopsy is necessary during the DGF.

When postoperative renal function appears to be lower than expected, it may suggest potential other lesions, such as BK virus infection, acute tubular injury, or calcineurin inhibitor (CNI) toxicity, which require pathological examination for prognosis.

Because the kidney has a strong reserve function, changes in serum creatinine are usually seen later than in kidney disease. However, the increase in creatinine basically suggests a decrease in renal filtration rate. Excluding laboratory testing errors, kidney function may be considered to change when creatinine continues to increase by 25–50%. There are many factors that cause a decline in kidney function. After excluding nonrenal factors such as urinary tract obstruction, dehydration, and CNI toxicity (which can be monitored by blood concentration), unexplained creatinine elevation should be determined by renal biopsy, such as BK virus infection, rejection, or de novo or recurrent kidney disease.

3 Banff Classification

The Banff classification is a pathological classification of kidney transplantation established in 1991 by a group of renal clinicians and pathologists, including Kim Solez and Lorraine C. Racusen, in Banff, Canada. It has now been expanded to other vital organs. Following revision in 2007, the 2013 Banff classification has again modified the classification of antibody-mediated rejection by adding C4d-negative antibody-mediated rejection (Table 7.2).

Table 7.2 Banff pathological classification [23, 24]

1	Normal biopsy or nonspecific changes
2	Acute antibody-mediated changes (all three features must be present for diagnosis)
	1. Histological evidence of acute tissue injury, including one or more of the following
	Microvascular inflammation ($g > 0$ in the absence of recurrent or de novo glomerulonephritis, and/or ptc > 0)
	Intimal or transmural arteritis ($v > 0$)
	Acute thrombotic microangiopathy in the absence of any other cause
	Acute tubular injury in the absence of any other apparent cause
	2. Evidence of current/recent antibody interaction with vascular endothelium, including at least one of the following
	Linear C4d staining in peritubular capillaries (C4d2 or C4d3 by IF on frozen sections or C4d >0 by IHC on paraffin sections)
	At least moderate microvascular inflammation ([g + ptc] ≥ 2), although in the presence of acute T cell-mediated rejection (TCMR), borderline infiltrate, or infection; ptc ≥ 2 alone is not sufficient, and g must be ≥1
	Increased expression of gene transcripts in the biopsy tissue indicative of endothelial injury, if thoroughly validated
	3. Serological evidence of DSAs (HLA or other antigens)
	Chronic active antibody-mediated rejection (ABMR) (all three features must be present for diagnosis)
	1. Histological evidence of chronic tissue injury, including one or more of the following
	TG (cg > 0), if no evidence of chronic thrombotic microangiopathy; includes changes evident by EM only
	Severe peritubular capillary basement membrane multi-layering (requires EM)
	Arterial intimal fibrosis of new onset, excluding other causes
	2. Evidence of current/recent antibody interaction with vascular endothelium, including at least one of the following
	Linear C4d staining in peritubular capillaries (C4d2 or C4d3 by IF on frozen sections, or C4d >0 by IHC on paraffin sections)
	At least moderate microvascular inflammation ([g + ptc] ≥ 2), although in the presence of acute TCMR, borderline infiltrate, or infection, ptc ≥ 2 alone is not sufficient and g must be ≥1
	Increased expression of gene transcripts in the biopsy tissue indicative of endothelial injury, if thoroughly validated
	3. Serological evidence of DSAs (HLA or other antigens)
	C4d staining without evidence of rejection (all three features must be present for diagnosis)
	1. Linear C4d staining in peritubular capillaries (C4d2 or C4d3 by IF on frozen sections, or C4d >0 by IHC on paraffin sections)
	2. $g = 0$, ptc = 0, cg = 0 [by light microscopy and by electron microscopy (EM) if available], $v = 0$; no TMA, no peritubular capillary basement membrane multi-layering, no acute tubular injury (in the absence of another apparent cause for this)
	3. No acute cell-mediated rejection or borderline changes

(continued)

Table 7.2 (continued)

3	Borderline changes suspicious for acute TCMR
	Foci of tubulitis (t1, t2, t3) with minor interstitial inflammation (i0 or i1) or interstitial inflammation (i2, i3) with mild (t1) tubulitis; retaining the i1 threshold for borderline from Banff 2005 is permitted although this must be made transparent in reports and publications
4	TCMR
	Acute TCMR
	IA Significant interstitial inflammation (>25% of nonsclerotic cortical parenchyma, i2 or i3) and foci of moderate tubulitis (t2)
	IB Significant interstitial inflammation (>25% of nonsclerotic cortical parenchyma, i2 or i3) and foci of severe tubulitis (t3)
	IIA Mild to moderate intimal arteritis (v1) with or without interstitial inflammation and tubulitis
	IIB Severe intimal arteritis comprising >25% of the luminal area (v2) with or without interstitial inflammation and tubulitis
	III Transmural arteritis and/or arterial fibrinoid change and necrosis of medial smooth muscle cells with accompanying lymphocytic inflammation (v3)
	Chronic active TCMR
	Chronic allograft arteriopathy (arterial intimal fibrosis with mononuclear cell infiltration in fibrosis, formation of neointima); note that such lesions may represent chronic active ABMR as well as TCMR; the latter may also be manifest in the tubulointerstitial compartment
5	Interstitial fibrosis and tubular atrophy
	I Mild interstitial fibrosis and tubular atrophy (≤25% of cortical area)
	II Moderate interstitial fibrosis and tubular atrophy (26–50% of cortical area)
	III Severe interstitial fibrosis and tubular atrophy (>50% of cortical area)
6	Other changes not considered to be caused by acute or chronic rejection

4 C4d Staining

After antigen–antibody complex deposition or antibody binding to vascular endothelial cell-surface antigen (HLA or other), complement is activated, in which C4 is split into C4a and C4b, and C4b is converted to C4d. C4d can be covalently bound to the basal membrane of vascular endothelial cells to avoid degradation, which can be detected by immunohistochemistry or immunofluorescence. C4d can also be detected in glomerular mesangial membranes of normal allografts, indicating that there may be complement activity under normal conditions within the tolerance of the body.

4.1 Significance of C4d Staining in Organ Transplantation

The relationship between C4d staining and early graft failure was first reported by Feucht et al. in 1993 and confirmed by subsequent studies [25, 26]. C4d deposits in peripheral capillaries of transplanted kidneys have therefore been documented in the Banff 2007 classification scheme and is a necessary condition for antibody-regulated rejection. However, with the discovery of both C4d-positive normal kidney morphology and C4d-negative antibody rejection, C4d became an unnecessary requirement in the 2013 version of the antibody rejection index (see Banff pathological classification). The diagnostic specificity of C4d for ABO-compatible (ABOc)-KT antibody-mediated rejection (AMR) is about 90%, but the sensitivity is low (about 30%) [26, 27]. Protocol biopsy found that some patients had fluctuations in C4d staining scores at 3 months and 1 year post-operative biopsy [28, 29], but both microvascular inflammation and class II DSA were better predictors of AMR [30]. In addition, factors of both HLA antibodies and C4d are involved in AMR.

4.2 C4d Deposition in ABOi-KT

The significance of positive C4d with no histological evidence of rejection in a small proportion of ABOc-KT patients remains to be determined. Positive C4d staining can be detected in about 70–90% of ABOi patients, frequently on the glomerular basement membrane or tubular basement membrane. However, most of these cases were negative for AMR [31]. Moreover, the overall incidence of chronic rejection of C4d-positive ABOi-KT recipients within 1 year after surgery is still lower than that of C4d-negative ABOi-KT recipients. C4d deposition appears to be one of the markers of immune adaptation [32]. However, if C4d deposition is accompanied by other damage such as interstitial inflammation, it may have an adverse effect on prognosis [33].

4.3 C4d Deposition in Other Renal Tissue Compartment

Banff only scored perivascular capillary diffuse or focal linear C4d staining. Other sites such as glomerular endothelial cell basement membrane and mesangium, tubular basement membrane, arterial intima, and other forms such as granular deposition are not considered. Glomerular endothelial cells also express HLA antigen, but studies have found that glomerular endothelium may have more protective genes against complement activation, including CD35, CD46, CD55, and CD59, whereas perivascular capillaries express only CD59. Protective genes inhibit complement formation of membrane attack complexes, thus causing less damage, which may be the reason why more C4d deposits are seen on petitubular capillary (PTC) [34]. In ABOi-KT, C4d is often diffusely deposited, and more is deposited in other sites outside the PTC. Clinical studies have found no correlation between ABOc-KT glomerular and arterial C4d deposition, other forms of C4d deposition, and rejection [35, 36]. Therefore, only PTC diffuse or focal linear deposition is considered in the AMR diagnosis.

4.4 Other C4d-Related Diseases

Staining for C4d on PTC is relatively rare in other diseases, as may be the case in a small subset of patients with systematic lupus erythematosus (SLE). Thus, for patients with the primary disease of lupus nephritis (SLE), this factor should be considered in the diagnosis of rejection. The deposition of C4d in glomeruli and other places is relatively common, such as proliferative glomerulonephritis, anti-neutrophil cytoplasmic antibody (ANCA)-related glomerulonephritis, SLE [37], C4 glomerular nephropathy, and complement-mediated glomerulonephritis. The clinical manifestations are proteinuria and hematuria; renal function is normal, and serum complement levels are not low. Pathological manifestations are mesangial proliferative or membrane proliferative glomerular nephropathy, positive glomerular basement membrane C4d staining, C1q, C3, and immunoglobulin negative. By these criteria, common infections and immune diseases can be ruled out [38].

5 Rejection

5.1 T Cell-Mediated Rejection

T cell-regulated rejection is mainly caused by the binding of effector T cells and specific antigens (mainly HLA antigens), followed by the release of inflammatory factors, including tumor necrosis factor and perforin, and mononuclear cell infiltration. Mild T cell-mediated rejection such as Banff grade I is mostly reversible, although severe grade III is difficult to reverse. Therefore, pathological biopsy not only can confirm the diagnosis but also is an important factor guiding treatment and prognosis. Cell rejection can be separated into acute and chronic from the aspect of time-course dependency. The main pathological manifestations of the former are metamorphism, exudation, and necrosis, and the latter is mainly characterized by hyperplastic changes of chronic inflammation.

Acute T cell-regulated rejection is mainly evidenced by interstitial inflammation of the transplanted kidney tissue, inflammatory cells infiltrating the renal tubular epithelium, renal tubular dermatitis, or infiltration of the arterial endothelium, endotheliitis, or endarteritis in T-cell rejection. Tubulitis is the most common; infiltrating cells are monocytes, lymphocytes, or macrophages, but there are no B cells and plasma cells. Light microscopy showed that lymphocytes had invaded the renal tubular epithelial cytoplasm; the epithelium was damaged, and the cytoplasm and nucleus had degenerated. In severe cases, the glomerular basement membrane was broken. Cortical inflammation is more common than medulla. Immunohistochemical staining with CD4 and CD8 showed positive cells. There are fewer or no CD19 positive-staining cells. Granular C3 deposition can be seen in the basement membrane of the renal tubule. According to the Banff classification of the severity of renal tubular inflammation, those patients with lower scores responded better to treatment. Repeated tubular inflammation will lead to chronic damage and fibrosis.

Arteritis is another manifestation of acute T-cell rejection, which can be separated into endarteritis or transarteritis based on its severity. Endometritis refers to the infiltration of subendothelial lymphocytes and macrophages in the renal parenchyma, and some cellulose-like necrosis is observed. Endometritis is a more severe rejection with tubular epithelial inflammation. Intimal inflammation spreads to the media and affects the outer membrane, resulting in partial or complete occlusion of the lumen. Nickeleit et al. reported the prognosis of vascular rejection. The 1-year renal allograft failure rate without endometritis was 21%, with endarteritis was 28%, and with cellulose-like necrosis was 100% [39].

Most of the tubular inflammation or arteritis is accompanied by interstitial inflammation, that is, interstitial lymphocyte infiltration. Glomerulitis, which is relatively rare in acute rejection, is mainly manifested as swelling of endothelial cells and lymphocyte infiltration.

Chronic T cell-regulated rejection is mainly characterized by tubulointerstitial, vascular, or glomerular fibrosis.

5.2 Antibody-Regulated Rejection

Based on the Banff classification, AMR diagnosis requires all the following criteria: morphology, digital subtraction angiography (DSA), and evidence on DSA of binding to the endothelium. Kidney damage caused by AMR is diverse. The clinical demonstrations of antibody-regulated rejection are also renal failure, oliguria, and elevated creatinine levels.

Acute antibody-regulated rejection usually appears several weeks after surgery. However, it can also occur several months or years after surgery, such as with sudden withdrawal of immunosuppressive drugs or other causes. It manifests as glomerular or perivascular capillary mononuclear cell infiltration. Endarteritis, the infiltration of inflammatory cells in the submedial space, can invade endothelial cells in severe cases, and can also be seen as aneurysmal necrosis. Acute tubular injury is also a manifestation of antibody-regulated rejection, showing the disappearance of brush borders of renal tubular epithelial cells and even epithelial cell shedding. Immunofluorescence has showed IgG, IgM, and C3 deposition. Perivascular capillaries were positive for C4d staining.

Chronic antibody-mediated rejection (AMR) begins several months or years after surgery, resulting in persistent irreversible damage. It is the main factor for chronic kidney allograft failure. The main clinical manifestations are gradual deterioration in renal function, hypertension, and proteinuria. The main pathological signs are arterial intimal thickening, inflammatory cell infiltration, luminal stenosis, GBM thickening, double-track sign formation, and glomerular sclerosis.

References

1. Fogo A, Cohen AH, Colvin RB, et al. Fundamentals of renal pathology. Berlin: Springer; 2014.
2. Gaber LW, Moore LW, Alloway RR, et al. Glomerulosclerosis as a determinant of posttransplant function of older donor renal allografts. Transplantation. 1995;60:334–9.
3. Haas M, Segev DL, Racusen LC, et al. Arteriosclerosis in kidneys from healthy live donors: comparison of wedge and needle core perioperative biopsies. Arch Pathol Lab Med. 2008;132:37–42.
4. Koo DD, Welsh KI, Roake JA, et al. Ischemia/reperfusion injury in human kidney transplantation: an immunohistochemical analysis of changes after reperfusion. Am J Pathol. 1998;153:557–66.

5. Haas M, Ratner LE, Montgomery RA. C4d staining of perioperative renal transplant biopsies. Transplantation. 2002;74:711–7.
6. Takahashi K, Saito K. ABO-incompatible kidney transplantation. Transplant Rev (Orlando). 2013;27:1–8.
7. Kanetsuna Y, Yamaguchi Y, Horita S, et al. C4d and/or immunoglobulins deposition in peritubular capillaries in perioperative graft biopsies in ABO-incompatible renal transplantation. Clin Transplant. 2004;18(Suppl 11):13–7.
8. Rigotti P, Ekser B, Furian L, et al. Outcome of renal transplantation from very old donors. N Engl J Med. 2009;360:1464–5.
9. Remuzzi G, Grinyo J, Ruggenenti P, et al. Early experience with dual kidney transplantation in adults using expanded donor criteria. Double Kidney Transplant Group (DKG). J Am Soc Nephrol. 1999;10:2591–8.
10. Remuzzi G, Cravedi P, Perna A, et al. Long-term outcome of renal transplantation from older donors. N Engl J Med. 2006;354:343–52.
11. Snanoudj R, Rabant M, Timsit MO, et al. Donor-estimated GFR as an appropriate criterion for allocation of ECD kidneys into single or dual kidney transplantation. Am J Transplant. 2009;9:2542–51.
12. Edwards EB, Posner MP, Maluf DG, et al. Reasons for non-use of recovered kidneys: the effect of donor glomerulosclerosis and creatinine clearance on graft survival. Transplantation. 2004;77:1411–5.
13. Wang CJ, Wetmore JB, Crary GS, et al. The donor kidney biopsy and its implications in predicting graft outcomes: a systematic review. Am J Transplant. 2015;15:1903–14.
14. Naesens M. Zero-time renal transplant biopsies: a comprehensive review. Transplantation. 2016;100(7):1425–39.
15. Lee AL, Kim YS, Lim BJ, et al. The impact of time-zero biopsy on early graft outcomes after living donor kidney transplantation. Transplant Proc. 2013;45:2937–40.
16. Furness PN, Philpott CM, Chorbadjian MT, et al. Protocol biopsy of the stable renal transplant: a multicenter study of methods and complication rates. Transplantation. 2003;76:969–73.
17. Henderson LK, Nankivell BJ, Chapman JR. Surveillance protocol kidney transplant biopsies: their evolving role in clinical practice. Am J Transplant. 2011;11:1570–5.
18. Rush D, Arlen D, Boucher A, et al. Lack of benefit of early protocol biopsies in renal transplant patients receiving TAC and MMF: a randomized study. Am J Transplant. 2007;7:2538–45.
19. Moulin B, Merville P, Renaudin K, et al. Evaluation of protocol biopsy utility 12 months after renal transplantation: a multicenter observational analysis. J Transplant. 2012;2012:781263.
20. Dorje C, Reisaeter AV, Dahle DO, et al. Total inflammation in early protocol kidney graft biopsies does not predict progression of fibrosis at 1 year post-transplant. Clin Transplant. 2016;30(7):802–9.
21. Choi BS, Shin MJ, Shin SJ, et al. Clinical significance of an early protocol biopsy in living-donor renal transplantation: ten-year experience at a single center. Am J Transplant. 2005;5:1354–60.
22. Setoguchi K, Ishida H, Shimmura H, et al. Analysis of renal transplant protocol biopsies in abo-incompatible kidney transplantation. Am J Transplant. 2008;8:86–94.
23. Solez K, Colvin RB, Racusen LC, et al. Banff 07 classification of renal allograft pathology: updates and future directions. Am J Transplant. 2008;8:753–60.
24. Haas M, Sis B, Racusen LC, et al. Banff 2013 meeting report: inclusion of c4d-negative antibody-mediated rejection and antibody-associated arterial lesions. Am J Transplant. 2014;14:272–83.
25. Feucht HE, Schneeberger H, Hillebrand G, et al. Capillary deposition of c4d complement fragment and early renal graft loss. Kidney Int. 1993;43:1333–8.
26. Correa RR, Machado JR, da Silva MV, et al. The importance of c4d in biopsies of kidney transplant recipients. Clin Dev Immunol. 2013;2013:678180.
27. Bohmig GA, Exner M, Habicht A, et al. Capillary c4d deposition in kidney allografts: a specific marker of alloantibody-dependent graft injury. J Am Soc Nephrol. 2002;13:1091–9.

28. Orandi BJ, Alachkar N, Kraus ES, et al. Presentation and outcomes of c4d-negative antibody-mediated rejection after kidney transplantation. Am J Transplant. 2016;16:213–20.
29. Sai K, Omoto K, Shimizu T, et al. The impact of c4d-negative acute antibody-mediated rejection on short-term prognosis among kidney transplant recipients. Nephrology (Carlton). 2015;20(Suppl 2):16–9.
30. Loupy A, Hill GS, Suberbielle C, et al. Significance of c4d Banff scores in early protocol biopsies of kidney transplant recipients with preformed donor-specific antibodies (DSA). Am J Transplant. 2011;11:56–65.
31. Brocker V, Pfaffenbach A, Habicht A, et al. Beyond c4d: the ultrastructural appearances of endothelium in abo-incompatible renal allografts. Nephrol Dial Transplant. 2013;28:3101–9.
32. Haas M, Segev DL, Racusen LC, et al. C4d deposition without rejection correlates with reduced early scarring in ABO-incompatible renal allografts. J Am Soc Nephrol. 2009;20:197–204.
33. Couzi L, Perera R, Manook M, et al. Incidence and outcome of c4d staining with tubulointerstitial inflammation in blood group-incompatible kidney transplantation. Transplantation. 2015;99:1487–94.
34. Collins AB, Schneeberger EE, Pascual MA, et al. Complement activation in acute humoral renal allograft rejection: diagnostic significance of c4d deposits in peritubular capillaries. J Am Soc Nephrol. 1999;10:2208–14.
35. Kikic Z, Kozakowski N, Regele H, et al. Clinicopathological relevance of granular c4d deposition in peritubular capillaries of kidney allografts. Transplant Int. 2014;27:312–21.
36. Kikic Z, Regele H, Nordmeyer V, et al. Significance of peritubular capillary, glomerular, and arteriolar c4d staining patterns in paraffin sections of early kidney transplant biopsies. Transplantation. 2011;91:440–6.
37. Cohen D, Colvin RB, Daha MR, et al. Pros and cons for c4d as a biomarker. Kidney Int. 2012;81:628–39.
38. Sethi S, Quint PS, O'Seaghdha CM, et al. C4 glomerulopathy: a disease entity associated with c4d deposition. Am J Kidney Dis. 2016;67(6):949–53.
39. Nickeleit V, Vamvakas EC, Pascual M, et al. The prognostic significance of specific arterial lesions in acute renal allograft rejection. J Am Soc Nephrol. 1998;9:1301–8.

8 Anti-ABO Antibody Elimination: Pre- and Post-ABO-Incompatible Kidney Transplantation

Daiki Iwami and Nobuo Shinohara

Abstract

The first reported successful ABO-incompatible kidney transplantation was performed by Alexandre and his colleagues who employed plasma exchange to eliminate ABO antibodies with intensive immunosuppression prior to transplantation. Thereafter, pretransplant desensitization therapy has allowed kidney transplantation across ABO blood type barriers. Most desensitization protocols consist of antibody-producing cells deprivation therapy anti-CD20 monoclonal antibody, rituximab, and/or splenectomy, intensive immunosuppressive treatment, and apheresis to eliminate ABO antibodies. Apheresis is also a treatment option for antibody-mediated rejection after ABO-incompatible kidney transplantation, and the combinational therapy produces excellent graft outcomes.

At present, there are three major apheresis modalities to remove ABO antibodies: therapeutic plasma exchange, double-filtration plasmapheresis, and immunoadsorption. Therapeutic plasma exchange is the basic modality of apheresis; however, it has potential adverse events associated with using fresh frozen plasma. Double-filtration plasmapheresis was introduced in Japan and aimed to remove molecules with sizes between the two pore sizes of different filtrating membranes. Immunoadsorption is the most selective of the three modalities to eliminate ABO antibodies without supplement fluid.

Keywords

ABO antibody · ABO-incompatible kidney transplantation · Antibody-mediated rejection · Antibody elimination · Apheresis · Therapeutic plasma exchange Desensitization therapy · Double-filtration plasmapheresis · Immunoadsorption

D. Iwami (✉) · N. Shinohara
Department of Renal and Genitourinary Surgery, Graduate School of Medicine, Hokkaido University, Sapporo, Hokkaido, Japan
e-mail: iwamidaiki@ybb.ne.jp; nozomis@mbj.nifty.com

Y. Wang (ed.), *ABO-incompatible Organ Transplantation*,
https://doi.org/10.1007/978-981-13-3399-6_8

1 Introduction

Because of an extreme shortage of compatible solid organs, the need for ABO-incompatible living-donor transplantation has been increasing. ABO incompatibility refers to the presence of natural antibodies against a donor's A and/or B blood group carbohydrate antigens (ABO antibody). For a long time, ABO-incompatible (ABO-i) kidney transplantation has been a contraindication because ABO antigens are strongly expressed on the surface of the endothelial cells and kidney parenchymal cells [1]. Natural antibodies against nonself ABO antigens are known as isoagglutinins, and IgG class ABO antibodies cause acute antibody-mediated rejection (AMR) in the early postoperative period. Subsequent graft loss by injury of endothelial cells occurs through activation of the complement system, while the pathogenic role of IgM antibodies is still undetermined [2].

The first reported successful ABO-i kidney transplantation was performed by Alexandre et al., who employed plasma exchange to eliminate such harmful isoagglutinins (i.e., ABO antibodies) in combination with intensive immunosuppression in advance of kidney transplantation [3]. Thereafter, improvements in such pretransplant conditioning (desensitization therapy) have allowed the transplantation of kidneys across ABO blood type barriers [4–7]. The largest amount of experience for ABO-i kidney transplantation exists in Japan [8, 9]. Most Japanese desensitization protocols consist of (1) antibody-producing cell deprivation with rituximab, and/or splenectomy, (2) intensive immunosuppressive treatment to prevent additional production of ABO antibodies, and (3) extracorporeal treatment with apheresis to remove ABO antibodies [4, 6, 7, 10]. In addition, apheresis is also a treatment option for AMR after ABO-i kidney transplantation, and the combinational therapy produces excellent graft outcomes [6]. A large body of promising evidence produced by Japanese institutions has promoted the spread of ABO-i kidney transplantation worldwide. Consequently, the graft outcome of ABO-i kidney transplantation has become comparable to that of ABO-compatible kidney transplantation in Japan [8, 9], Korea [11], Europe [12–15], and the United States [16].

In this chapter, we introduce principles of the apheresis modality to eliminate ABO antibodies and discuss advantages and disadvantages of various apheresis techniques to achieve successful outcomes effectively and safely in ABO-i kidney transplantation.

2 ABO Antibody Elimination Therapy in ABO-Incompatible Kidney Transplantation

2.1 Pretransplant Anti-ABO Antibody Elimination as a Part of Desensitization Therapy

Apheresis involves circulating blood through an external circuit made of artificial materials, altering its composition or function, to prevent or delay the progression of diseases [17]. The first technique to be introduced has become the conventional means of apheresis. It is known as therapeutic plasma exchange (TPE) with plasma separated by centrifugation. In the context of ABO-i kidney transplantation, the harmful substances are donor-reactive ABO antibodies, especially a subclass of immunoglobulin G (IgG), and potentially IgM. In addition, complements have supportive roles in the development of AMR in transplanted organs. In other words, these molecules are the targets of apheresis in the management of ABO-i kidney transplantation.

There have recently been three major apheresis modalities applied in the desensitization protocol of ABO-i kidney transplantation, as shown in Table 8.1. In TPE, the circulating blood is separated by a plasma separator with a pore size of 0.3 μm; then the filtrated portion is discarded and replaced by a crystalloid with albumin solution or fresh frozen plasma (FFP).

In the 1980s in Japan, to overcome major disadvantages of TPE associated with the use of FFP, an original method called double-filtration plasmapheresis (DFPP) with albumin replacement was introduced, which rendered FFP unnecessary [19–21]. In Japan, the plasma separator and plasma fractionator typically used are Plasmaflo OP-08W (Asahi Kasei Medical CO., LTD., Tokyo, Japan) and Cascadeflo EC-20W (Asahi Kasei Medical CO., LTD.), respectively.

Contrary to TPE and DFPP, immunoadsorption (IA) does not need replacement fluid; thus IA does not exhibit the adverse events caused by replacement fluid. In 2001, a Swedish group introduced a new mode of antibody elimination for ABO-i kidney transplantation in which isoagglutinins are removed using an antigen-specific IA device [22]. Anti-A or anti-B isoagglutinins are removed from the plasma using the sorbent, which has synthetic carbohydrate blood group A-trisaccharides [GalNAcα1-3(Fucα1-2)Gal] or B-trisaccharides [Galα1-3(Fucα1-2)Gal] covalently immobilized on Sepharose matrix (Glycosorb ABO-A or Glycosorb ABO-B columns, Glycorex Transplantation AB, Lund, Sweden) [23]. This IA column is considered to be the most selective for adsorption of ABO antibodies (antigen-specific IA).

A clinical experience using Immunosorba (Fresenius Medical Care, Bad Homburg, Germany) was also reported in 1994, in which the sorbent has *Staphylococcus aureus* protein A immobilized on Sepharose matrix. Furthermore, a novel method of nonantigen-specific IA (Ig-Therasorb, Miltenyi Biotec, GmbH, Germany) has a reusable sorbent involving a polyclonal sheep antihuman Ig-coated Sepharose matrix. Thus, Ig-Therasorb and Immunosorba are considered to be less selective IA than Glycosorb. However, in contrast to antigen-specific IA, these devices can adsorb ABO antibodies irrespective of A or B antigen by the same column. IA sorbent has several advantages as described in the following section. Becker et al. demonstrated a comparable Ig elimination profile of the nonantigen-specific and antigen-specific IA modalities [24].

In addition, a double-column technique was introduced in which antibodies adsorbed in one column are detached by acid eluent passed through that column while circulating plasma is passing through the other column to continuously adsorb antibodies. Thus, the "regenerated column" can adsorb ABO antibodies again by passing plasma through the column. In this novel system, the elimination rate of

Table 8.1 Advantages and disadvantages of various methods of antibody removal (modified from [18])

	Supplement fluid	Advantages	Disadvantages
TPE	FFP or crystalloid with albumin solution	– Simple – Readily available – Simultaneous elimination of ABO Abs and HLA Abs, immune complexes, and unknown circulating factors – Relatively low costs	– Nonselective elimination of other plasma components – Application of FFP is necessary with risk of subsequent infections or anaphylactic reactions
DFPP	Crystalloid with albumin solution	– Selective (only elimination of high molecular weight plasma fractions) – Simultaneous elimination of ABO Abs and HLA Abs, immune complexes, and unknown circulating factors – No application of FFP needed	– Elimination of other plasma components – Low biocompatibility of the cascade filter Evaflux 2A (Kuraray, Kurashiki, Japan)
Glycosorb IA (antigen-specific)	Unnecessary	– Most selective – Simple to use technique – Elimination of both IgG and IgM antibodies for ABO antigens – No replacement fluid is needed	– No elimination of HLA Abs – In blood type O recipients and AB donors, two different columns are needed – Short shelf life – High costs
Immunosorba IA (nonantigen-specific)	Unnecessary	– Selective but less than Glycosorb – Simultaneous elimination of ABO Abs and HLA Abs – No replacement fluid is needed	– Elimination of all Ig fractions – Different affinities for various Ig subtypes (insufficient removal of IgG3 and IgM) – Rarely anaphylactic reactions triggered by *Staphylococcus* protein A – High costs
Ig-Therasorb IA (nonantigen-specific)	Unnecessary	– Selective but less than Glycosorb – Simultaneous elimination of ABO Abs and HLA Abs – Elimination of all Ig fractions – 36 months shelf life – High removal capacity – No replacement fluid is needed	– Removal of all Ig fractions – High costs, but less costs with double-column system

ABO Abs ABO antibodies, *DFPP* double-filtration plasmapheresis, *FFP* fresh frozen plasma, *HLA Abs* human leukocyte antigen antibodies, *IA* immunoadsorption, *Ig* immunoglobulin, *TPE* therapeutic plasma exchange

ABO antibody was improved to 59% compared with 28% in the single-column blood group antigen-specific IA [25].

To what titer should ABO antibody be reduced before ABO-i kidney transplant? Although the variance of the procedure and results of titration need to be considered, generally pretransplant ABO antibody titers are proposed to be less than 1:16 to permit engraftment of ABO-i kidney transplant [16, 26]. Tobian et al. demonstrated that a higher titer of ABO antibody in the early posttransplant period was associated with a higher incidence of AMR after ABO-i kidney transplantation; however, the positive predictive value of a high titer for AMR was poor [27]. A meta-analysis comparing pre-ABO-i kidney transplant desensitization protocols demonstrated that median peak ABO antibody IgG titers were 1:64 (interquartile range, 1:32–1:256) and those at post-desensitization therapy were 1:4 (interquartile range, 1:2–1:8) [28].

2.2 Therapeutic Apheresis for Antibody-Mediated Rejection After ABO-Incompatible Kidney Transplantation

AMR is defined by kidney tissue injury following antibody binding to endothelial cells and subsequent activation of the complement system. This leads to glomerular and peritubular capillary inflammation [29]. Complement activation is also detected by complement C4d deposition on peritubular capillaries. Anti-ABO antibody injures renal endothelial cells and causes endothelial damage, loss of capillary patency, ischemia, and proliferation of myofibroblasts, which results in interstitial fibrosis of the graft. In an ABO-i kidney transplant setting, almost all AMR develops within 2 weeks after kidney transplant [20]. Available tools for treating AMR are removal of ABO antibodies by apheresis, neutralization of the antibodies by intravenous immunoglobulin (IVIG), B-cell depletion by rituximab, and intensive immunosuppression. A recent trial demonstrated that a comprehensive approach, including apheresis, was superior to high-dose IVIG alone for treating AMR [30].

3 Apheresis for ABO Antibody Elimination

3.1 Therapeutic Plasma Exchange

TPE is recommended in the guidelines proposed by the American Society for Apheresis (ASFA) to reduce anti-ABO blood antibodies to achieve better graft prognosis with recommendation grade 1B [31]. The replacement fluid for TPE is albumin with a crystalloid or FFP (the plasma should be compatible with both the recipient and the donor), depending on the presence or absence of coagulopathy. The treated volume is usually set 1–1.5 times that of the calculated plasma volume.

In TPE, whole blood in the extracorporeal circuit is divided into two fractions, the blood cell fraction and protein-rich fraction, including graft injurious Ig (Fig. 8.1a). Then, the protein-rich fraction is discarded and replaced with supplemental fluid, albumin solution, or FFP. The advantage of TPE is that it can remove

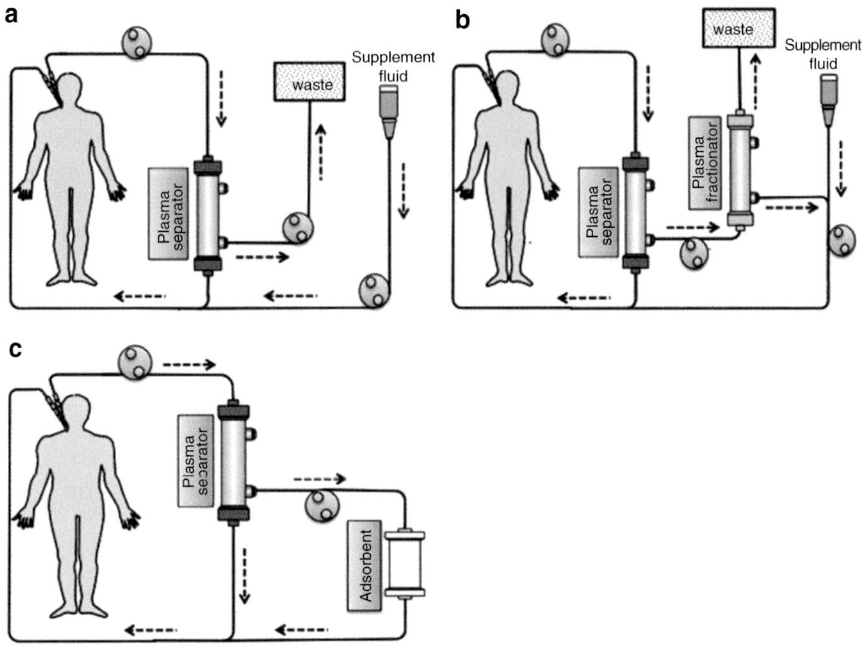

Fig. 8.1 Three major modalities of apheresis for ABO antibody elimination. (**a**) Therapeutic plasma exchange. Plasma is separated from whole blood by filtration or centrifugation and then discarded. The whole plasma volume is replaced by Ringer's solution and albumin and/or fresh frozen plasma. (**b**) Double-filtration plasmapheresis. Plasma is separated from whole blood by filtration. The plasma is then passed through a second filter where substances with molecular weights of 170,000 (IgG) and 1,000,000 (IgM) are filtered out and discarded. Only the volume of the discarded immunoglobulin fraction is replaced by Ringer's solution and albumin. (**c**) Immunoadsorption. Plasma is separated from whole blood by filtration or centrifugation. The plasma is then processed through an immunoadsorbent column and reinfused to the patient. There are no volume losses and thus no need for replacement fluids

unknown pathogenic components other than IgG and IgM, such as circulating factors, immune complexes, or complement regulatory factors. In addition, Won et al. demonstrated that FFP was better than albumin solution alone as a replacement fluid in terms of efficacy in removing ABO antibodies when donor-type or AB blood type FFP was used [32]. The improved antibody eliminating capacity was explained by the presence of soluble ABO group substances in the replaced plasma that neutralize ABO antibodies against the donor blood type. Thus, FFP is preferable to albumin solution as a supplemental fluid when TPE is performed [32].

Adverse events are determined by the replacement fluid composition, that is, when FFP is used, anaphylaxis, allergic reaction, hypocalcemia induced by citrate sodium (a preservative in FFP), and microorganism transmission can occur. In addition, the massive consumption of blood-derived products cannot be overlooked. When a crystalloid with or without albumin solution is used, drifting blood pressure caused by dilution or condensation in circulating plasma can occur.

3.2 Double-Filtration Plasmapheresis

In Japan, to overcome major disadvantages and complications of TPE associated with the use of FFP, an original method called double-filtration plasmapheresis (DFPP) with albumin solution replacement was introduced in which FFP is unnecessary. DFPP was first developed by Agishi et al. in the early 1980s [33], and it was intended to remove molecules with sizes between the pore sizes of the first membrane (plasma separator) and second membrane (plasma fractionator). Since the introduction of DFPP, the characteristics of the modality, including molecular eliminating profiles and clinical complications, have been well evaluated in Japan [19]. In DFPP, the plasma separated from whole blood by the same membrane that TPE uses (i.e., OP-08W) is further processed through a plasma fractionator where substances with molecular weights of 170,000 (IgG) and 1,000,000 (IgM) are filtrated and eliminated (Fig. 8.1b). The remaining plasma is returned to the patient together with a supplemented albumin solution. The membrane can remove both IgG and IgM molecules while allowing albumin, with a molecular weight of approximately 70,000, to pass through. However, in practice, the filtration process may remove considerable amounts of albumin, and 5–8% of albumin Ringer's solution is therefore used as replacement fluid.

Yeh et al. sought to determine the incidence of bleeding complications and coagulation abnormalities after serial DFPP treatment during a short period in myasthenia gravis patients [34]. They divided the patients into two groups, serum fibrinogen <70 and >70 mg/dL (18 and 14 patients, respectively) after five sessions of DFPP, and found that there was no difference in the incidence of bleeding complications. (Oozing at the central venous catheter site occurred in four and two cases, respectively, suggesting that simply reducing coagulation factors may not result in serious bleeding [34]). However, the modality is no longer described in ASFA as an apheresis modality for desensitization therapy before ABO-i kidney transplantation.

3.3 Immunoadsorption

In 2001, a new technique of ABO antibody elimination was introduced by a Swedish group in which isoagglutinins were removed using an antigen-specific IA device [22] (Fig. 8.1c). In this antigen-specific IA, anti-A or anti-B isoagglutinins were eliminated from the plasma using Glycosorb ABO-A or Glycosorb ABO-B columns (Glycorex Transplantation AB, Lund, Sweden) [12, 22, 23, 35]. The ABO antigen-specific columns adsorbed anti-A or anti-B antibodies regardless of Ig class or subclass [36].

In the sorbent of Immunosorba, protein A, a ligand for adsorption of ABO antigen, is covalently immobilized to a Sepharose matrix [37]. Protein A constitutes a component of the bacterial membrane of *Staphylococcus aureus*, which has an affinity for the fixed region of Ig antibodies [36, 37]. The column can be used to remove not only Ig but also immune complexes and other proteins bound to Ig [36]. The plasma is separated from whole blood by filtration or centrifugation and returned to the patient after being processed through the column. Wilpert et al. treated 11 recipients with two plasma volumes and achieved a lowering from initial titers higher than 1:128 to the intended ABO antibody titer threshold of <1:8 in eight patients, who thereafter underwent successful ABO-i kidney transplantation [38].

More recently, a novel technique, double-column device, was introduced that eliminated donor-reactive antibodies in a less antigen-specific manner using Ig-Therasorb IA columns (Fig. 8.2). In this technique, the sorbent was a reusable polyclonal sheep antihuman Ig immobilized to a Sepharose matrix (Miltenyi Biotec, Germany) [18, 24, 39]. The used columns of absorbent were patient-specific and allowed up to 20 single treatments per patient [18]. The use of nonantigen-specific IA has several advantages: (1) in addition to blood group ABO antibodies, potentially existing donor-specific HLA alloantibodies may also be eliminated from the recipient's circulation during the treatment [40], (2) nonantigen-specific IA is performed by a reusable double-column device that allows for multiple treatments, and (3) it is associated with reduced cost compared with desensitization by single-use blood group antigen-specific IA columns [39]. Becker et al. demonstrated comparable Ig elimination profiles between nonantigen-specific (using double-column system) and antigen-specific IA (single use of the column) with less cost in nonantigen-specific IA [24].

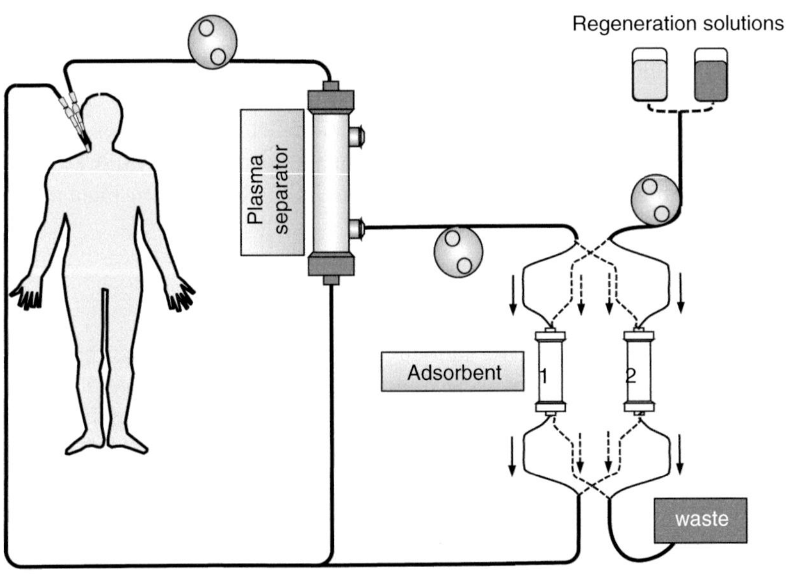

Fig. 8.2 Double-column technique to remove antibodies more efficiently during immunoadsorption. In the technique, first (solid lines and arrows), antibodies are adsorbed in one column (column 1 in the figure). Next (dashed lines and arrows), the adsorbed antibodies in the column 1 are detached by acid eluent passed through the column while circulating plasma is passing through the other column (column 2) to continuously adsorb antibodies. Then, the "regenerated column 1" can adsorb ABO antibodies again by passing plasma through the column

Unfortunately, none of these IA [12] techniques have yet been approved in Japan for health insurance coverage as a desensitization protocol in ABO-i kidney transplantation.

4 Selection of Apheresis Modality to Eliminate ABO Antibodies

It is important to know which apheresis technique is effective and safe for the ABO-i transplant recipient; however, there are few randomized controlled studies comparing apheresis modalities. In addition, it has not been determined whether the elimination of complements has additional benefits on the prevention and/or treatment of AMR in ABO-i kidney transplant recipients. Thus, in the clinical setting, the selection of apheresis modalities is discussed mainly based on their influence on the coagulation system and their eliminating efficacy of IgG and IgM.

Agishi et al. demonstrated a comparative study between DFPP and IA, Biosynsorb, which employed *N*-acetyl-D-galactosamine and D-galactosamine as ligands for A and B antigens, respectively. In the study, they demonstrated that DFPP removed both IgG and IgM ABO antibodies more effectively than IA [41].

It is also important that DFPP should be avoided in the perioperative phase because DFPP eliminates coagulation factors together with antibodies [42]. Accordingly, ASFA recommends using either TPE or IA for desensitization protocols in ABO-i kidney transplantation [31].

Comparing antibody eliminating efficacy between antigen-specific (Glycosorb) and nonantigen-specific IA (Immunosorba and Ig-Therasorb) techniques, Morath et al. demonstrated a better titer drop of ABO IgG antibody in double-column nonantigen-specific IA than in single-use antigen-specific IA (average titer drop: 1.2 and 1.7, respectively) with a reasonable cost [39]. Wahrmann et al. also showed similar superiority in the eliminating efficacy of antibody in nonantigen-specific IA than in antigen-specific IA; however, nonantigen-specific IA was inferior to antigen-specific IA in eliminating IgG3 and IgM subclasses [25, 39]. An additional potential advantage of TPE, DFPP, and nonantigen-specific IA is that, in contrast to antigen-specific IA, these simultaneously remove all the various antibodies reactive to donor HLA, as well as non-HLA molecules such as MHC class I polypeptide-related sequence A (MICA), angiotensin II receptor type 1, and collagen type V on the vascular endothelial cells of the kidney graft. Nevertheless, although there are differences in the eliminating characteristics among apheresis modalities, no difference in graft outcome, such as the AMR rate or graft survival, has been shown.

Regarding the potential influences on the complement system, Biglarnia et al. demonstrated that antigen-specific IA, Glycosorb, interferes with the complement system and that the reduction in complements, in particular C3a and the C3a/C3 ratio, may disturb antibody-induced complement activation leading to AMR [43]. Similarly, DFPP, but not TPE replaced with FFP rich in complements, can also be expected to have the same effects because DFPP can remove complements.

A recently published meta-analysis of 83 studies comparing pre-ABO-i kidney transplant desensitization protocols of 4810 recipients revealed that 3041 (63.2%) transplant recipients underwent apheresis to eliminate ABO antibodies and 1294 (26.9%) received IA as a part of the desensitization protocols [28]. The authors also suggested that apheresis to remove ABO antibodies, as well as the B cell-depleting reagent, rituximab, and a high dose of IVIG, is an essential part of the desensitization protocol before ABO-i kidney transplant [28]. In their review, an average of four sessions of apheresis before transplantation were used. Extra sessions of apheresis were required if the pretransplant ABO antibody titers were high among recipients with initial titers greater than 1:256 or 1:512 [44, 45]. Moreover, additional apheresis was needed if ABO antibody titers remained higher than 1:8 just after the standard number of apheresis sessions in the desensitization protocol [46, 47]. However, recent studies suggested higher cutoff titers, such as 1:32 or 1:64, to determine the necessity of additional apheresis sessions.

5 Conclusion

Pre-ABO-i kidney transplant desensitization therapy and treatment for posttransplant AMR have developed in combination with progress in apheresis modalities, which have sought to eliminate ABO antibodies more efficiently and more selectively with fewer adverse events. Currently, nonantigen-specific IA seems to be a widely accepted mode of antibody elimination in ABO-i kidney transplantation as it does not compromise the recipient's hemostatic system. However, TPE or DFPP can be still selected in settings where other antibodies need to be removed, such as the ABO IgM antibody and anti-donor HLA antibodies.

References

1. Breimer ME, Molne J, Norden G, Rydberg L, Thiel G, Svalander CT. Blood group A and B antigen expression in human kidneys correlated to A1/A2/B, Lewis, and secretor status. Transplantation. 2006;82(4):479–85.
2. Bohmig GA, Farkas AM, Eskandary F, Wekerle T. Strategies to overcome the ABO barrier in kidney transplantation. Nat Rev Nephrol. 2015;11(12):732–47.
3. Alexandre GP, De Bruyere M, Squifflet JP, Moriau M, Latinne D, Pirson Y. Human ABO-incompatible living donor renal homografts. Neth J Med. 1985;28(6):231–4.
4. Bentall A, Cornell LD, Gloor JM, Park WD, Gandhi MJ, Winters JL, et al. Five-year outcomes in living donor kidney transplants with a positive crossmatch. Am J Transplant. 2013;13(1):76–85.
5. Higgins RM, Daga S, Mitchell DA. Antibody-incompatible kidney transplantation in 2015 and beyond. Nephrol Dial Transplant. 2015;30(12):1972–8.
6. Takahashi K, Saito K, Takahara S, Okuyama A, Tanabe K, Toma H, et al. Excellent long-term outcome of ABO-incompatible living donor kidney transplantation in Japan. Am J Transplant. 2004;4(7):1089–96.
7. Ishida H, Miyamoto N, Shirakawa H, Shimizu T, Tokumoto T, Ishikawa N, et al. Evaluation of immunosuppressive regimens in ABO-incompatible living kidney transplantation—single center analysis. Am J Transplant. 2007;7(4):825–31.

8. Takahashi K, Saito K. Present status of ABO-incompatible kidney transplantation in Japan. Xenotransplantation. 2006;13(2):118–22.
9. Fuchinoue S, Ishii Y, Sawada T, Murakami T, Iwadoh K, Sannomiya A, et al. The 5-year outcome of ABO-incompatible kidney transplantation with rituximab induction. Transplantation. 2011;91(8):853–7.
10. Lawrence C, Galliford JW, Willicombe MK, McLean AG, Lesabe M, Rowan F, et al. Antibody removal before ABO-incompatible renal transplantation: how much plasma exchange is therapeutic? Transplantation. 2011;92(10):1129–33.
11. Yu JH, Chung BH, Yang CW, Korean Organ Transplantation Registry Study Group. Impact of ABO incompatible kidney transplantation on living donor transplantation. PLoS One. 2017;12(3):e0173878.
12. Genberg H, Kumlien G, Wennberg L, Tyden G. Long-term results of ABO-incompatible kidney transplantation with antigen-specific immunoadsorption and rituximab. Transplantation. 2007;84(12 Suppl):S44–7.
13. Genberg H, Kumlien G, Wennberg L, Berg U, Tyden G. ABO-incompatible kidney transplantation using antigen-specific immunoadsorption and rituximab: a 3-year follow-up. Transplantation. 2008;85(12):1745–54.
14. Opelz G, Morath C, Susal C, Tran TH, Zeier M, Dohler B. Three-year outcomes following 1420 ABO-incompatible living-donor kidney transplants performed after ABO antibody reduction: results from 101 centers. Transplantation. 2015;99(2):400–4.
15. Wilpert J, Fischer KG, Pisarski P, Wiech T, Daskalakis M, Ziegler A, et al. Long-term outcome of ABO-incompatible living donor kidney transplantation based on antigen-specific desensitization. An observational comparative analysis. Nephrol Dial Transplant. 2010;25(11):3778–86.
16. Montgomery RA, Locke JE, King KE, Segev DL, Warren DS, Kraus ES, et al. ABO incompatible renal transplantation: a paradigm ready for broad implementation. Transplantation. 2009;87(8):1246–55.
17. Nishio-Lucar A, Balogun RA, Sanoff S. Therapeutic apheresis in kidney transplantation: a review of renal transplant immunobiology and current interventions with apheresis medicine. J Clin Apher. 2013;28(1):56–63.
18. Hickstein H, Koball S, Lehmann R, Protzel C, Stein K, Mitzner S, et al. AB0 incompatible kidney transplantation using unspecific immunoadsorption. Transfus Apher Sci. 2014;50(2):263–6.
19. Agishi T, Kaneko I, Hasuo Y, Hayasaka Y, Sanaka T, Ota K, et al. Double filtration plasmapheresis. Trans Am Soc Artif Intern Organs. 1980;26:406–11.
20. Takahashi K, Saito K. ABO-incompatible kidney transplantation. Transplant Rev (Orlando). 2013;27(1):1–8.
21. Tanabe K. Double-filtration plasmapheresis. Transplantation. 2007;84(12 Suppl):S30–2.
22. Tyden G, Kumlien G, Fehrman I. Successful ABO-incompatible kidney transplantations without splenectomy using antigen-specific immunoadsorption and rituximab. Transplantation. 2003;76(4):730–1.
23. Rydberg L, Bengtsson A, Samuelsson O, Nilsson K, Breimer ME. In vitro assessment of a new ABO immunosorbent with synthetic carbohydrates attached to sepharose. Transpl Int. 2005;17(11):666–72.
24. Becker LE, Siebert D, Susal C, Opelz G, Leo A, Waldherr R, et al. Outcomes following ABO-incompatible kidney transplantation performed after desensitization by nonantigen-specific immunoadsorption. Transplantation. 2015;99(11):2364–71.
25. Wahrmann M, Schiemann M, Marinova L, Kormoczi GF, Derfler K, Fehr T, et al. Anti-A/B antibody depletion by semiselective versus ABO blood group-specific immunoadsorption. Nephrol Dial Transplant. 2012;27(5):2122–9.
26. Tobian AA, Shirey RS, Montgomery RA, Tisch DJ, Ness PM, King KE. Therapeutic plasma exchange reduces ABO titers to permit ABO-incompatible renal transplantation. Transfusion. 2009;49(6):1248–54.
27. Tobian AA, Shirey RS, Montgomery RA, Cai W, Haas M, Ness PM, et al. ABO antibody titer and risk of antibody-mediated rejection in ABO-incompatible renal transplantation. Am J Transplant. 2010;10(5):1247–53.

28. Lo P, Sharma A, Craig JC, Wyburn K, Lim W, Chapman JR, et al. Preconditioning therapy in ABO-incompatible living kidney transplantation: a systematic review and meta-analysis. Transplantation. 2016;100(4):933–42.
29. Colvin RB. Antibody-mediated renal allograft rejection: diagnosis and pathogenesis. J Am Soc Nephrol. 2007;18(4):1046–56.
30. Lefaucheur C, Nochy D, Andrade J, Verine J, Gautreau C, Charron D, et al. Comparison of combination Plasmapheresis/IVIg/anti-CD20 versus high-dose IVIg in the treatment of antibody-mediated rejection. Am J Transplant. 2009;9(5):1099–107.
31. Schwartz J, Padmanabhan A, Aqui N, Balogun RA, Connelly-Smith L, Delaney M, et al. Guidelines on the use of therapeutic apheresis in clinical practice-evidence-based approach from the Writing Committee of the American Society for Apheresis: The Seventh Special Issue. J Clin Apher. 2016;31(3):149–62.
32. Won DI, Ham JY, Kim CD, Suh JS, Kim BC. Benefits of fresh-frozen plasma as a replacement fluid to neutralize ABO antibodies. J Clin Apher. 2015;30(5):288–96.
33. Agishi T. Selective removal of pathogenetic macromolecules directly from whole blood by double filtration technique. Int J Artif Organs. 1986;9(5):355–8.
34. Yeh JH, Chiu HC. Coagulation abnormalities in serial double-filtration plasmapheresis. J Clin Apher. 2001;16(3):139–42.
35. Norden G, Briggs D, Cockwell P, Lipkin G, Mjornstedt L, Molne J, et al. ABO-incompatible live donor renal transplantation using blood group A/B carbohydrate antigen immunoadsorption and anti-CD20 antibody treatment. Xenotransplantation. 2006;13(2):148–53.
36. Tyden G, Kumlien G, Efvergren M. Present techniques for antibody removal. Transplantation. 2007;84(12 Suppl):S27–9.
37. Belak M, Borberg H, Jimenez C, Oette K. Technical and clinical experience with protein A immunoadsorption columns. Transfus Sci. 1994;15(4):419–22.
38. Wilpert J, Geyer M, Teschner S, Schaefer T, Pisarski P, Schulz-Huotari C, et al. ABO-incompatible kidney transplantation-proposal of an intensified apheresis strategy for patients with high initial isoagglutinine titers. J Clin Apher. 2007;22(6):314–22.
39. Morath C, Becker LE, Leo A, Beimler J, Klein K, Seckinger J, et al. ABO-incompatible kidney transplantation enabled by non-antigen-specific immunoadsorption. Transplantation. 2012;93(8):827–34.
40. Morath C, Beimler J, Opelz G, Scherer S, Schmidt J, Macher-Goeppinger S, et al. Living donor kidney transplantation in crossmatch-positive patients enabled by peritransplant immunoadsorption and anti-CD20 therapy. Transpl Int. 2012;25(5):506–17.
41. Agishi T, Takahashi K, Ota K, Yagisawa T. Comparative evaluation of immunoadsorption and double filtration plasmapheresis for removal of anti-A or -B antibody in ABO-incompatible kidney transplantation. Jpn Biosynsorb Res Group Transpl Proc. 1992;24(2):557–8.
42. Hanafusa N, Hamasaki Y, Kawarasaki H, Kido R, Shibagaki Y, Ishikawa A, et al. The effect of different apheresis modalities on coagulation factor XIII level during antibody removal in ABO-blood type incompatible living related renal transplantation. Transfus Apher Sci. 2013;49(2):254–8.
43. Biglarnia AR, Nilsson B, Nilsson Ekdahl K, Tufveson G, Nilsson T, Larsson E, et al. Desensitization with antigen-specific immunoadsorption interferes with complement in ABO-incompatible kidney transplantation. Transplantation. 2012;93(1):87–92.
44. Uchida J, Iwai T, Machida Y, Kuwabara N, Kabei K, Murao M, et al. ABO-incompatible kidney transplantation in elderly patients over 60 years of age. Int Urol Nephrol. 2012;44(5):1563–70.
45. Chung BH, Lee JY, Kang SH, Sun IO, Choi SR, Park HS, et al. Comparison of clinical outcome between high and low baseline anti-ABO antibody titers in ABO-incompatible kidney transplantation. Ren Fail. 2011;33(2):150–8.

46. Oettl T, Halter J, Bachmann A, Guerke L, Infanti L, Oertli D, et al. ABO blood group-incompatible living donor kidney transplantation: a prospective, single-centre analysis including serial protocol biopsies. Nephrol Dial Transplant. 2009;24(1):298–303.
47. Tyden G, Kumlien G, Genberg H, Sandberg J, Sedigh A, Lundgren T, et al. The Stockholm experience with ABO-incompatible kidney transplantations without splenectomy. Xenotransplantation. 2006;13(2):105–7.

9 Rejection After ABO-Incompatible Organ Transplantation

Ming Cai

Abstract

Antigen variety, especially HLA discrepancies between the recipients and donors, can cause rejection reaction, which is a complex and hazardous immunological reaction involving multiple cell- and antibody-mediated processes. Similarly for ABOi transplants, previous studies have confirmed that minimization of HLA mismatch is a key to the success of solid organ transplant (Holgersson et al., Transplantation 84:S48–S50, 2007). Allograft rejections are similar to other immunological responses except they are mainly mediated by alloreactive T cells that specifically recognize alloantigen and exert their destructive functions through direct cytotoxicity, NK cell-mediated cytotoxicity, ADCC, complement activation, a variety of pro-inflammatory cytokines, etc. (Holgersson et al., Transplantation 84:S48–S50, 2007 and Subramanian et al., Int J Immunogenet 39:282–290, 2012).

Due to the different underlying mechanisms, rejection reactions can be classified as described in the following chapters and vary on their clinical manifestations as well as managements.

Keywords

HLA · Rejection · NK cell · Management

M. Cai (✉)
Department of Urology PLA No. 309 Hospital, Heishanhu Rd. Number 17, Haidian, Beijing, China

Y. Wang (ed.), *ABO-incompatible Organ Transplantation*,
https://doi.org/10.1007/978-981-13-3399-6_9

1 Classification and Mechanism of Rejection of ABO-Incompatible Organ Transplant

Rejection reactions are a board of recipient's immunological responses mounted against the alloantigens carried by the allografts, including humoral and cellular rejections and the mixture of both, which vary in their etiology and pathological and clinical manifestations.

Humoral rejection is mediated by the existing alloantibodies in recipient serum. These antibodies are capable of binding complements and activate this system in the transplanted organ once exposed to specific alloantigen from donor, leading to the formation of immune complex; aggregation of RBCs, neutrophils, and platelets; and, consequently, ischemic necrosis of the allograft [1]. Humoral response plays important role in hyperacute rejection, accelerated rejection, acute rejection, and chronic rejection.

Cellular immune response requires T cells undergoing antigen recognition, priming, and proliferation before they exert effector functions; it is the major cause of acute rejection.

Based on different mechanisms of development and pathological findings, rejections can be classified into four types: hyperacute rejection, accelerated rejection, acute rejection, and chronic rejection. The rejection that happens within minutes to the first 24 h posttransplant is defined as hyperacute rejection. Accelerated rejection usually appears on 2–5 days posttransplant but can also arise within the first week. Acute rejection happens several days to months after transplant, and chronic rejections commonly develop after 6 months or years.

1.1 Hyperacute Rejection

Hyperacute rejection is termed as the rejection response which develops within few minutes to the first 24 h after bloodstream is opened to the allograft. This type of rejection is most commonly seen in second transplantation cases and recipients with history of repeated blood transfusion, multiple gestations, long-term hemodialysis, and/or multiple organ transplants. It is caused by the preexisting antibodies against alloantigen from recipients including ABO hemagglutinin, platelet antigen, HLA, as well as VEC antigens, belonging to type III hypersensitivity reactions. Once antigen-antibody complex is formed, complement system is activated which can destroy target cells directly and activate cascade to increase permeability of vasculature and neutrophil infiltration by bioactive fragments, finally leading to severe capillary and vascular endothelial injuries along with fibrin deposit and platelet aggregation. The outcome of this process is an irreversible catastrophic allograft damage which is characterized by diffuse arteritis, thrombosis, and massive tissue necrosis.

Aside from the immunological causes, sub-optimally infused organ and long ischemia time may also attribute to the development of hyperacute rejection.

Clinical and pathological manifestations: Hyperacute rejection is an irreversible humoral response. On gross examination, shortly after restoration of blood supply, the color of transplanted organ gradually turns out from bright red to dark red or blue. The consistency is also softened with possible hemorrhagic necrosis, enlarged size, and mottled appearance. Biopsy findings may include small vessel vasculitis with thrombosis formation, neutrophil infiltration, and fibrinoid necrosis of vascular wall as well as the presence of IgG, IgM, and complements.

Diagnosis and management: It is important to have surgical situations on the list of differential diagnosis, which include blood vessel tortuosity, arterial or venal thrombi, anastomosis stricture, or hypotension of the recipient. These factors may cause perfusion impairment and allograft injury which is similar to hyperacute rejection. Since hyperacute rejection is an irreversible, rapid, and intense immunological response, physicians should prevent its onset with their best effort. Nowadays, the measures to prevent hyperacute rejection include preconditioning with immunosuppressants before surgery, ABO typing and HLA matching, and crossmatch testing between the donor and recipient to exclude the presence of preformed donor-specific antibodies [2]. PRA test and CTL can provide information of recipient's sensitization status and HLA antibody level. Plasmapheresis and immunoglobulin infusion can be effective on ameliorating hyperacute rejection when recognized at early stage, but resection of the allograft is inevitable in most instances to prevent further lethal complications.

1.2 Accelerated Rejection

Accelerated rejection is also termed as vascular rejection of delayed hyperacute rejection which is attributed to the repeated immunological response caused by alloantigen 2–5 days before transplantation. Due to the recipient's T cells already primed during the first transplant, immunological response comes up rapidly after second transplantation, leading to the accelerated destruction of the allograft.

Clinical and pathological manifestation: Accelerated rejection also belongs to humoral rejections. It usually happens 2–5 days posttransplant but can also develop within the first 1 month after transplant. Biopsy examination mainly includes vessel vasculitis and fibrinoid necrosis, accompanied by parenchymal hemorrhage or infarction. Clinically, allograft undergoes function deterioration or even loss, accompanied by constitutional symptoms including spiking fever, chills, fatigue, appetite loss, and leukocytosis. It has a rapid progress and may ameliorate to bolus steroid therapy; nevertheless it tends to recur and lead to irreversible injury of the allograft.

For example, accelerated rejections in kidney transplant patients often happen 2–5 days posttransplant, manifested by hematuria, significant oliguria and even anuria, and impairment of already restored kidney allograft function; other symptoms like spiking fever, weakness, abdominal distention, and throbbing pain in the allograft area may also appear [3]. Swelling and petechial hemorrhages maybe noted on gross examination of the graft. Immunofluorescent and microscopic examination can show similar results of hyperacute rejection, including severe microvasculature damage with intimal edema, endothelial sloughing, and thrombosis. Granular deposit of IgG and C3 along the arteriole intima and in glomerulus and interstitial infiltration by monocytes and lymphocytes are also characteristic pathological changes. Living-related donor transplant may develop this type of rejection when the recipient has antibodies specific to the donor's HLA I and II antigen which are expressed on T cells and vascular endothelial, respectively [4, 5].

Diagnosis and treatment: Accelerated rejection should be highly suspected when above symptoms and/or signs are presented, and multiple diagnostic modalities are necessary for diagnosis. Doppler US can reveal reduced blood perfusion with increased resistance index and allograft size. For ABOi kidney transplant, ECT is especially useful to demonstrate impaired blood supply and delayed excretion. However, biopsy and pathological study are still the golden standard.

Treatment of accelerated rejection is difficult in the ABOi transplant. If steroid bolus therapy is not effective, lymph-depletive antibodies and plasmapheresis should be applied as soon as possible and there is still a high risk of recurrence of rejection. This temporary potent immunosuppression is associated with increased risk of life-threatening complications, including infection, congestive heart failure, GI bleeding, etc. Early resection of kidney graft needs to be performed without hesitation if conservative management failed. Accelerated rejection is a common cause for delayed or even loss of allograft.

1.3 Acute Rejection

Acute rejection (AR) is the most common type of rejection in solid organ transplants. Most ARs occur in the first month posttransplant. Biopsy examination demonstrates enormous MRP and T cell infiltration, caused by activation and proliferation of T cells. In typical cases, the patient may suffer from tenderness and/or distention over the kidney graft. Other characteristic symptoms are oliguria, anuria, azotemia, decreased plasma compliment level, and platelet count. Acute rejection can be completely relieved by proper treatment. AR is predominantly mediated by cellular response and belongs to type IV hypersensitivity response, in which Th1 cells play pivotal role to enhance the response of CD8+CTL and CD4+CTL T cells and activated macrophages as well as NK cells which impose injury on the allograft. The incidence of AR is high, and its clinical manifestation varies with the alloantigen discrepancies, immunosuppression regimen strategy, and precipitation factor such as infections [5]. ARs that happen at early stage after transplant are usually more serious, while late-onset ARs tend to develop more slowly and present with less severe clinical symptoms.

Pathological and clinical manifestations: Typical pathological findings of ARs are abundant T cell infiltration with parenchymal damage, with CD4+ T cell predominance in the initial phase and CD8+ T cell dominance later. If treated improperly or delay, ARs can cause irreversible graft injury and function loss. Pathological findings are significant inflammatory cell infiltration that consists of lymphocytes, monocytes, plasma cells, and sometimes neutrophils and eosinophils. AR is a DTH response mainly mediated by cellular arm of immune response. Except isograft transplant, AR can occur in both living related and deceased donor transplant, especially when the immunosuppression is insufficient or withhold. Most AR episodes develop within the first month posttransplant; however they can also occur in later time points. Mild ARs lack typical clinical features and need to be differentiated from primary kidney insufficiency, immunosuppressant adverse effects, infectious diseases, etc. Typical symptoms and signs of AR are fever, chills, malaise, graft pain, or tenderness with function impairment. For example, AR episodes in kidney transplant lead to sudden increase in blood pressure, enlargement of kidney graft with pain or tenderness on palpation, oliguria or anuria, bouncing of serum creatinine, and BUN levels after restoration to baselines. Doppler ultrasound may present increased kidney graft size, reduced blood perfusion, and higher arterial resistance index. There is no single lab test or imaging study that can determine the diagnosis alone, and the golden standard is still biopsy diagnosis.

Diagnosis and treatment: When under suspicion of ARs, graft biopsy and pathological examination should be exerted on time if diagnosis of ARs cannot be confirmed by clinic. It is of critical importance to recognize and treat ARs in time, otherwise ARs will cause irreversible damage to the grafts. Most AR episodes respond effectively to steroid bolus therapy, and the patient is expected to have a complete recovery. Nonetheless, some AR episodes are refractory and can cause permanent function impairment or even graft loss despite being managed aggressively with lymph-depletive strategies.

1.4 Chronic Rejection

Chronic rejection commonly occurs several months to years after transplantation. Its onset is insidious and progressive, accompanying chronic graft function impairment and eventually graft loss. Humoral response is the main process involved in chronic rejections. Low-level but persistent alloantibodies in the recipient's plasma will cause perivasculitis, smooth muscle proliferation, and allograft capillary stenosis, leading to the progressive graft function loss. The precise mechanism of chronic rejection still remains unclear, though hypothesis has been proposed, including continuation process of subclinical AR, chronic inflammation caused by inflammatory cells, antibody- and cell-mediated vascular endothelial damage, thickening of vascular wall, and interstitial fibrosis.

Clinical and pathological manifestation: Chronic rejection is mainly due to humoral immune response. It usually occurs 4 months after transplantation with a very insidious progression. The hallmarks of chronic rejection are perivasculitis, fibrosis, and atherosclerosis of arterioles. Microscopic findings reveal concentric intimal thickening and intimal smooth muscle proliferation. These lesions narrow the lumen of both the main artery and arterioles, leading to eventual vascular blockage and chronic allograft ischemia with apparent fibrosis and atrophy. For example, graft with chronic rejection can show significantly reduced size, pale color, and hard consistency. Pathological features may show infiltration of vascular wall by inflammatory cells, interstitial fibrosis, and scarring accompanied by vascular sclerosis. Immunofluorescence may reveal deposition of IgG and C3 along the arteriole walls. The clinical abnormalities are progressive, with the presence of proteinuria, hematuria, hypertension, anemia, and worsening renal insufficiency. Chronic rejection is an irreversible process, and there is no efficacious treatment for this condition so far, and it is one of the major causes of graft loss and negative factor for long-term survival of the transplant recipient.

Diagnosis and treatment: Diagnosis of chronic rejection is primarily determined by biopsy and pathology. Because of the irreversibility of CR, efforts are focused on optimal immunosuppression regimen strategy to delay the progress and to prolong the survival of the allograft. Recently, a clinical trial in Austria has reported initial experience of bortezomib in treating chronic rejections caused by alloantibodies, and the result is promising, greatly advancing our knowledge in the management of CR [6].

2 Differential Diagnosis and Experiences of Rejections

2.1 Thrombotic Microangiopathy vs. Accelerated Rejection

Thrombotic microangiopathy (TMA) is a range of disorders characterized by thrombi formation in the microcirculation, thrombocytopenia, hemolytic anemia, and erythrocyte destructions underpinned by abnormal aggregation of platelets and endothelial injuries, usually involving multiple vital systems including the lungs, brain, kidneys, liver, and skin with impaired perfusion and function of a single or multiple organs. TMA spectrum diseases contain disseminated intravascular coagulation (DIC), transient ischemic attack, thrombotic thrombocytopenic purpura (TTP), hemolytic uremic syndrome (HUS), as well as diabetic nephropathy (DN). These disorders share similar etiological feature, which is the formation of platelet- and fibrin-rich thrombus within microcirculation.

Platelet is a major component of the microthrombi. Alwayn et al. had suggested that in the transplant setting, TMA could be caused by the following:

1. Neutrophils and platelets in the allograft capable of activating the recipient's complement system that subsequently releases thrombin and leads to platelet aggregation [7]
2. Upregulation of P-selectin and beta2-integrin which activate donor's neutrophils to conjugate with recipient's platelets resulting in their aggregation [8]
3. Pro-inflammatory cytokines secreted by monocytes, such as TNF-alpha, that can both activate neutrophils and promote platelet aggregation [9]

Lin et al. had shown that antigen-antibody reactions are also competent to induce endothelial cells to express tissue factor and fibrinogen mimics like Fgl-2, VWF, ADP, and ATP, which can promote platelet activation directly or indirectly [10].

Accelerated rejection commonly happens within 2–5 days posttransplant, but it was reported to occur anytime in the first month. Accelerated rejection presents as allograft function deterioration or loss, and constitutional symptoms like high fever, chills, weakness, and decreased appetite are common. Lab tests reveal leukocytosis. This type of humoral rejection tends to be recurrent and can cause irreversible damage to allograft.

It is difficult to differentiate accelerated rejection from TMA because:

1. Similar clinical symptoms include oliguria, anuria, pain over the kidney graft, and decreased blood perfusion of allografts in Doppler ultrasonic scan.
2. Overlapped time of onset in the first week posttransplant.
3. No specific test for diagnosis.
4. Early diagnosis and intervention can be effective for both.

2.2 Coagulopathy

The incidence of nonsurgical hemorrhage associated with coagulopathy is 0.4–3%. Etiology of coagulopathy in the ABOi transplant setting includes conditioning before transplant, changes in coagulation, anticoagulation factors, and platelet numbers. Clinical presentations are (1) persistent thrombocytopenia without clear causes, (2) reduced plasma fibrinogen and increased fibrinolytic product like D-dimer, and (3) obvious hemorrhagic diathesis and lethargy [10].

Studies have pointed out that tissue factor expressed by platelets is the main cause of coagulopathy after ABOi transplant and the development was not immunological dependent. Several mechanisms have been suggested:

1. Platelets can be activated by chemokines, activated monocytes, and vWF factor expressed by vascular endothelial that possesses an A1 domain [11, 12].
2. Functional TF is also produced by platelets via alternative mRNA splicing in a similar manner with neutrophils involved in sepsis [13, 14].
3. Other chemokines (TNF-α, IL-1, IFN-γ) and TF released from platelets further stimulate endothelium and induce abnormal coagulation cascades, which in turn activates platelets, fueling a vicious circle [15, 16].

In order to prevent coagulopathy in the ABOi transplant, it is critical to balance the homeostasis between anticoagulation and hemostasis in accordance with different clinical scenarios. These approaches contain optimizing treatment to remove hemagglutinin, timely tipping anticoagulation, and hemostasis medications on an individualized basis. It is also prudent to correct coagulation deficiency by infusing specific coagulation factors pretransplantation. Sufficient hemodialysis to normalize electrolyte imbalances and other metabolic disorders has also been proven crucial. Preventive measures are needed in the transplant procedures to minimize blood loss. In the immediate postoperative period, maintenance of slightly lower-than-normal coagulation status and close monitoring of coagulation parameters with prompt adjustment in hemostatic medications are all crucial to the prevention of coagulopathy [17].

References

1. Tyden G, Kumlien G, Fehrman I. Successful ABO-incompatible kidney transplantations without splenectomy using antigen-specific immunoadsorption and rituximab. Transplantation. 2003;76:730–1.
2. Tobian AA, Shirey RS, Montgomery RA, et al. ABO antibody titer and risk of antibody-mediated rejection in ABO-incompatible renal transplantation. Am J Transplant. 2010;10:1247–53.
3. Montgomery RA, Hardy MA, Jordan SC, et al. Consensus opinion from the antibody working group on the diagnosis, reporting, and risk assessment for antibody-mediated rejection and desensitization protocols. Transplantation. 2004;78:181–5.
4. Singh N, Pirsch J, Samaniego M. Antibody-mediated rejection: treatment alternatives and outcomes. Transplant Rev (Orlando). 2009;23:34–46.
5. Madan AK, Slakey DP, Becker A, et al. Treatment of antibody-mediated accelerated rejection using plasmapheresis. J Clin Apher. 2000;15:180–3.
6. Schwaiger E, Regele H, Wahrmann M, et al. Bortezomib for the treatment of chronic antibody-mediated kidney allograft rejection: a case report. Clin Transpl. 2010:391–6.
7. Peerschke EI, Jesty J, Reid KB, et al. The soluble recombinant form of a binding protein/receptor for the globular domain of c1q(gc1qr) enhances blood coagulation. Blood Coagul Fibrinolysis. 1998;9:29–37.
8. Brown KK, Henson PM, Maclouf J, et al. Neutrophil-platelet adhesion: relative roles of platelet P-selectin and neutrophil beta2(dc18) integrins. Am J Respir Cell Mol Biol. 1998;18:100–10.
9. Lin CC, Cooper DK, Dorling A. Coagulation dysregulation as a barrier to xenotransplantation in the primate. Transpl Immunol. 2009;21:75–80.
10. Lin CC, Ezzelarab M, Shapiro R, et al. Recipient tissue factor expression is associated with consumptive coagulopathy in pig-to-primate kidney xenotransplantation. Am J Transplant. 2010;10:1556–68.
11. Schulte am Esch J II, Cruz MA, Siegel JB, et al. Activation of human platelets by the membrane-expressed A1 domain of von Willebrand factor. Blood. 1997;90:4425–37.
12. Cantu E, Balsara KR, Li B, et al. Prolonged function of macrophage, von Willebrand factor-deficient porcine pulmonary xenografts. Am J Transplant. 2007;7:66–75.
13. Panes O, Matus V, Saez CG, et al. Human platelets synthesize and express functional tissue factor. Blood. 2007;109:5242–50.
14. Holgersson J. Can ABO-incompatible organ transplantation pave the way for clinical xenotransplantation? Transplantation. 2007;84:S48–50.
15. Subramanian V, Ramachandran S, Klein C, et al. ABO-incompatible organ transplantation. Int J Immunogenet. 2012;39:282–90.
16. Zhang Q, Liang LW, Gjertson DW, et al. Development of posttransplant anti-donor HLA antibodies is associated with acute humoral rejection and early graft dysfunction. Transplantation. 2005;79:591–8.
17. Racusen LC, Colvin RB, Solez K, et al. Antibody-mediated rejection criteria—an addition to the Banff 97 classification of renal allograft rejection. Am J Transplant. 2003;3:708–14.

Experience with ABO-Incompatible Heart Transplantation

10

Haihao Wang and Qiannan Guo

Abstract

There is no great progress in ABO-incompatible heart transplantation in adults, and only a few cases are reported about the ABO-incompatible heart transplantation in children. Currently, ABO-incompatible heart transplantation remains at the basic stage. However, we believe that with the rapid development and gradual maturity of ABO-incompatible cardiac transplantation in infants and young children, we will make a breakthrough and progress of the research and application of ABO-incompatible cardiac transplantation in adults in the future.

Keywords

ABO-incompatible heart transplantation · Infants and young children · Adults

1 Introduction

Heart transplantation is an effective treatment for terminal-stage heart disease. It includes all kinds of severe cardiomyopathy, congenital heart disease, coronary heart disease, and valvular heart disease, which cannot be treated by routine surgery. Heart transplantation can be divided into orthotopic heart transplantation and allograft heart transplantation.

Heart transplantation is not a routine treatment for heart disease but rather a means of saving the lives of terminally ill heart patients and improving their quality of life. On the basis of the traditional heart transplantation, attempts have been made

H. Wang (✉) · Q. Guo
Department of Cardiothoracic and Vascular Surgery and Department of Heart-Lung Transplantation Center, Tongji Hospital, Huazhong University of Science and Technology, Wuhan, Hubei Province, China
e-mail: hhwang@tjh.tjmu.edu.cn; 936163754@qq.com

Y. Wang (ed.), *ABO-incompatible Organ Transplantation*,
https://doi.org/10.1007/978-981-13-3399-6_10

to get through the blood disorders, and some achievements have been made, especially widely used in infants, so this chapter will briefly discuss the experience with ABO-incompatible cardiac transplantation.

2 The Selection and Therapeutic Regimens of the Patients

2.1 The Selection of Patients

2.1.1 The Age Factor

The Transplantation of Infants

At present, there is no big progress about the ABO-incompatible heart transplantation of adults, but studies suggest that newborns and infants who have received the donor heart are relatively safe; its curative effect has been confirmed, yet the long-term efficiency remains to be observed. Whether the heart should be accepted or not, the age, clinical condition, history of blood transfusion and donor quality must be taken into consideration carefully for children over 1 years old. Patel ND has studied 35 cases of ABO-incompatible heart transplantation under 1 year, and no hyperacute rejection occurred. There was no significant difference about the 3-year survival rate, all above 75%, compared to the blood type matching group. It is suggested that this may be related to the immature development of the immune system in infants and the lack of or only very low concentration of ABO antibodies in the body and the possibility of inducing immune tolerance. However, the age of ABO-incompatible heart transplant recipients is still uncertain. In Britain, 9-year-old and 5-year-old children have been treated successfully with ABO-incompatible donor hearts, and no long-term complications have been reported. Some scholars believe that the combination of blood antibody titer detection and age can provide guidance, and the survival rate of such children can be improved through plasma replacement.

The Transplantation of Adults

The ABO-compatible heart transplantation of adults is widely used around the world, but the number of grafts is still less than that of other organs such as liver and kidney transplantation. For the application of incompatible heart transplantation in adults that is rarely reported at home and abroad, the transplantation has huge risks, and the main reason for it is the heart may play a crucial role in the body's blood circulation; once early rejection occurred, the hemodynamic abnormalities caused by it may have great impact on all organs of the body. The uniqueness of the heart belongs to the non-symmetry of the organ in human body. Under Chinese law and ethical system, the application of heart transplantation is far fewer than other organ transplantation. However, we firmly believe that with the rapid development and gradual maturity of ABO-incompatible cardiac transplantation in infants and young children, the research and application of adult ABO-incompatible heart transplantation will have a breakthrough and progress in the future.

2.1.2 Assessment of Coagulation Function in Heart Transplant Recipients

The patient's history of bleeding (including detailed family history, prior trauma, or excessive bleeding after surgery) and the history of the use of the drugs that affect coagulation were needed to be asked. Coagulation function must be measured before transplantation, including prothrombin time, activated partial thromboplastin time, and platelet count. The activated coagulation time should be examined many times during transplantation, and the effect of heparin on each period is measured. Optional: Intraoperative monitoring of thrombelastogram is helpful to further clarify the recipient's blood coagulation state; we can assess the platelet function through the platelet agglutination test and platelet function test (PFA-100); during the postoperative time, we can make the detection of fibrinogen and D-dimer of two other fibrinolytic indexes, and these indexes are related to the risk of bleeding after transplantation. After the transplantation, the blood coagulation status of recipients was monitored by thrombus graph.

2.1.3 Immune System Factors

Tissue-Specific Antigen

Endothelial cell-specific antigen is a specific antigen system expressed on the surface of endothelial cell. It is neither HLA antigen nor ABO antigen. The antigen system was discovered in the early 1970s and has attracted much attention by many scholars in recent years. Endothelial cells are the first contact between the donor tissue and the recipient's immune system. Recent studies have shown that primate endothelial cells can express class II antigens, which have the function of antigen-presenting cells, and can elicit immune responses through indirect pathways and can express a variety of cytokines and adhesion molecules. Once an immune response is presented at this site, it may affect graft blood supply, cause graft injury, and ultimately result in graft loss. A retrospective study showed that the rate of rapid and slow onset increases in patients with positive endothelial cell antibodies, irrespective of their HLA type. The evaluation of HLA matching and clinical effects has been controversial in the transplant community, and it has been found that about 10% of the patients have irreversible rejection even though HLA is the same living relatives' donor kidney. The reason may also be related to immune damage caused by tissue-specific antigens.

Immune Effect

Many factors can cause graft injury, such as cytokines, antibodies, activation of coagulation process, and activation of complement pathway. People often pay attention to the complex cytokine network when analyzing rejection and pay little attention to the coagulation process, complement pathway, hypertension, and other factors. With further investigation of the role of antigen-independent factors in rejection, it is increasingly noted that these factors play an important role.

The Factor of High Immune Sensitization

The multipara people accepted the specific donor heart (such as males receive females' donor heart) and recipients who have multiple blood transfusions and some special types such as the recipients of HBV infection. The incompatible donor heart should be avoided as far as possible to choose in heart transplantation.

Donor Status and the Quality of Donor Organs

Experiments have shown that many factors associated with organ donors have an influence on the long-term graft survival. Takada and his colleagues noted that the graft survival rate of brain death donors was significantly lower than that of living donors. The hypothesis is that the inflammatory mediators and surface molecules on the cells in the donor organs increased significantly after brain death, which was confirmed by the experimental model in rats. It is found that the severe increase of intracranial pressure can obviously increase the MHC antigen, costimulatory molecules, cytokines, and chemical factors in cardiac organs. The study of the brain-dead rat which accepted cross-circulation (cross-circulation, that is to say, the abdominal aorta of the experimental animal is communicated with the inferior vena cava of the normal animal, and the abdominal aorta of the normal animal is communicated with the inferior vena cava of the experimental animal) showed similar results. This suggests that this change is related to some soluble factor. This process can be inhibited by the recombinant soluble selectin P (P-selectin), glycoprotein ligand-Ig (ligand-Ig), or cytotoxic T lymphocyte (CTL) A4-Ig. The latter may block the B7-mediated T cell costimulatory pathway. If this method is feasible in humans, it can greatly improve the quality of donor organs and enlarge the donor's range. Data show that the incidence of acute rejection of brain death donor organs has increased significantly, so further research on the effect of brain death on chronic rejection is necessary.

2.1.4 Indications for ABO-Incompatible Cardiac Allograft Surgery

(More details on Chap. 5.)

2.1.5 Contraindications of ABO-Incompatible Heart Transplant

Absolute Contraindication

1. There has active infection focus in the whole body.
2. Suffering from malignant tumors outside the heart recently.
3. The lung, liver, and kidney have irreversible functional failure.
4. People who have severe systemic diseases (such as systemic connective tissue disease) and the survival time is limited.
5. After a complete medical treatment, the mean pressure of pulmonary artery was measured >8.0 kPa (60 mmHg), and the pulmonary vascular resistance (PVR) >8 Woods unit was measured.
6. Positive serum HIV.
7. People who is not subject to treatment or abuse of drugs or alcoholism.
8. People who suffer from psychosis or mentally ill.
9. There is a history of severe pulmonary infarction recently.

Relative Contraindication

1. People whose age beyond 65 years old
2. People who has a history of old pulmonary infarction
3. Patients with diabetes
4. Cerebrovascular and peripheral vascular disease
5. Chronic hepatitis
6. Peptic ulcer disease and diverticulitis
7. Active myocarditis; giant cell myocarditis
8. Cardiogenic fluid (such as poor constitution, anemia, low blood protein, emaciation, etc.)

2.2 Therapeutic Regimens

2.2.1 Immunosuppressive Treatment in Perioperative Period

Standard (triple) immunosuppressive regimens (CNI, antiproliferative agents, and corticosteroids) can be used for ABO-incompatible heart transplantation in children, without increasing the risk of rejection after transplantation. The immunosuppressive regimen after surgery is the same as that of a blood-compatible pediatric heart transplant, so we will not introduce much here.

2.2.2 Intraoperative Treatment

ABO-incompatible heart transplantation can be performed by extracorporeal circulation for plasma exchange and removal of donor-specific allogeneic blood cell antibodies. No preoperative immunosuppression or splenectomy is required.

2.2.3 Blood Product Transfusion

Children who receive ABO-incompatible heart transplants should not be transfused with whole blood, and their family members should be educated about this, and medical workers should be reminded when doing emergency or surgical procedures in the future. Type O red blood cells and type AB plasma are safe for all types of blood grafts. If the recipient is transfused with red blood cells, the transfused red blood cell type should match the recipient's ABO blood type. If the recipient requires transfusion of platelets or plasma, the transfused blood product should be matched with the donor ABO blood group.

2.2.4 Anticoagulant Therapy in Recipients

There is no anti-platelet factor 4-heparin complex antibody should be identified in the recipient. The use of unfractionated heparin is limited to the surgical procedure itself, and the use of low molecular weight heparin is not recommended because its half-life is longer than unfractionated heparin and is not completely neutralized by protamine. For patients with a history of heparin-induced thrombocytopenia, if the platelet count has returned to normal, the antiplatelet factor 4-heparin complex antibody remains, and alternative anticoagulant drugs may be used before and after surgery. The lepirudin, danaparoid, or fondaparinux can be selected by patients who have abnormal liver function and normal renal function. Patients who have abnormal renal function and normal liver function should choose the routine dose of argatroban or reduction of lepirudin. Patients with abnormal liver and kidney function should be treated with reduced doses of tramadol or a prescribed version of atorvastatin.

2.2.5 Extracorporeal Membrane Oxygenation (ECMO) in the Treatment of Primary Graft Failure of Children after Heart Transplantation

If all corrective factors are excluded during transplantation, ECMO should be used as early as possible when the patient cannot seperate from the cardiopulmonary bypass or get progressive graft failure after transplantation. The flow of ECMO should provide adequate systemic perfusion and tissue oxygen supply to await myocardial recovery. The problem of left ventricular dilation during ECMO support should be actively corrected because it can affect lung function and impede the recovery of left ventricular function. The clinical symptoms were closely monitored, and the echocardiographic parameters were continuously monitored to assess whether the myocardium was recovering. Improvement of objective indicators is used to guide the discontinuation and removal of ECMO. If the objective evidence of no muscle recovery within 3–5 days remains to be considered, long-term mechanical circulatory support should be used to support the transition to rehabilitation or secondary heart transplantation or to abandon life extension therapy.

3 Diagnosis and Treatment of Postoperative Complications

3.1 Monitoring of Rejection

3.1.1 Clinical Symptoms

The clinical symptoms of rejection after heart transplantation are often atypical and nonspecific. But the researchers believe that careful clinical observation and a series of noninvasive monitoring can well identify rejection. Patients with rejection should be treated with methylprednisolone as early as possible so as not to delay the treatment. The rejection reaction except the hyperacute rejection can be identified from the following clinical symptoms: systemic discomfort including fatigue, anxiety, drowsiness, loss of appetite, low fever, shortness of breath and the reduced capacity of activity, at the same time, enlarged heart, jugular vein enlargement, low heart sounds, galloping horse rhythm, arrhythmia, unexplained hypotension and increased peripheral blood lymphocyte count can also be the signs.

3.1.2 Endomyocardial Biopsy

Rejection is an important factor related to the rehabilitation and prognosis of patients after cardiac transplantation. Therefore, timely and effective monitoring is needed to provide evidence for early diagnosis and early treatment. Endomyocardial biopsy is a sensitive and reliable diagnostic method for acute rejection, but it's also a method that is invasive and expensive and sometimes can cause cardiac conduction system damage, arrhythmia, and even cardiac perforation. Three months after heart transplantation is the peak frequency of rejection, and frequent examinations are required, and EMB is restricted for these reasons. Kuhn and so on followed 1108 long-term heart transplant patients and found that 8–10% of the patients had moderate rejection after 10 years. Rejection monitoring should be combined with clinical symptoms and signs, comprehensive understanding of the patient's situation, careful observation, and comprehensive analysis of the condition, and the number of invasive cardiac biopsy can be effectively reduced. Olivier and other researchers [1] believe that real-time ultrasound combined with EMB examination is of great value; it can improve the safety of EMB, improve the success rate of puncture, make the material more accurate, and reduce complications. The combination of EMB and other monitoring methods can make up for their shortcomings and will be a future direction of development.

3.1.3 Imaging Monitoring

ECG

ECG diagnosis is important before the application of cyclosporine (CsA), but the ECG is not typical after CsA application, so the diagnosis is not of great value. In acute rejection, we can see heart rate increases, arrhythmia, and other phenomena, and the phenomena such as low voltage have not been seen. In recent years, the electrocardiogram in diagnosis of acute rejection reaction is of great value and even can replace the endomyocardial biopsy; What the principle is to connecting the two modified electrodes which implanted in the left and right ventricular epicardial just like the pacing leads to the pacemaker after the donor heart transplanted to the patient. This allows recording of the internal ECG of the myocardium, and by observing the changes in the amplitude of the R wave, it is possible to determine whether the rejection occurs. The daily internal ECG R wave amplitude was recorded 3 days after surgery, which was used as a baseline for future comparisons. After that, the amplitude of R wave recorded daily should be recommend. The rejection was indicated when the amplitude of R wave decreased more than 10%, at the same time, the symptoms, signs, body surface electrocardiogram, echocardiography and serum myocardial enzymatic indicators are also should be taken into accout. EMB examination should be performed if necessary to make a definite diagnosis. The QRS wave group represents the process of ventricular excitation, especially the amplitude of the R wave, which directly reflects the systolic function of the ventricles. A large number of experimental and clinical studies have shown that the amplitude of R waves decreases during the early days of rejection. This early rejection can reduce both left and right ventricular R wave amplitudes or can also reduce the amplitude of a ventricular R wave.

Chest X-Ray Examination

In the early stage of acute rejection, the chest radiograph has not changed, but if the pericardial effusion increases rapidly, the enlargement of the heart image can be seen, which can be used as an auxiliary diagnostic tool. Taking bedside chest X-ray once a day within 1 week after operation. The examination required the staff to wear isolation clothing, masks, and hats, change shoes, and wash hands and then enter the isolation room. The instruments should be disinfected with chlorine disinfectant to prevent infection.

Echocardiography

As a noninvasive method, echocardiography is of great value for the diagnosis of rejection after cardiac transplantation. When acute rejection occurred, the left ventricular hypertrophy increased significantly, especially the thickening of interventricular septum. It is all suggesting the acute rejection reaction that including the shortened time of the left ventricular isovolumic diastolic, right ventricle increased rapidly to 30–40 mm, tricuspid regurgitation increased significantly, pericardial effusion increased abruptly, left ventricular myocardial weight exceeded 236 g+51 g (excluding hypertensive left ventricular hypertrophy after immunosuppressive therapy), and E/A ratio increased significantly and so on. Some studies have shown that intravascular ultrasound can be very sensitive and specific to observe the changes of the whole vascular wall. It can calculate the cross-sectional area of the intima and the intima index (the cross-sectional area of the intima/the area of the intima+lumen) to reflect the changes of the vascular wall, and then diagnose the occurrence of rejection. But intravascular ultrasound is also an invasive method, and it can not observe all the changes of the blood vessels [2]. Echocardiography is a kind of ultrasonic tomography; it is able to use acoustic reflection characteristics of free shuttle in the microcirculation of the inflatable microbubbles as red blood cell tracer and contrast to the inactive tracer flow microbubble and directional microbubble adhesion to specific epitopes of the endothelial cell; for ultrasonic detection of these epitopes, however, cardiac ultrasound angiography for the diagnosis of rejection after heart transplantation is limited to animal experiments. It has also been reported that ultrasonic deformation imaging (strain S and strain rate SR) can sensitively detect subclinical abnormalities in local systolic function and can sensitively detect myocardial deformation induced by allograft rejection. Myocardial deformation assessed by S/SR may become a clinical indicator of acute rejection monitoring and diagnosis in cardiac transplant recipients and improve the quality of life of the recipients by reducing the number of biopsies [3]. The myocardial performance index can be used as a noninvasive index for the diagnosis of chronic rejection. The myocardial performance index is equal to the sum of the cardiac isometric contraction time and the equal diastolic time and the ejection time of the heart. It can well reflect the contractile and diastolic functions of the myocardium. In the early stage of chronic rejection, the myocardial performance index can often show abnormalities, thus helpful to the early diagnosis [4].

3.1.4 Immunological Monitoring

Rejection is a complex immune pathological lesion mediated by cellular and humoral immunity. The application of immunological indicators, cardiac markers, and other serum markers of relatively noninvasive index prediction estimate the incidence and severity of rejection; it is helpful to the early detection and control of transplant rejection, and it also contributes to improve the effect of heart transplantation.

C-reactive protein (CRP), synthesized by liver cells, is an acute phase characteristic protein, and inflammation and tissue damage can cause its plasma concentration to rise. The CRP should be examined from the peripheral venous bloodonce or twice before transplantation, once a day to one month after transplantation. Simultaneous examination with endocardial myocardial biopsy should be considered during patient reexamination. After observing the dynamic changes of serum CRP in patients with heart transplantation, it was found that the detection of CRP had no specificity for the diagnosis of diseases, but its rising concentration was an indicator of inflammation and tissue damage caused by various causes, and it is a marker of increased immune or inflammatory reactivity in patients with heart transplantation. Monitoring showed that the CRP value decreased with the recovery of surgical trauma in the early stage of transplantation, but in some patients the CRP value fluctuated greatly. CRP can be used as an indicator of the health or lesion status of heart transplant recipients and is also a marker of the early survival quality of heart transplant recipients.

3.1.5 Monitoring and Diagnosis of Molecular Level

At present, some researchers have studied the relationship between cytokines and rejection at the molecular level and attempted to diagnose the rejection by monitoring the expression of some cytokines in the recipient. Hammond thinks that after transplantation the vascular endothelial cell swelling, vasculitis, endothelial immune complexes, and complement deposition can prompt the occurrence of rejection; Crespo-Leiro et al. [5, 6] found that acute rejection was mainly mediated by humoral immunity. The endocardial myocardial biopsy (EMB) confirmed that when there was no obvious cellular immunity, the detection of the level of C4d in myocardial endometrium was very useful for the diagnosis of rejection. Once diagnosed, plasma exchange therapy could achieve good results. Other studies have shown that phosphorylation of S6 ribosomal protein after transplantation is closely related to antibody-mediated humoral immune response, which is a very useful biochemical marker for the diagnosis of humoral immune response [7]. Although animal experiments have shown that serum creatine kinase (CK) is a marker for the diagnosis of acute rejection after cardiac transplantation, monitoring of serum CK may indicate rejection, but further studies are needed to confirm it. Another study showed that, compared with CK, cardiac troponin T has strict myocardial specificity, and intracellular concentration is high, once the damaged cells can be quickly released, but the sensitivity and specificity of cardiac troponin T are not enough to separate for the diagnosis of rejection. Deng [8] found that peripheral blood mononuclear cells by using microarray analysis and real-time PCR for the detection of cardiac transplant recipients of the gene expression level can be good to the early diagnosis of rejection, little trauma; this conclusion needs to be confirmed by multicenter-controlled clinical study. Some researchers found that TOAG-1, A-1 and 2-mannosidase gene markers were down-regulated before the occurrence of rejection, which had high specificity and reproducibility and could be used to predict the occurrence of rejection [9]. The high expression of transforming growth factor β1 codon 10–25 is closely related to acute rejection and graft vasculopathy [10].

The expression of IL-12 and IL-15 is positively related to the occurrence and development of acute rejection after cardiac transplantation and can be used as a monitoring indicator for acute rejection after cardiac transplantation. IL-12 is a multifunctional cytokine with many biological activities. It is known to directly regulate the proliferation, cytotoxicity and lymphokine production of T cells and NK cells, such as inducing T cells and NK cells to produce INF-C, TNF-A, IL-2, etc.IL-15 can activate T lymphocyte to produce chemotaxis, induce the proliferation of T lymphocyte , enhance the toxic activity of T cells and NK cells, and promote T cells and NK cells to produce Th1 cytokines such as INF-C and TNF-A. Its effect is stronger than that of traditional Thl major factor IL-2. It can also stimulate peripheral blood monocytes by binding with IL-2 receptor and IL-15 receptor A chain, and produce cytotoxicity and cytotoxicity to transplants. It also stimulates the proliferation, differentiation and DNA synthesis of B lymphocytes. Studies have also found that IL-15 has synergistic effects with IL-2 and IL-12 in anti-graft rejection.

The expression of CTLA4, CD40, and CD40L costimulatory pathway molecules in peripheral blood is closely related to the rejection. Dynamic monitoring of these molecules helps to evaluate the state of rejection. CD28 is a non-inducible molecule, showing a high density expressed on the surface of resting T cells, which means that the activation of CD28 expression may have no direct relationship of the activation state of T cells; therefore, peripheral blood T cells positive expression rate of CD28 molecules did not change with the change of rejection.

The upregulation of local vascular cell adhesion molecule 1 in transplanted myocardium is related to the positive feedback regulation of cell receptor interaction; the local inflammation can have sustainable development, leading to fibrosis and heart transplant arteriosclerosis. Therefore, the determination of the level of vascular cell adhesion molecule 1 can predict the functional status of the transplanted heart, thus providing the basis for the early diagnosis and prevention of chronic rejection.

3.2 Pathological Histology of Rejection in Early and Late Transplantation

3.2.1 Ischemia-Reperfusion Injury

Although there are some myocardial protective measures to the transplanted heart taken from transplant to completion, it is inevitable to undergo a period of long or short ischemia and hypoxia, and the blood supply to the heart (reperfusion) is completed after transplantation. In this process, the damage is caused by ischemia-reperfusion injury, although this injury occurs at the reperfusion stage when the donor heart is removed and the transplant is completed, but its damage effects will last until a considerable period of time after the operation, with several hours to several days, which vary depending on the degree of injury; minor injuries are reversible, while severe injuries are attributed to myocardial necrosis and scarring as a result. The morphology of myocardial ischemic injury is similar to that of acute myocardial infarction without reperfusion; initially, we can only see the eosinophilic enhancement of cardiac muscle cells; however, after the reperfusion, the state of the cells changed dramatically, namely, cell edema, nuclear chromatin aggregation, mitochondrial swelling, and rupture of myofibrils, condensation, etc. Vascular capillary endothelium was extremely swollen, with sparse cytoplasm, and the lumen is almost occluded. Its morphological manifestation is similar to that of myocardial infarction.

3.2.2 Rejection Reaction

According to the time of the rejection reaction and the mode of reaction, it is generally divided into two categories: acute rejection and chronic rejection. Acute rejection was manifested by infiltration of myocardial inflammatory cells and/or myocardial necrosis. Chronic rejection was mainly manifested by coronary artery lesions, rehypertrophy of myocardium, markly decrease of cardiac output and lymphocyte proliferation.

Acute rejection after transplantation in 5~7 days, the highest incidence within 3 months after operation, showed congestive heart and dark red, myocardial interstitial edema, infiltration, and swelling due to significant, hard texture, pericardial fibrinous inflammation, and near endocardial myocardial hemorrhage. Microscopically, there is an interstitial inflammation of the myocardium and necrosis of the myocardial cells. During moderate response, there is a mass of inflammatory cell infiltration in the interstitium and around the blood vessels. The severe cases were accompanied by vasculitis, swelling of endothelial cells, platelet and fibrin deposits on the intima, and necrosis and edema in the middle of small arteries. The degree of rejection is mainly reflected in the degree of myocardial interstitial inflammatory infiltration and the accompanying degree of myocardial necrosis: mild reaction only endocardial and/or myocardial interstitial edema, perivascular lymphocytes; moderate reaction of myocardial interstitial and perivascular stacks of inflammatory cell infiltration, accompanied by myocardial necrosis; the emergence of a large number of inflammatory cell infiltration and severe reactions, neutrophil and eosinophil, accompanied by myocardial necrosis; and the damaged vessel wall, microthrombosis, and interstitial hemorrhage. The pathomorphological development of acute rejection after heart transplantation indicates that the initial stage of rejection is mainly myocardial interstitial edema, lymphocyte infiltration around small vessels, the degeneration and necrosis of cardiac myocytes occur with the aggravation of the reaction, accompanied by infiltration of inflammatory cells such as neutrophils and eosinophils, cellulose-like degeneration and necrosis of blood vessels occur when rejection is more severe.

Chronic rejection usually occurs one year after heart transplantation, manifested as infiltration of lymphocyte in the intima of coronary artery (endocarditis). Subsequently, smooth muscle cells proliferated in the intima and thickened the arterial wall, narrowed lumen, extracellular lipids and calcium salts into it, showing typical atherosclerosis. But this atherosclerosis is diffuse and can involve large, medium and small arteries. Infection is another manifestation of transplanted heart and one of the main causes of death. Because of the suppression of immune system, besides bacteria, there are also viruses, fungi and protozoa infection. In addition, heart transplanters are prone to lymphoproliferative disorders, especially lymphoma.

The pathological criteria of acute rejection of cardiac allograft (2004) points are as follows:

1. Acute Cellular Rejection
   - Grade 0R (no acute rejection): There were no mononuclear cell invasion and myocardial cell damage in myocardial biopsy.
   - Grade 1R (mild acute rejection): Myocardial biopsy, focal or interstitial inflammation of the perivascular or interstitial tissue of the myocardium, can have a single focal myocardial cell injury.
   - Grade 2R (moderate acute rejection): In myocardial biopsies, focal or interstitial inflammatory inflammation of the tissue is present, and there are two or more focal myocardial cell injuries in single or multiple biopsy tissues.
   - Grade 3R (severe acute rejection): Diffuse and/or mixed inflammatory cells invade the interstitium of the myocardium, and myocardial cell damage is seen in multiple biopsy blocks, accompanied by interstitial edema, hemorrhage, and/or intimal inflammation.
2. Acute Humoral Rejection
   - AMR level 0 (no acute humoral rejection): No histological changes of rejection
   - AMR 1 (with acute humoral rejection): Capillary endothelial edema; capillary between macrophage infiltration; interstitial edema; hemorrhage; microthrombosis in blood capillary; myocardial cell necrosis; capillary endothelial C3d, C4d, and C1q deposition; and vascular CD68-positive cells

3.2.3 The Pathology of Coronary Artery Bypass Grafting

Coronary artery bypass graft includes saphenous vein, internal mammary artery, and gastroepiploic artery; the blood flow and blood vascular wall will be changed in the high state of hypertension; some are adapted to a changing environment, but some changes can lead to injury to the transplanted blood vessel, which is pathological. Endothelial cell injury in transplanted blood vessels can cause platelet adhesion, which release mitogenic factors in smooth muscle cells or fibromuscular hyperplasia caused by the vein exposed in the artery. Fibromuscular hyperplasia generally starts within 3 days after the operation; most of the patients reached a steady state within a month. A small number of patients may have lumen obstruction due to severe intimal hyperplasia. The same vein in the same patient has different degrees of lesion in different segments. In severe cases, the middle part of the lesion may be lost and replaced by fibrotic tissue. Some of the patients died in 1 week due to the presence of necrosis of the middle membrane. Early fibrous myogenic hyperplasia of transplanted vein often has no atheromatous lesion, but some years later there may be atheromatous lesions. Therefore, it is a time related phenomenon. Foam cells accumulate in the most superficial layer without endothelial cells. Scattered plaques are distributed at the branches of ligature. Over time, the destruction of the intima was covered by foam cells, endothelial cells, collagen fibers, and fibrin thrombi, and finally grafts were blocked with lipid and thrombus. Some clinical data show that the reduction of hyperlipidemia and normal levels of HDL can accelerate the development of atherosclerotic lesions in vein grafts. The study also showed that the ability of the internal mammary artery to protect against atherosclerotic lesions is greater than that of the veins.

3.2.4 The Blood Type Change of the Transplant

A patient with a blood type O died of graft vasculopathy nearly 5 years after receiving a heart transplant of type B donor unexpectedly; it was reported. In the period of 4 months after transplantation, monoclonal antibody technique of immunohistochemistry was applied. The ABO blood group antigen expressed in vascular endothelial cells of allograft heart was monitored. The results showed that blood group antigen of graft endothelial cells changed from B type to type O gradually. The blood group antigen changes in grafts were found 14 months after surgery, and this change was particularly pronounced in the later part of the observation period. The observation showed that the blood group substance of the same cardiac endothelium in the implanted patients began to change from B type to O type in 1 year after transplantation and finally completely transformed into type O at 4 months after transplantation.

Recent studies have shown that infants undergoing tolerance to ABO-incompatible heart transplants do not undergo any changes in the antigen of the graft endothelial cells. It is not clear whether different results are caused by the immaturity of the immune system or because the time of observation is too short. However, in ABO-incompatible kidney transplantation (from A2 blood kidney to 0 blood kidney), similar studies have reported that transplantation of kidney function has maintained for 4 years, but in the end renal failure occurs due to chronic rejection, and a large number of antigen-positive cells were found in the resected kidney. But no expression of O antigen was analyzed.

3.3 Special Complications

3.3.1 Immunosuppressive Drug-Associated Complications

Infection

Because a large number of immunosuppressive agents are used after operation, the patient's immune function is low and infection is easy to occur. Infection can be caused by bacteria, fungi, viruses and protozoa. Infection can affect any organ, especially lung and urinary tract infections. Infection can affect any organ, especially lung infection and urinary system infection. Strict monitoring of early infection is very important, and taking positive measures, timely diagnosis, and treatment of various infections, all related to the survival of patients. Chest X-ray examination and blood and urine examination in the postoperative period are especially important. Although there are not many ways to prevent the posttransplant infection, there are still some effective measures. For example, we can use sulfamethoxazole and trimethoprim to prevent pneumocystis carinii infection and use ganciclovir to prevent cytomegalovirus infection.

Malignant Tumor

Long-term immunotherapy is associated with the risk of malignancy, which most commonly is the lymphoproliferative diseases and skin cancers, which account for 11% of deaths after cardiac transplantation. An analysis of 173 questionnaires from the heart transplant center in the United States and Canada revealed 24 cases of primary cardiac malignancies after heart transplantation; after resection, chemotherapy, or combined chemotherapy, the 12-month survival rate of the patients was 54%, the 24-month survival rate was 45%, and the survival rates were 35% at 36 months, 48 months, and 60 months, respectively. The authors emphasize t0068 at early diagnosis and resection can lead to better results.

3.3.2 Coronary Atherosclerotic Heart Disease

Up to date, more and more ABO-incompatible heart transplant patients have been affected by diffuse coronary atherosclerotic disease. Currently, ischemic sequelae are a major threat to long-term survival in heart transplant recipients and are one of the leading causes of death among transplant recipients, accounting for approximately 39% of deaths after cardiac transplantation [11]. Coronary angiography was performed 1 year after operation, and coronary artery damage was seen in 10% of the patients, up to 50% after 5 years. This vascular lesion is limited to the blood vessels transplanted into the heart, which is associated with reduced endothelial oxide (NOS3) activity. In addition to immunization, many scholars generally believe that there are many nonimmune factors combined to accelerate the development of this disease. These factors include traditional risk factors, such as dyslipidemia, obesity, diabetes mellitus, smoking, etc. In recent years, some scholars have found that the vascular lesion of the transplanted heart is related to cytomegalovirus infection [12]. Early vascular disease is associated with a poor prognosis.

In the form of heart transplantation, artery disease is a concentric, longitudinal diffuse lesion, involving all epicardial coronary artery and its branches, which occasionally appear proximal focal lesions, but is extremely rare, and few corresponding collateral circulation can be developed. This dispersion allows angiography that can only depict lumen contours, underestimating the severity of the lesion. Intravascular ultrasound can make up for the lack of angiography and has become a sensitive method to detect and follow the same heart allograft vascular disease. The clinical manifestation of coronary artery obstruction is usually myocardial ischemia, which is manifested by left ventricular failure, ventricular arrhythmia, and sudden death. Lack of angina is the characteristic of the disease. The lesion was diagnosed by angiography, especially in one case of ischemic stroke, and the prognosis was poor. In one set of reports, any coronary artery lesion was 40%, with a 1-year survival rate of 63%, and one with congestive heart failure, with a survival rate of only 23%.

In the field of treatment, classic transcatheter intervention and surgical coronary artery bypass surgery are rarely used in patients with heart transplant vascular disease, because vascular lesions are too dispersed and at the end of the heart. An analysis of data on coronary artery interventional therapy in US cardiac transplant recipients showed that transcatheter intervention was safe and successful; however, during follow-up, lesions continued to develop and lead to corresponding consequences. Therefore, the authors emphasize that these interventions have only short-term palliative effects. Some scholars also conducted coronary artery bypass grafting, and the results showed that coronary artery bypass grafting was effective in the treatment of coronary artery occlusion in cardiac transplantation, but the mortality rate was higher.

3.3.3 Renal Insufficiency

Long-term chronic heart failure before cardiac transplantation is associated with decreased renal output and decreased renal reserve function. The blow of extracorporeal circulation during the surgery, the low cardiac output after operation, and the damage of CsA to the kidney are all the causes of renal dysfunction after transplantation. Especially in ABO incompatible heart transplantation, anti-blood group antibody immune complexes are easily accumulated in kidney tissues, leading to kidney injury. CsA has a great toxic effect on the kidney, and the nephrotoxicity of FK506 is theoretically smaller than that of CsA, but its nephrotoxicity is not small in actual use. Therefore, some scholars have adjusted and modified the rejection program and cancelled the use of CsA or FK506 1 day before and after the operation. Induced by monoclonal antibodies and added with methylprednisolone, 2 days after surgery, CsA (or FK506) plus MMF plus corticosteroid triple immunosuppressant was initiated. With this adjusted procedure, most of the transplant patients did not develop early postoperative renal failure. For patients with renal failure, hemodialysis filtration replacement therapy should be applied as soon as possible.

4 Clinical efficacy and experience

Heart transplantation has been the standard treatment for end-stage heart failure. In January 1996, the first pediatric ABO-incompatible heart transplant was performed at a hospital in Toronto, Canada, for 25 days in children with hypoplastic left ventricular syndrome. It is reported that the transplant is successful, and there is no postoperative complications or need to undergo a heart transplant [13–17]. It is reported that by 1996, the mortality rate of children waiting for heart transplantation in Toronto was 58%. This high mortality rate is largely due to donor heart size and blood group compatibility limitations [18]. Since the ABO-incompatible organ transplant has developed, the mortality rate for patients waiting for heart transplants has dropped from 10% to 7% [14–17].

However, the comparison between the efficacy of ABO-incompatible cardiac transplantation and ABO-compatible cardiac transplantation remains the focus of most scholars; next, we analyze and discuss the clinical results and related statistical data reported by foreign scholars.

The overall survival rate of 4 years after pediatric heart transplantation was 70% and dropped to 55% after 10 years [18]. Less than 1-year-old infants in children after heart transplantation is the highest risk receptor in transplantation group; their 30-day mortality rate was 40%; however, as long as these patients can survive in the first year after surgery, their 4-year survival rate will be 90% [14]. Patel reported that the mortality rate of children with ABO-incompatible heart transplantation 30 days and 1 year after operation was 5.9% and 14.7%, respectively; the blood compatibility was 8.8% and 16.6%, respectively. Between 1999 and 2007, the 3-year survival rate for ABO-incompatible and ABO-compatible heart transplants was close to 70% [18], Kaplan-Meier said. It can be seen that ABO-incompatible cardiac transplantation and blood compatibility cardiac transplantation in children have little difference in postoperative mortality and survival rate, and even the former is better than the latter.

West et al. compared the rejection between ABO-incompatible and ABO-compatible heart transplantation, but none of the two patients experienced hyperacute rejection. In the ABO-incompatible group, an acute cellular rejection occurred in six patients within 6 months after the operation. The response time was short, and after a large dose of glucocorticoid shock treatment, the effect was better; yet in the ABO blood compatibility group, seven patients experienced acute cellular rejection many times. Each patient experienced one or more rejection reactions within 6 months after operation and became more frequent 6 months after the operation. From the data above, we can conclude that the incidence of postoperative rejection in ABO patients is higher than that in patients with incompatible blood type. The difference in the incidence of this rejection may be due to a different immunosuppressive regimen. For example, patients who are incompatible with the ABO blood group usually undergo rigorous tacrolimus and mycophenolate mofetil combined with immunosuppressive therapy [15].

During the 1999~2006 period, 35 pediatric ABO-incompatible heart transplants were performed in the United States, accounting for 6% of the total pediatric heart transplant [17]. However, since the ABO-incompatible heart transplant was carried out in Toronto, the local child mortality rate has been below 15% for 1999–2006 years. In addition, Irving et al. compared patients' waiting time of ABO-incompatible and ABO-compatible heart transplant; they found that the waiting time for ABO-incompatible heart transplants was less than 2 weeks longer than for ABO-compatible heart transplants.

There is still a lot of debate about the maximum age limit for ABO-incompatible cardiac transplant recipients. The United States Organ Resource Sharing Center (UNOS) stipulates that the recipient is less than 2 years old and the antibody titer is less than 1:4 [13]. The maximum age of recipients of ABO-incompatible heart transplantation in Britain is 40 months, and the antibody titer is less than 1:16 [13]. Some British scholars even reported that ABO-incompatible heart transplantation with 9-year-old recipient, 1:16 anti-B antibody and 5-yearold recipient and 1:126 anti-A antibody was carried out [16]. Among them, 5-year-old receptor before transplantation, its anti-A antibody titer reached 1:0, and 9 years old appeared antibody-mediated rejection after the recipient but after strengthening treatment recovered well, and there was no long-term complications [16]. Therefore, the age limit and antibody titer of ABO-incompatible cardiac transplantation are still at the exploratory stage.

In conclusion, the use of incompatible ABO heart transplants has broken the traditional logic of heart transplant. The ABO-incompatible heart transplant will be more feasible through multidisciplinary development and technological advances. There was no significant difference in recipient survival or rejection between ABO-incompatible and ABO-compatible cardiac allograft recipients [19]; at the same time, the use of incompatible ABO heart transplants shortened the recipient's waiting time and helped reduce mortality in such recipients [17].

References

1. Olivier AF, Copeland JG. Real-time sonography in central venous access for endomyocardial biopsy in cardiac transplantation patients. J Am Coll Surg. 2007;205:13–8.
2. Kass M, Haddad H. Cardiac allograft vasculopathy: pathology, prevention and treatment. Curr Opin Cardiol. 2006;21:132–7.
3. Marciniak A, Eroglu E, Marciniak M, et al. The potential clinical role of ultrasonic strain and strain rate imaging in diagnosing acute rejection after heart transplantation. Eur J Echocardiogr. 2007;8:213–21.
4. Tona F, Caforio AL, Piaserico S, et al. Abnormal total ejection isovolume index as early non-invasive marker of chronic rejection in heart transplantation. Transpl Int. 2005;18:303–8.
5. Crespo-Leiro MG, Veiga-Barreiro A, Dompenech N, et al. Humoral heart rejection (severe allograft dysfunction with no signs of cellular rejection or ischemia) : incidence, management, and the value of C4d for diagnosis. Am J Transplant. 2005;5:2560–4.
6. Uehara S, Chase CM, Cornell LD, et al. Chronic cardiac transplant arteriopathy in mice: relationship of alloantibody, C 4d deposition and neointimal fibrosis. Am J Transplant. 2007;7:57–65.
7. Lopin EJ, Zhang Q, Zhang X, et al. Phosphorylated S6 ribosomal Protein a novel biomarker of antibody-mediated rejection in heart allografts. Am J Transplant. 2006;6:1560–71.
8. Deng MC, Eisen HJ, Mehra MR, et al. Noninvasive discrimination of rejection in cardiac allograft recipients using gene expression profiling. Am J Transplant. 2006;6:150–60.
9. Sawitzki B, Bushell A, Steger U, et al. Identification of gene markers for the prediction of allograft rejection or permanent acceptance. Am J Transplant. 2007;7:1091–102.
10. Di Filippo S, Zeevi A, McDade KK, et al. Impact of TGF beta1 gene polymorphisms on acute and chronic rejection in pediatric heart transplant allografts. Transplantation. 2006;81:934–9.
11. Valli PV, Puga Yung G, Fehr T, et al. Changes of circulating antibody levels induced by ABO antibody adsorption for ABO-incompatible kidney transplantation. Am J Transplant. 2009;9(5):1072–80.
12. Toki D, Ishida H, Setoguchi K, et al. Acute antibody-mediated rejection in living ABO-incompatible kidney transplantation: long-term impact and risk factors. Am J Transplant. 2009;9(3):567–77.
13. Roche SL, Burch M, O'Sullivan J, et al. Multicenter experience of ABO-incompatible pediatric cardiac transplantation. Am J Transplant. 2008;8:208–15.
14. Foreman C, Gruenwald C, West L. ABO-incompatible heart transplantation: a perfusion strategy. Perfusion. 2004;19:69–72.
15. West LJ, Pollock-Barziv SM, Dipchand AI, et al. ABO-incompatible heart transplantation in infants. N Engl J Med. 2001;344:793–800.

16. Irving C, Gennery A, Kirk R. Pushing the boundaries: the current status of ABO-incompatible cardiac transplantation. J Heart Lung Transplant. 2012;31:791–6.
17. Dipchand AI, Pollock BarZiv SM, Manlhoit C, et al. Equivalent outcomes for pediatric heart transplantation recipients: ABO-blood group incompatible versus ABO-compatible. Am J Transplant. 2010;10:389–97.
18. Hageman M, Michaud N, Chinnappan I, et al. ABO-incompatible heart transplants. Perfusion. 2015;30(3):209–12.
19. Patel ND, Weiss ES, Scheel J, et al. ABO-incompatible heart transplantation in infants: analysis of the United Network for Organ Sharing Database. J Heart Lung Transplant. 2008;27:1085–9.

Experience with ABO-Incompatible Liver Transplantation

11

Lin Wei

Abstract

Though the possibility of super acute and acute rejection of ABO-imcompitable organ transplantation in liver is smaller than in kidney due to no blood group antigen expression on hepatocellular surface, but as a result of bile duct epithelial cells express blood group antigen, caused by the bile duct damage is relatively serious, therefore, the authors suggest that conventional plasma desensitization treatment must be done before ABOi-liver transplant. In this chapter, the indications, plasma desensitization scheme, and postoperative management of ABOi-liver are described.

Keywords

ABOi-liver transplantation · Transplantation indications · Plasma desensitization scheme · Postoperative management

Liver transplantation has been one of the most effective therapeutic methods for the treatment of end-stage liver diseases. With increasing number of hepatopaths who are waiting for liver transplantation, the shortage of organ donantion has become the challenge for medical workers. Although living donor liver transplantation has relieved this discrepancy a little, but ABO incompatibility between the donor and the recipient has always encountered. In the early stage, due to the immaturity of surgical technique and the limitation of immunosuppresive agents, ABO-incompatible liver transplantation performed only in special conditions and the recipient always died of fatal antibody mediate rejection. Therefore, ABO

L. Wei (✉)
Beijing Friendship Hospital, Capital Medical University, Beijing, China

Y. Wang (ed.), *ABO-incompatible Organ Transplantation*,
https://doi.org/10.1007/978-981-13-3399-6_11

incompatibility was a contraindication for liver transplantation in that time. With the development and improvement of ABO-incompatible kidney transplantation, ABO-incompatible liver transplantation has been developed greatly, which provides more selections for recipient of liver transplant.

1 Donor and recipient Selection and Therapeutic Scheme

Liver transplantation is one of the most efficient methods for the treatment of end-stage liver diseases. However, due to the shortage of donors, many hepatopaths have died during the waiting time therefore ABO-incompatible liver transplant is considered, which will greatly relieve organ shortage. But in order to continuously improve the survival rate of ABO blood group incompatible liver grafts or recipients, it will be very important to carefully prepare patients for the perioperative period and make reasonable selection of patients as well as adequate treatment.

1.1 Selection of Recipient

1.1.1 Blood Types

1. ABO blood type

   Human's ABO antigen not only exists on the surface of red blood cells but also on the surface of vascular endothelial cells, biliary epithelial cells, and liver sinusoidal endothelial cells of transplanted livers. According to the ABO blood group coordination of donor and recipient, it can be divided into three types: ABO blood group identical, ABO blood group compatible and ABO blood group incompatible. Therefore, after liver transplantation with ABO blood group incompatibility, antibody mediate rejection is likely to occur, which attack the above target cells and cause complications such as biliary tract, blood vessels and liver necrosis, resulting in significantly lower graft survival rate than those with blood group compatibility. Sanchez-Urdazpal et al. reported that in 18 cases of ABO-incompatible liver transplantation, the incidence rate of biliary tract complications was 82% (6% in the group with the compatible blood type), that of hepatic artery thrombosis was 24%, and that of cellular rejection was 65% (28% in the group with the compatible blood type). In addition, compared with that of 78% in the group with compatible blood type, 1 year survival rate in the group with incompatible blood type was only 44%. However, the liver, as a privileged organ of immunity, has a good tolerance to antibody-mediated injury and rarely produces hyperacute rejection. Although survival rates are lower than in cases of blood group compatibility, liver transplantation with ABO incompatibility in emergency situations is acceptable. Multiple center studies have found that the donor blood type A, especially the A2 subtype, and the recipient blood type O have A high survival rate in the selection of donor and recipient [1]. The donor of A2 blood subtype only expresses a few A-antigens; thus it has better effect to the receptor with O blood type. The antibody titer in pediatric receptors (less than 2 years old) is quite low; the prognosis is better.

2. Rh blood type
   Studies have shown that liver and biliary tract complications of recipients with different Rh blood types are higher than those with the same Rh, especially those with Rh (+) given to Rh (−) [2].

1.1.2 Transplantation Indications

1. Liver parenchyma diseases caused by nonpathogenic microorganisms
   It includes alcoholic liver cirrhosis, ACLF induced by drugs and chemical poisons, congenital hepatic fibrosis, liver cystic fibrosis, huge liver cyst, Budd-Chiari syndrome, Severe refractory trauma, autoimmune hepatitis, and so on.
2. Hepatic failure and portal hypertension caused by hepatitis and liver cirrhosis induced by various pathogenic microorganisms
   It includes acute and chronic severe hepatitis, cirrhosis caused by hepatitis B virus and hepatitis C virus, schistosomiasis, liver hydatid disease, etc.
3. Congenital metabolic disorder
   It includes Wilson's disease, glycogen accumulation, hyperaminemia, anti-trypsin deficiency, familial non-hemolytic jaundice, tyrosinemia, etc. This kind of disease, due to the abnormal metabolism of certain substances in patients, can lead to the early death of children or abnormal development, is a common indication of pediatric liver transplantation.
4. Cholestatic liver diseases
   It includes biliary atresia, primary biliary cirrhosis (PBC), primary sclerosing cholangitis (PSC), secondary biliary cirrhosis, calroie's disease, progressive familial intrahepatic cholestasis disease (Byler disease) and so on, this kind of disease, patients with cholestasis as the main clinical manifestations, and most of these patients bilirubin are tall, but normal liver function can keep for a long time. Among them, PBC and PSC are at risk of recurrence after transplantation.
5. Liver tumors
   Liver malignancy without extrahepatic metastasis or invasion of large blood vessels can also be used as an indication of liver transplantation. In 2000, when the world transplantation conference was held in milan, Italy, the conference recommended that liver transplantation of hepatocellular carcinoma should be carried out according to the milan standard, that is, the diameter of single tumor should not exceed 5cm, the diameter of multiple tumors should not exceed 3cm, and the maximum size should not exceed 3cm, without major vascular invasion. According to this standard, the 5-year tumor-free survival rate of liver transplantation for hepatocellular carcinoma can reach 80%, which is significantly better than the traditional treatment methods.

1.2 Therapeutic Scheme

There is no difference in the technique between ABO incompatible liver transplantation and ABO compatible liver transplantation. The key is to timely and effectively prevent and treat the pre-stored antibodies and possible complications during the perioperative period. If there are no complications during the perioperative period, the long-term curative effect will not be affected. ABO incompatible liver transplantation can be treated in perioperative period according to its characteristics and possible complications.

1.2.1 Perioperative management

Plasma exchange and plasma immunoadsorption: Preoperative plasma exchange or immunosorption for the removal of anti-blood type antibodies has been successfully applied in kidney transplantation patients, so that ABO incompatible kidney transplantation patients can survive for a long time after surgery. Immunosorption in ABO incompatible liver transplantation is also applicable [3]. Studies have shown that same volume total plasmapheresis can remove 67% of immunoglobulin and double volume total plasmapheresis can remove 90% of antibodies. In general, type AB fresh frozen plasma (FFP) should be used for plasmapheresis. The duration and frequency of total plasmapheresis vary from person to person, mainly based on changes in antibody levels and individual responses to plasmapheresis. It is generally believed that maintaining serum antibody titers less than or equal to l: 8 within 2 weeks after liver transplantation can effectively reduce the occurrence of antibody-mediated rejection, and antibody titers greater than or equal to 1:16 can increase the risk of ABO-incompatible antibody-mediated rejection after liver transplantation. Hanto et al. reported that 3 of the 14 patients underwent multiple total plasma exchange within 2 weeks after surgery, but the titer was still high, but no antibody-mediated rejection occurred [4], which was explained as follows: plasma exchange removed most antibodies and complement components; Second, the liver itself seems to be able to tolerate environments with high titer antibodies. After 2 weeks, antibody mediated rejection rarely occurs even if there is a high level of antibody titer. This immune phenomenon is called "adaptive regulation", which refers to the ability of allograft to survive in the environment of antibodies and complements against the donor. This is related to the function of endothelial cells, the target cells of antibody mediated rejection. Endothelial cells can up-regulate the expression of certain protective genes, including the genes encoding heme oxygenase, A20, bcl-2, bcl-x, etc., and block the pre-inflammatory response related to endothelial cells, thereby inhibiting the occurrence of rejection.

1.2.2 Intraoperative Treatment

1. Selection of donors

   To ensure the quality of donor liver, the warm ischemia time should be within 5 min, and the cold ischemia time should be within 8 h. The recognized high-risk factors which affect the quality of donor liver include hypotension time, CPR history, fatty liver, applied time and dose of terlipressin, primary diseases of patients, and whether DCD or hypernatremia.

2. Splenectomy
   Splenectomy can reduce the production of relevant antibodies, thereby reducing the antibody mediated rejection reaction and improving the survival rate of patients and grafts. However, splenectomy will cause injury to the body. If the operation time is prolonged and intraoperative bleeding occurs, postoperative complications are more likely to occur. The greatest risk of splenectomy in transplant patients is an increased incidence of infection, associated with thrombocytopenia and hypercoagulation, and increased risk of portal thrombosis. Splenectomy as a standard treatment has played a positive role in the early stage of cross blood type transplantation, but with the widespread use of rituximab, splenectomy has not been recommended as a treatment to prevent rejection associated with blood type incompatibility.
3. Portal perfusion and hepatic artery perfusion
   Prostaglandin E, gaberidate or hormone can improve microcirculation by dilating blood vessels, inhibiting platelet and leukocyte adhesion. Gabeate is a serine protease inhibitor, which mainly inhibits thrombin, thrombin Xa and platelet aggregation. Studies have shown that this method can increase the 2-year survival rate of liver transplantation with blood type incompatibility to 70% [5]. Tallabe et al. reported that in addition to conventional immunosuppressive agents, methylprednisolone, prostaglandin El and gabelate mesylate were injected through portal vein catheterization, and 2 patients survived for 30 months and 12 months respectively, without rejection and vascular complications, and had good liver function. Although continuous perfusion of blood vessels has reduced the occurrence of rejection due to blood type incompatibility to a certain extent, it has not been widely accepted and popularized due to its difficulties in perioperative monitoring and maintenance.
4. Specific white blood cells isolated from donor whole blood were injected through portal vein
   Sato et al. reported that in the treatment of acute severe hepatitis with liver transplantation due to blood type incompatibility, specific white blood cells isolated from the whole blood of the donor were injected through the patient's portal vein, and the recipient was cured and discharged after surgery without humoral or cellular rejection. Immunological analysis showed that 54.6% of the large chimera in the liver one month after surgery were donor CD56 +T cells, and il-1 and Th2 cytokines were increased one day after surgery. Say, blood type is not the adult liver transplantation can be via the portal vein infusion of donor specific whole blood separation of white blood cells that new immunosuppressive scheme to improve the survival rate receptors, and has a lower risk of AMR, for the size of CD56 + NKT cells (natural killer T cells) system or individual genotype inducing immune tolerance, liver transplantation can be through the strategy of blood type is improved.

1.2.3 Immunosuppression

The addition of il-2 receptor monoclonal antibodies or OKT3 on the basis of conventional triple immunosuppressant (FK506 / cyclophenolate A, mycophenolate, hormone) can effectively inhibit the antibody-mediated rejection after ABO incompatible liver transplantation. CD20 monoclonal antibody plays a very important role in the development of organ transplantation with blood type incompatibility. For planned liver transplantation, the application of rituximab in advance can effectively reduce the production of new anti-blood type antibodies after surgery, basically replacing the treatment method of splenectomy. The application of rituximab not only simplifies the treatment of organ transplantation with blood type incompatibility, but also significantly improves the prognosis of patients. In recent years, it has been repeatedly reported that the simplified pretreatment regimen with rituximab and plasma exchange as the main pretreatment methods has achieved satisfactory results in the clinical observation of liver transplantation with blood type incompatibility. Morioka et al. treated antibody-mediated rejection with globulin (IVIG) and plasma exchange, and the results were satisfactory. The 2 patients survived for 6 months and 35 months respectively.

1.2.4 Anhepatic Phase and Its Treatment

Without liver stage, multiple cytokines can be increased, especially il-6, which leads to injury of transplanted liver cells. In addition, metabolic product accumulation and hemodynamic disorder caused by metabolic disorder in the absence of liver can all have a significant impact on the function of the transplanted liver. In the nonhepatic stage, due to the decrease of hemodynamics, there is obvious deficiency of effective circulating blood volume, obvious congestion of gastrointestinal tract, kidney and lower limbs, decreased average arterial pressure, and accelerated heart rate. At this time, patients are prone to shock if not properly treated. The disorder of hemodynamics in the non-hepatic stage will lead to a series of pathophysiological changes, such as metabolic acidosis caused by the massive accumulation of lactic acid, water and electrolyte imbalance caused by gastrointestinal congestion disorder.

1.2.5 Postoperative Management

1. Improve oxygen supply

   Postoperative comprehensive measures such as mechanical ventilation, oxygen absorption, timely drainage of pleural effusion, control of fluid volume, diuresis and prevention of pulmonary infection can be adopted to improve pulmonary function, and oxygen saturation can be maintained at > 95% to ensure oxygen supply to liver cells and bile duct epithelial cells.

2. Postoperative anticoagulant therapy

   In order to avoid microcirculation thrombosis after operation, moderate fluid infusion and anticoagulation therapy can be given. Heparin has a short half-life and can be antagonistic to protamine. Prostaglandin E1 also improves microcirculation. Postoperative non-bloody fluid in the abdominal drainage tube should be given 500ml/d of low-molecular-dextran, and aspirin and low-molecular-weight heparin should be added for anticoagulation treatment after the recovery of coagulation function of the patient, so as to prevent the formation of microthrombi.

3. Anti-infection
   Since the high dose of quadruple anti-rejection treatment after surgery increases the chance of infection, especially for patients with severe liver diseases, in addition to strengthening the anti-bacterial infection treatment, preventive anti-fungal and antiviral treatment should also be given. Closely monitor the clinical test of pathogen microorganism infection and timely adjust the anti-infection program according to the results of pathogen test.
4. Ancillary measures
   Early removal of catheters and reduction of invasive procedures. In addition, increase nutrition to improve systemic condition also nots allow to ignore, still should enable gastrointestinal tract as early as possible and the exercise that strengthens the function such as respiratory tract.

1.2.6 Rituximab

Rituximab is a mouse chimeric anti-CD20 antibody that uses rituximab in the early prophylactic removal of B cells, including memory B lymphocytes, to reduce the incidence of antibody-mediated rejection and replace intraoperative splenectomy. Rituximab is primarily based on the experience of kidney transplantation with blood type incompatibility.Kawagishi, such as 2000 years ago in children in liver transplantation, blood type without the use of rituxan can still achieve very good effect, until January 2000 cases fatal humoral rejection that they changed the point of view, they began to use rituxan, and successfully treated other medication invalid rejection in 1 case.Intravenous infusion of thymus globulin can reduce anti-abo blood group IgG and IgM titers [6], and combined intravenous infusion of immunoglobulin for 2 weeks can avoid agglutinin titer rebound [7, 8]. In addition, the occurrence of acute rejection (AMR) can be reduced by specific white blood cells isolated from the whole blood of the donor via portal vein infusion [9].Plasma exchange combined with high-dose immunoglobulin and in vitro photodynamic effects can also reduce the occurrence of AMR [10].Although there are many postoperative complications in liver transplantation patients with ABO blood group incompatibility, targeted preventive treatment during the perioperative period can reduce the occurrence of complications and effectively improve the efficacy of liver transplantation with ABO blood group incompatibility.

1.2.7 Intravenous Infusion with Immunoglobulin and ATG

Testa et al. believed that plasma removal and intravenous infusion of immune globular eggs (150mg/kg) were accepted for all receptors before surgery, and antithymoglobulin 1 ~ 5mg/kg during transplantation could reduce anti-ABO blood group IgG and IgM titers. Urbani and Ikegami et al. believed that humoral rejection was mainly reflected by the rebound of the same lectin titer. In order to prevent humoral rejection, immunoglobulin was used for 2 weeks. The dosage is 1.0 ~ 1.5g/(kg·d).

2 Diagnosis and Treatment of Postoperative Complications

2.1 Detection of Rejection

ABO blood group incompatible rejection after organ transplantation, including acute rejection in the early stage and chronic rejection in the later stage, will seriously affect the function and long-term survival of the graft, and is still one of the thorny problems in the field of transplantation. Simply increase the dosage of immunosuppressant to prevent or reduce the occurrence of rejection reaction, not only the effect is not good, but also increase the possibility of liver and kidney function damage due to high drug concentration , at the same time excessive immunosuppression leads to infection and malignant tumors and other toxic side effects.

Therefore, objective and accurate monitoring of the changes in the immune function of patients after transplantation, early detection and intervention of rejection reaction are the prerequisites to prevent graft function damage. Currently, the plasma drug concentration detection of immunosuppressive agents commonly used in clinical practice only reflects the absorption and metabolism of immunosuppressive agents in vivo, which can only be speculated indirectly and cannot truly reflect the immunosuppressive status of patients after transplantation.

2.1.1 Triphosadenine Activity Determination

The determination of adenosine triphosphate activity in CD4 T lymphocytes by Cylex ImmuKnow assay reflects the level of immune cell function, which can more accurately assess the immune status of patients and has a higher reference value for cell-mediated rejection.Rejection after organ transplantation is often accompanied by increased adenosine triphosphate in CD4 T lymphocytes. However, patients with high adenosine triphosphate after transplantation have strong immune cell activity and are prone to cellular rejection. One study showed that adenosine triphosphate values in CD4 T lymphocytes were different between the rejection group and the non-rejection group. Further analysis showed that the incidence of rejection was different under different immune response states, and the rejection was more likely to occur in the high immune response group.

Meanwhile, it has been found that the dynamic change of ATP value of $CD4^+$ T cell during the perioperative period after liver transplantation is related to the acute rejection of liver transplantation. The ATP value of the patients with acute rejection after the liver transplantation reached the peak in the first week, higher than non-rejection patients, which will drop down after patients receiving the corticosteroid impulse therapy for the revision of rejection. Foreign researchers believe that among kidney transplant patients, the incidence of postoperative rejection in patients with preoperative adenosine triphosphate level of >375mg/ml is 3.67 times higher than that in patients with <375mg/ml. Studies have also shown that adenosine triphosphate is prone to rejection when it is greater than 525mg/ml, infection when it is less than 225mg/ml, and immune stability between 225 and 525mg/ml.

2.1.2 Th1/Th2

The incidence of acute rejection after liver transplantation ranges from 20% to 40%, often within 1 month after surgery, and Th cells play an important role. Currently, it is believed that Th1 cells are important effector cells mediating graft rejection, and IL-2 secreted by Th1 cells is an important cytokine in acute rejection. Wang et al. found that the level of IL-2 in peripheral blood increased when acute rejection (AR) occurred after transplantation, while Gibelli et al. used the IL-2 receptor blocker baliximab to effectively reduce the incidence of postoperative acute rejection.

Unlike Th1, which is involved in acute rejection, Th2 is believed to be related to chronic rejection and immune tolerance. Th2 cells down-regulate the rejection driven by Th1 cells and promote the immune tolerance of transplantation.

Studies have shown that Th1/Th2 in patients with rejection is significantly higher than that in patients without rejection, suggesting that the function of Th1 cells is enhanced, leading to immune rejection in the body. At the same time, the increase of Th1/Th2 has occurred before the occurrence of clinical rejection. However, after the application of immunosuppressive shock therapy, the activity of Th1 cells is inhibited, resulting in the decrease of Th1/ Th2 and the control of immune rejection. Therefore, it is believed that the change of Th1/ Th2 is closely related to the occurrence of acute rejection after liver transplantation. At the same time, changes in Th1/ Th2 can more sensitively reflect the immune status of the body.

Th1/Th2 in peripheral blood reaches the highest level after liver transplantation, which is consistent with pathological examination results of liver puncture, so it has a good predictability. It can be effectively used to monitor the immune status after liver transplantation and guide the dosage of immunosuppressant.

2.1.3 Bile and Biochemical Monitoring

It has been reported abroad that the blood antibody titer is related to the incidence of postoperative rejection, and almost all ABO incompatible liver transplantation rejection is effective for hormone shock therapy, Therefore, hemagglutinin titer was not monitored, but changes in liver function and color and volume of postoperative t-tube bile drainage were closely monitored. Once transaminase and bilirubin rapidly increased in clinical consideration of rejection, liver biopsy and timely treatment were performed.

2.1.4 Monitoring of Kidney Function

The increase of serum creatinine is related to the classic non-shunt operation and intraoperative vena cava occlusion. In addition, the renal dysfunction caused by the deposition of antigen-antibody complex in the glomeruli cannot be excluded, and the specific mechanism needs to be further studied. Therefore, postoperative renal function monitoring and application should be avoided.

2.1.5 Color Doppler Ultrasound Monitoring

1. Rejection After Liver Transplantation: Dynamical observation of hepatic arterial resistance index and blood flow velocity change of portal is of great significance to confirm the rejection of liver transplantation after transplantation. Normally,

the earlier hepatic arterial resistance index after the liver transplantation is on the rise (about 0.7), which will be close to normal after 1–2 weeks. If the high resistance (above 0.8) stay still, the vascular color is in poor filling or the frequency spectrum of hepatic artery blood flow cannot be detected, it may be considered as the rejection after the liver transplantation; the earlier portal blood flow after the liver transplantation appears compensatory acceleration, and the color fill of blood vessel is displayed with multicolor mosaic blood flow. As the hepatic artery blood supply returns to normal, the portal venous blood flow rate should be reduced to normal. Rejection should be considered if the portal vein continues to experience high blood flow; meanwhile, the waveform of venous blood becomes blunt or shows one-direction wave. Its formation mechanism lies in the cellular edema and liver enlargement due to cellular infiltration in portal area. At the same time, the increase of strain in the liver but being limited by Glisson's capsule brings about the compliance decrease of the liver which gives rise to the pulsatory reduction of hepatic vein and blunt frequency spectrum.

2. Changes of Bile Duct After Liver Transplantation: The inner diameter of bile duct mainly ranges from 0.4 to 0.6 cm. Some patients show unclear images of bile duct, which is related to the surgery, but they will recover gradually after 1–2 weeks. The possibility of rejection or HAT should be taken into consideration once the bile duct fail to recover together with jaundice and persistent fever occur or increased jaundice index (which is shown by laboratory exam).

2.1.6 Histopathology the Earlier Period of Transplantation and the Later Rejection

ABO antigens not only exist on the surface of erythrocyte but also on the surface of vascular endothelium, bile duct epithelium and hepatic sinus endothelial cells of the transplanted liver, and can exist until about 150 days after transplantation. Therefore, ABO blood group incompatible liver transplantation is prone to antibody mediated immune response, which attacks the above target cell causing complications, such as the biliary tract, blood vessel, and hepatic necrosis, thus resulting in the lower survival rate of transplanted organs than compatible blood type cases. When incompatible blood type liver is implanted into patients, whose natural A and B antibody in the body directly combining with antigen on the vascular endothelial cell of the transplanted organs to produce the antigenantibody complex ,which will induce a series of complement reactions that activate complement system and rapidly damage vasoganglion in the transplanted organ, resulting in wide range of thrombus that will disable the transplanted organ. In addition, if the antibody titer of the anti-A and anti-B of the transplanted organs is too high, then the rejection damage of acute humoral immunity response will occur. The A and B antigen in the transplanted organs can also stimulate recipient, causing hemolytic anemia and thrombocytopenia.

1. Inflammatory Cell Infiltration in Portal Area: In portal area, the infiltration of the most of the lymphocytes, transformative macrolymphocytes, monocytes, neutrophilic granulocytes, and eosinophils gather around bile duct and blood vessels. When the rejection reaction is severe, the inflammatory cell will bring injury to

liver parenchyma around portal area and further give rise to expansion of portal area.
2. Biliary Epithelia Injury in Lobule of the Portal Area: The increase of nucleu/cytoplasm ratio for most of the biliary epithelial cell, overlapping and polymorphic nucleus, karyopyknosis, cytoplasm vacuolar degeneration, cell poloidal disorder, and other degenerative changes, resulting in lumen deformation. It presents bile duct inflammatory lesion: lymphocyte, monocyte, neutrophilic granulocyte, etc. invade bile duct epithelium which give rise to the incompleteness of the Lumen basement membrane. When the rejection is too severe and the lumen in bile duct is significantly damaged, the sporadic biliary epithelial cell can be seen in portal area with the application of CK-19 immunohistochemical staining.
3. Central phlebitis and/or interlobular phlebitiss of the portal area: In portal area, the lymphocytes, transformative macrolymphocytes, and monocytes are infiltrated under interlobular vein endothelia, thus giving rise to elevation of endothelial cells and inflammatory cell pavementing and blood vessel endothelium swelling in lumen. When the rejection is too severe, it presents the damage of local vascular wall, pipe wall discontinuity, and inflammatory cell infiltration in the damaged vascular. Few inflammatory cell infiltration with lymphocyte and monocyte is shown around the central vein, which presents slight congestion; when the rejection is too severe, there shows the loss and necrosis of hepatocyte around the central phlebitis.
4. Hepatic Cell and Bile Capillaries Cholestasis: Hepatic cell and bile capillaries get mild to moderate cholestasis being focally distributed. For few cases, bile thrombus is formed in bile capillaries. While the rejection is severe, hepatic cell is represented with feathery degeneration occasionally accompanied by focal cholestatic degeneration of hepatic cell.
5. Hydropic Degeneration and Ballooning Degeneration of Hepatic Cell: Hydropic degeneration and ballooning degeneration of hepatic cell featured as hepatic acinus appear small vacuous in the cytoplasm of hepatic cells in some cases.
6. Acidophilic Degeneration, Point Degeneration, and Focal Degeneration of Hepatic Cell: The sporadic acidophilic degeneration and acidophilic body in hepatic cell have formed (most of them are in vocal shape and seldom in anomalous shape); few of them get point degeneration and focal in hepatic cell. When the rejection is severe, hepatic acinus will be involved by the above lesions.

2.2 Special Complication and Its Solution

During the clinic exploration, the earlier reports believed that the incidence of acute rejection after ABO-incompatible liver transplantation, hepatic necrosis, and biliary and vascular complications is really high. Meanwhile, the transplanted organs show low survival rate. In recent years, due to the improvement of many therapies, including plasma exchange therapy, preoperative or postoperative immunotherapy, splenectomy, intravascular drug infusion, etc. whose clinical effect has been widely accepted, many scholars hold that their clinical effect is equivalent to blood type incompatibility liver transplantation. It can be learnt from the literatures that the occurrence of biliary tract and blood vessel complication will increase after ABO-incompatible liver transplantation. The reason lies in the recipient's antibody acts on the endothelial cells and biliary epithelial cell of the donor's antigen, causing the damage of the above structure. Immunoreaction attacks biliary endothelial cells causing the damage of inner membrane in biliary tract and then showing the clinical manifestation of obstruction of biliary tract that can be removed through placing intra- or extrahepatic drainage tube support. Rejection is also one of the postoperative complications.

2.2.1 Hepatic Artery-Related Complications

1. Hepatic artery thrombosis (HAT): Hepatic artery supplies intrahepatic bile duct branch with blood. Therefore, HAT is usually related to biliary complications. The risk factors of HAT include hepatic artery insufficiency (HAI) and vessel ligation compression which are relevant to atherosclerosis of coeliac trunk artery. And anastomotic biliary strictures (ABS) are one of other technological factors. Routinely ligating gastroduodenal artery (GDA) of the recipient can prevent the bypass flow of GDA from the transplant. Once HAT is confirmed, treatment such as thrombolysis and thrombectomy by ways of hepatic artery catheterization should be performed as early as possible. Pro re nata, thrombectomy surgery or re-transplantation could be carried out.

2. Hepatic artery stenosis (HAS): Hepatic artery stenosis refers to the reduction of blood vessel diameter that is over 50% in accordance with the indication of angiography. With early diagnosis made after transplantation, HAS can be restored successfully through the surgery. Hepatic artery stenosis can be successfully repaired by surgery. Once HAS is confirmed, intravascular balloon artery should be expanded, and stent should be placed in it to achieve the purpose of expanding hepatic artery. But the major complications of this method are arteriorrhexis or the formation of pseudoaneurysm.

2.2.2 Hyperacute Rejection

After donor liver with incompatible blood type is transplanted into the recipient, anti-A or anti-B agglutinin naturally occurring in the recipient can combine with specific antigen in transplanted intrahepatic vessels and at the surface of bile duct endothelial cells to form immune complex and further activate complement system, blood cells, and inflammatory cells so as to cause the damage of vascular endothelial cells and therewith turn into disseminated intravascular coagulation (DIC) in transplanted liver. And all of those will work together to cause the damage or necrosis of hepatic parenchymal cells and intrahepatic bile duct, to put it another way, antibody-mediated rejection (AMR). The clinical manifestations include: liver enzyme shows an evident rise, so does bilirubin; imaging indicates hepatonecrosis; cholangiography presents sclerosing changes of intrahepatic bile duct; immunohistochemical test indicates antibody and complement C4d [9, 10] deposit extensively in area vasculosa, among which the AMR of blood type can observe the rebound of blood group antibody; remedial plasmapheresis and immunoglobulin are conducive to the reversal of AMR.

2.2.3 Biliary Complications (BC)

Biliary complications (BC) are a common complication in liver transplantation, and according to the report of foreign scholars, the incidence rate of BC ranges from 15 to 50%. BC is related to many factors including ischemia, immunologic injury, preservation injury, infection, ABO-incompatibility, etc. ABO-incompatible liver transplantation will lead to the evident rise of the incidence rate of hepatic artery and biliary complications. Luis reported a group of cases about liver transplantation recipients who received the livers from donors with mismatched blood type. And according to his report, the incidence rate of BC was 41% [11]. Cholangiography via T-tube indicates biliary tract stenosis, biliary silt, recurrent infection of biliary tract, and hyperbilirubinemia. As to liver transplantation with incompatible blood type, controlling the occurrence of AMR in perioperative period is the key to avoid BC. In addition, other matters should be paid attention in order to reduce BC:

1. When the donor liver is being trimmed, biliary tract should be rinsed with organ preservation solutions, gallbladder should be cut off, and it's inappropriate to weed out too many adipose tissues around hepatic portal and bile duct so as to avoid the injury of the blood circulation in bile duct.
2. Reducing the cold ischemia time and warm ischemia time, especially the latter one. It's reported that over 5 min of warm ischemia will cause the evident shape change of biliary tract after the operation.
3. Ensuring that the hepatic artery is unobstructed and avoiding the constant ischemia of biliary tract after the operation.
4. Strengthening the postoperative management of biliary tract and preventing the infection of biliary tract and the prolapse of T tube.

2.2.4 Bone Disease

Bone disease is one of the long-term complications of orthotopic liver transplantation after the operation, which includes osteoporosis and ischemic necrosis. Osteoporosis refers to a systemic skeletal disease with the features of osteopenia and degradation in bone microstructure for a variety of causes, which can lead to an increased risk of skeletal fractures with the increasing fragility and decreasing strength of bone. Osteoporosis after liver transplantation mainly has something to do with preoperative osteopenia and postoperative rapid bone loss. And ischemic necrosis is commonly related to corticosteroid hormone treatment, and most cases are found in caput femoris. After conducting the ABO-incompatible liver transplantation, the risk of bone disease will increase for the dosage of hormone is increased and its duration is prolonged.

2.2.5 Infectious Complications

Infection is a vital reason for early death of recipients after ABO-incompatible liver transplantation. Due to the poor physical status of patients before the liver transplantation, the opportunities of various pathogen infections will increase for operation wound, low resistance after liver transplantation, and the immunosuppression state. Sometimes, it's easy to confuse infection with rejection reaction and surgical complications. Once infection is suspected to exist, it should be ascertained in time and given treatment. When infection is taken into consideration, immunosuppressant should be stopped to use selectively, and if necessary, immunopotentiator should be increased to use. As pulmonary infection becomes more serious, windpipe should be cut open timely, and bronchofiberscope can be used to aspirate sputum. Meanwhile, enteral nutrition should be ensured in early stage, and intestinal mucosal barrier should be protected to prevent the translocation of bacterial flora. A research indicates that it is conducive to reduce the incidence rate of pulmonary complications after transplantation by adopting inverse perfusion in venae cava inferior, controlling infusion quantities (<10 L) and reducing the infusion of blood products (<4 L) in the process of transplantation, and achieving the negative balance of liquid intake and output volume as early as possible after transplantation (≤ -300 mL). In view of that, the incidence rate of infectious complications can be effectively reduced through the following methods: attaching great importance to pulmonary diseases exiting before the liver transplantation, controlling the infection of ascitis well, improving the nutritional status, correct hypoproteinemia, reducing infusion quantities and the infusion of blood products in the process of transplantation, more aggressive tracheotomy indications, using bronchofiberscope to aspirate sputum, keeping the negative balance of liquid intake and output volume in the early stage of posttransplantation, choosing antibiotics in accordance with culture results, early posttransplant isolation enhancement, etc.

3 Clinical Experience

3.1 Experience Worthy of Learning from

Currently, in the context that the number of patients waiting for the liver transplantation mounts up constantly, and the shortage of donor liver has been a growing problem, it may take patients several weeks or even several months to wait for suitable donors. And as for patients with hepatic failure and hepatocellular carcinoma of middle-later stage, the prolongation of waiting time is likely to result in the further deterioration of the condition and thus opportunities losing. (Patients with hepatic failure may suffer from irreversible infection, hepatorenal syndrome, etc., and liver cancer patients may undergo tumor enlargement, distant metastasis, and so on.) In order to reduce the waiting time for donor liver and making such patients gain opportunities of transplantation as soon as possible and then achieve the possibility of long-term survival, literature in recent years has suggested that the graft survival rate of ABO-incompatible liver transplantation has been close to that of blood type compatible transplantation. Though properly ABO-incompatible liver transplantation has relevant complications, more approving clinical effect is able to be achieved with strict selection of recipients, appropriate management in perioperative period, and strict postoperative monitoring. On the basis of referencing treatment experience at home and abroad in recent years, and from the point of actual conditions of the test, appropriately enhancing the plasma concentration of Tacrolimus can control potential complications after the operation. The plasma concentration of Tacrolimus should be maintained at around 10 μg/L within 1 month after surgery, about 8 μg/L between 1 and 3 months, 7 μg/L or so between 3 and 6 months, and about 6 μg/L over 6 months after operation. For liver is an immunologically privileged organ with a low repellency, patients accepting ABO-compatible liver transplantation are generally given single Tacrolimus to resist rejection, whereas the recipients who accept blood type-incompatible liver transplantation have both the specific antibody of anti-donor HLA and ABO-incompatible antigen antibody in their bodies. Hence, after the operation, MMF and hormone can be applied to the antirejection therapy on the basis of taking Tacrolimus, which has achieved quite good clinical effect. It was reported by Sato that DST (donor-specific leukocyte) was injected into portal vein of liver transplantation recipient for immunosuppression, which got a commendable effect [12]. Donor natural killer T (NKT) cells may play a regulatory role, and DST can be guided to produce neutralizing antibody, can induce the immune tolerance of cells and body fluid, and can be taken as the hypurgia of ABO-incompatible organ transplantation. In China, the 1-year survival rate of liver transplantation recipients has risen from 40% in 1993 to 80% at present, which is more ideal for living donor liver transplantation (LDLT). At the same time, after the liver transplantation, the 3-year survival rate has risen to about 75%, 5-year survival rate has increased from 56.1 to 65.9%, but the specific circumstances should be decided in accordance with patients' condition. The 10-year survival rate of patients accepting liver transplantation has reached 57%, and the long-term quality of life in "posttransplantation era" can be greatly enhanced through intervening comprehensively and formulating individualized nursing scheme. Nowadays, the longest survival time of patients accepting liver transplantation has reached 30 years. And the constant improvement of medical technology is sure to bring a much longer survival time for those accepting organ transplantation. Informed consents from the patients for publication have been obtained.

4 Case Report

Case 1

A 10-month-old baby boy was found to have some clinical manifestations in half a month after his birth: Skin jaundice, stools were in pale color, etc. The local hospital had been unable to identify the cause of jaundice, so he was transferred to the superior hospital. With improving relevant examination, he underwent laparoscopic exploration under general anesthesia. As a result, the baby boy was diagnosed with biliary atresia (BA) definitely, so Kasai Procedure was performed on him. After the operation, the jaundice that appeared in the skin decreased gradually, the color of stools turned into yellow, and initial success had been made in biliary drainage. In the following 3 months after operation, the patient suffered from the jaundice that appeared in skin once again, and the condition aggravated progressively; the color of stools whitened again; his abdominal perimeter increased gradually; and indexes of liver function were in a constant deterioration. In view of that, liver transplantation was advised to perform.

Before the operation, ABO blood type match should be conducted on donor and recipient. The baby boy was type O blood, while both of his parents were type B blood. Due to the incompatibility of blood type, living donor liver transplantation (LDLT) with his parents as the donors had to be conducted just under the condition of ABO incompatibility. The baby less than 1 year old had an imperfect humoral immunity; the titer of ABO antibody was quite low as well. Anti-A antibody and anti-B antibody of recipient were detected for several times before the operation, and both the titer of anti-A and that of anti-B were lower than 1:8. In view of that, the conclusion that the recipient had not yet established anti-A antibody and anti-B antibody could be drew. Preoperative examinations indicated that the indicators of liver transplantation surgery were evident and no special contraindications appeared; thus the living donor liver transplantation with his mother providing left lateral lobe was implemented. Finally, both the donor and the recipient underwent the operation safely, and the donor recovered uneventfully and dishcarged from hospital a week later.

Case 2

An 8-month baby boy has received Kasai procedure 60 days after the birth for biliary atresia. After surgery, jaundice didn't subside obviously, accompanying by intermittent cholangitis. After conservative treatment, the baby gradually developed into cholestatic cirrhosis which obviously limited his growth and development. He sought further diagnosis and treatment in a transplant center. Assessment results showed that he had met the requirements of the liver transplantation indications, and the MELD score was 23. The preoperative ABO blood type examination showed that the recipient was O, while his mother was B. Since there was no other suitable donor, relevant tests were given for further assessment. The results showed that his anti-blood antibodies were IgM 1:8 and IgG 1:16. Considering the lower anti-blood antibody and younger age (less than 1 year old), the preoperative preparation was done gradully. Without special intervention, the left lateral lobe in living-related liver transplantation surgery was performed successfully, and routine FK506 combined with hormone antirejection treatment were given after the surgery, monitoring the changes of his liver function and anti-blood antibody titer which indicated that his liver function recovered well. The IgM titer decreased to 1:2 on the third day, and IgG titer decreased to 1:8 on the seventh day. After that, intermittent monitoring was performed to the third week after surgery. The anti-blood antibodies were maintained at IgM 1:2 and IgG 1:8, and all indexes of liver function were maintained at normal level. Up to now, it was over 2 years since the patient had undergone surgery, and the liver was functioning normally. The patient recovered well and was followed up for more than 2 years. The results showed that the liver function was stable and normal which was similar to the results of several other cases of children under the age of 1 year in our center. It was also consistent with the foreign clinical results of incompatible blood type liver transplantation in children. Statistical results of current large samples showed that the long-term graft survival rate and patient's survival rate of incompatible blood type liver transplantation have no difference with compatible blood type liver transplantation for children under the age of 1, and no special perioperative management was required.

Case 3

A 57-year-old man was admitted to hospital for hepatitis B cirrhosis and hepatocellular carcinoma. The assessment results showed that the patient, in addition to the end-stage liver cirrhosis, still had a hepatocellular carcinoma (within Hangzhou criteria), but the tumor location was near the right hepatic veins, although treatment was given, the waiting time should not be too long. Since the blood type of the patient was O, there was still no suitable livers after 1 month of waiting, and his anti-B antibodies were IgM 1:32 and IgG 1:128. After obtaining the consent of the patient and his family, cross-blood transplant surgery of type B donor was given to the patient. He was given a single-dose of 375 mg/m^2 rituximab on the day of surgery and an injection of 600 mg/kg gamma immunoglobulin before the reperfusion of transplanted liver in surgery. After the surgery, in addition to monitoring the changes of anti-blood antibodies and liver function, daily injection of 400 mg/kg gamma immunoglobulin was given to the patient for a week, combining with postoperative routine anticoagulation (Early heparin was changed to warfarin 1 week later) and prostaglandin E1 of microcirculation improvement (2 weeks). Immunosuppressants were routine FK506, mycophenolate mofetil (MMF), and hormone. After the surgery, the liver function of the patient recovered well. Anti-blood antibody monitoring showed that on the first day after surgery, IgM was 1:4, while IgG was 1:32, and on the seventh day after surgery, IgM was 1:4, while IgG was 1:16, followed by weekly monitoring to the third week when the anti-blood antibodies were maintained at IgM 1:4 and IgG 1:16. Up to now, it was 2 years since the patient had undergone surgery, and the liver was functioning normally. In terms of the incompatible blood type liver transplantation of adult recipient, the long-term graft survival rate was still lower than that in patients with the same blood type, and the specific pretreatment regimen and monitoring standard of centers at domestic and overseas are not the same. Our center's regimen which combined rituximab with gamma immunoglobulin had achieved initial satisfactory result in clinical practice, but further clinical studies and observations were needed to estimate the effect objectively. For liver transplantation itself, there were numerous factors affecting the recovery of patients. It was necessary to take a comprehensive consideration and judgment for the selection of donor and recipient, perioperative management, and numerous related factors in long-term follow-up monitoring to ensure the maximum benefit of patients in receiving incompatible blood type liver transplantation.

References

1. Skogsberg U, Breimer ME, Friman S, et al. Adult abo-incompatible liver transplantation, using a and b donors. Xenotransplantation. 2006;13:154–9.
2. Busquets J, Castellote J, Torras J, et al. Liver transplantation across rh blood group barriers increases the risk of biliary complications. J GastrointestSurg. 2007;11:458–63.

3. Hanto DW, Fecteau AH, Alonso MH, et al. Abo-incompatible liver transplantation with no immunological graft losses using total plasma exchange, splenectomy, and quadruple immunosuppression: Evidence for accommodation. Liver Transpl. 2003;9:22–30.
4. Usui M, Isaji S, Mizuno S, et al. Experiences and problems pre-operative anti-cd20 monoclonal antibody infusion therapy with splenectomy and plasma exchange for abo-incompatible living-donor liver transplantation. Clin Transplant. 2007;21:24–31.
5. Lee CF, Cheng CH, Wang YC, et al. Adult living donor liver transplantation across abo-incompatibility. Medicine (Baltimore). 2015;94:e1796.
6. Urbani L, Mazzoni A, De Simone P, et al. Treatment of antibody-mediated rejection with high-dose immunoglobulins in abo-incompatible liver transplant recipient. Transpl Int. 2007;20:467–70.
7. Ikegami T, Taketomi A, Soejima Y, et al. Successful abo incompatible living donor liver transplantation in a patient with high isoagglutinin titer using high-dose intravenous immunoglobulin. Transplant Proc. 2007;39:3491–4.
8. Urbani L, Mazzoni A, Bianco I, et al. The role of immunomodulation in abo-incompatible adult liver transplant recipients. J Clin Apher. 2008;23:55–62.
9. Egawa H, Ohdan H, Haga H, et al. Current status of liver transplantation across abo blood-type barrier. J Hepatobiliary Pancreat Surg. 2008;15:131–8.
10. Haga H, Egawa H, Shirase T, et al. Periportal edema and necrosis as diagnostic histological features of early humoral rejection in abo-incompatible liver transplantation. Liver Transpl. 2004;10:16–27.
11. Sanchez-Urdazpal L, Batts KP, Gores GJ, et al. Increased bile duct complications in liver transplantation across the abo barrier. Ann Surg. 1993;218:152–8.
12. Sato Y, Yamamoto S, Oya H, et al. Adult abo-incompatible liver transplantation by intraportal transfusion of donor-specific antigen: a case report. Transplant Proc. 2008;40:2811–4.

Experience with ABO-Incompatible Kidney Transplantation

12

Yi Wang, Hongtao Jiang, and Luogen Liu

Abstract

Since the 1990s, more and more medical researchers all over the world have been studying ABO-incompatible kidney transplantation (ABOi-KT) and already made tremendous progress. The first ABOi-KT in mainland China was carried out by Professor Wang Yi in 2006. The whole treatments, including the strict selection of donors and recipients, the effective removal of antibodies, the perioperative managements, and the monitoring for rejection, have been optimized by Wang Yi and his team. This chapter will focus on the experience of ABOi-KT success as well as the comparative overview of ABOi-KT in different countries. All of the successful ABOi-KT experience not only provides other ABOi organ transplants with the specific methods to overcome the primary obstacle of ABO blood type incompatibility but also helps to relieve the organ shortage efficiently.

Keywords

ABOi-KT transplantation · Transplantation indications · Plasma desensitization scheme · Postoperative management

Y. Wang (✉) · H. Jiang · L. Liu
The Second Affiliated Hospital of Hainan Medical University, 48 Baishuitang Ave, Haikou City, Hainan Province 570100, China

The Second Affiliated Hospital, University of South China, Hengyang City, Hunan Province, China
e-mail: wy@usc.edu.cn

Y. Wang (ed.), *ABO-incompatible Organ Transplantation*,
https://doi.org/10.1007/978-981-13-3399-6_12

1 Brief History of ABO-Incompatible Kidney Transplantation

In 1901, Karl Landsteiner, the famous pathologist and physiologist at the University of Vienna, Austria, discovered the ABO blood group, for which he was conferred upon the 1930 Nobel Prize in Physiology or Medicine. In 1952, Hume et al. carried out the world's first operation of ABOi-KT, which failed because the transplanted kidney did not regain its function. In 1964, Starzl et al. carried out the ABOi kidney transplants for two patients, and the graft in one of the patients survived for a long period.

In 1967 Sonoda et al. completed a case of ABOi kidney transplant without special treatment before transplantation, but accidentally the patient attained long-term survival. In the same year, Gleason and Murray collected the statistical data of ABOi kidney transplant and summarized the dissatisfied transplant outcomes. After the report, ABOi kidney transplant was suspended.

In 1981, the acute rejections caused by the wrong match during kidney transplant accidentally help led Slapak et al. to the discovery of plasma exchange, which can effectively reduce the acute rejection after ABO-incompatible transplant. Since then, the treatments, such as removal of plasma, plasma exchange, splenectomy, immunosuppressive drugs, and immune adsorbent, have been used to reduce the level of ABO antibodies gradually, and ABOi transplants have been rapidly promoted.

In 1985, Alexandre used preoperative plasma exchange to remove ABO antibodies. Meanwhile, he emphasized the importance of splenectomy for the graft's long-term survival. In 1987, Cardella used plasma exchange postoperatively in ABOi transplant. In the same year, Bannett et al. used immune adsorbent to remove the pre-existing ABO antibodies selectively in the USA, and he noted the importance of splenectomy as well.

In 1989, Takahashi et al. used plasmapheresis with immune adsorption to remove the ABO antibodies before transplant and conducted splenectomy during the transplant surgery, for which the patient attained long-term survival after surgery. From 1989 to 1995, 67 cases of ABO-incompatible kidney transplants were conducted in the Urology Center of Tokyo Women's Medical University in Japan. The survival rate and the graft survival rate of the ABOi transplant were parallel to these rates of the ABOc transplant.

Since the association of ABOi kidney transplant was founded in Japan in 1998, ABOi kidney transplant has been leaping forward. In mainland China, the first ABOi kidney transplant was carried out by Professors Wang Yi, Luo Zhigang, et al. in the second affiliated hospital of Nanhua University on December 14, 2006, and the patient attained long-term survival without splenectomy. Since then, many ABO-incompatible kidney transplants were successfully conducted in the hospital, and the ABOi kidney transplant has developed in China. The treatments for the ABOi like plasma exchange have been optimized, and the therapeutic effect has been improved tremendously.

2 Selection of Donors and Recipients

The selection of donors and recipients, tissue match, and preoperative preparations are key to the long-term survival of patients.

2.1 Selection of Donors

Living kidney donors usually come from relatives or peoples who have no blood relationship but already voluntarily signed the donation documents as a legal basis. The donors must be specifically informed of the transplant risks and complications before the surgery.

2.1.1 Donor Age

People older than 55 years old usually have poor tolerance for surgery or potential diseases, such as cardiovascular diseases or renal insufficiency.

Health Assessment of the Donor

Those with mental disorder or chronic diseases, such as hypertension and cardiovascular disease, kidney disease, and hepatitis, will not be considered as the donors.

Routine Laboratory Examinations

Laboratory examinations of the donors like blood, urine, and stool routine tests must be normal.

Infection Examinations

Infection examinations like bacteria in urine, sputum, and stool should be done. Infection marks in blood such as CMV-IgG, IgM, EB virus, hepatitis virus, HIV, and PPD must be tested. It was reported that the donor organ with CMV virus increased the morbidity of the recipients. EB virus infection and the application of immunosuppressant can cause B-cell lymphoma.

Blood Biochemical Examinations

Biochemical examinations in blood include electrolytes (potassium, sodium, chloride, calcium, phosphorus, etc.), liver function (aminotransferase, alkaline, phosphatase), renal function (creatinine, urea nitrogen, creatinine clearance test), blood gas analysis (carbon dioxide binding force), blood sugar, etc.

Radiological Examinations

The X-ray examinations of the abdomen and chest, the ultrasound examination of the liver and kidney, and electrocardiogram (ECG) examination should be done.

Urinary System Examination

Urinary system examination can be used to estimate the function of the donor kidney and the remaining kidney, respectively. The tests include renal vein angiography, renal artery angiography, etc. Male donors generally use the left kidney as the graft because the left renal artery is exposed easily and the vein is longer. For nulliparous female donors, it is advisable to take the right kidney as the graft because hydronephrosis occurs more easily for the right kidney during pregnancy.

2.2 The Selection of the Recipients

2.2.1 The Age of the Recipient

The age of recipients has great influence on the long-term survival of recipients. At present the age range is wider than ever. The recommended ages are from 12 to 50 years old, but the survival rate of children aged 4–15 are similar to the younger. The risk of kidney transplant increases for the recipients more than 60 years old. The recent reports say that, due to the research progress of immunosuppressant, and mature surgical techniques, the success rate of kidney transplant for recipients aged over 60 has been increased.

2.2.2 Antibodies in Blood

ABO Antibodies

ABOi transplants were already carried out successfully in many countries, and the ABO antibodies are the key points for the transplant. The antigenicities are listed in the order of intensity, A_1B, A_2B, A_1, B, A_2, and O, from the strong to the weak. Therefore, people whose blood type is A_2 are the prior donors in light of the lower probability of transplant rejection. Blood type A_2 only accounts for less than 1% domestically, and the proportion in the white reaches 20%. As a result, the ABOi kidney transplants are mainly from the type A_2 to the type B or type O in the USA, and the 1-year survival rate is similar to that of the ABOc. The donors in Japan and China are mainly type A_1 and type B. The 8-year survival rate reaches 67%, and there are about 7% of the recipients with irreversible rejections in 1 year [1].

Rh Antibodies

Clinically, Rh-positive means D antigen in blood, and without D antigen is Rh-negative. Except a few ethnic minorities in China, the rate of Rh-positive accounts for 99%. Therefore, the Rh-blood-group-incompatible kidney transplant, which is rare, can be divided into two kinds: the donor Rh (+), the recipient Rh (−), and the donor Rh (−), the recipient Rh (+). Even though the antigenicity of Rh is weak and the rejection occurs rarely, we should exercise caution and lavage the graft organ completely [2].

2.2.3 The Primary Disease Types

The causes of chronic renal failure and uremia are a lot, but not all uremia patients can be considered as a recipient to do transplant; the primary disease types are the following.

Glomerulonephritis

In recent years, more and more uremia patients are suitable for kidney transplantation, but glomerulonephritis is also the most appropriate indication. If the kidney diseases tend to relapse after transplant, we suggest that the transplant should be delayed. For instance, the recipients with anti-glomerular basement membrane (GBM) disease shouldn't receive the transplant until the GBM antibody stays negative at least for 6 months. For patients with focal glomerular sclerosis, IgA nephropathy, mesangial hyperplastic glomerulonephritis, membranous glomerulonephritis, etc., the kidney transplant should be conducted when this disease is in a stable condition. In general, it's difficult for us to distinguish relapsing glomerulonephritis from chronic rejection.

Chronic Pyelonephritis

Chronic pyelonephritis must be completely controlled before transplant, and the two kidneys with relapsing pyelonephritis should be resected before transplant.

Interstitial Nephritis

We should find out the causes of interstitial nephritis, such as infection, drug allergy, toxic substances damage, ischemia, metabolic abnormalities, physical factors, urinary tract obstruction, tumors, or hereditary disease. The transplants are considered only when the primary diseases are under control and stop relapsing.

Hereditary Nephritis

The recipients with polycystic kidney diseases (PKD) should receive the transplant after the original kidney is resected, because PKD causes inflammation frequently. Furthermore, the survival rates of recipients are relatively low due to the onset age of PKD.

Vascular Diseases

According to the follow-up studies in recent years, the relapse of hypertensive nephrosclerosis occurs rarely after transplant.

Metabolic Diseases

The number of transplants for diabetic nephropathy in the past decades has increased, and the proportion may reach 25% according to some reports. Pancreas and kidney transplants are usually conducted at the same time in some transplant centers. The survival rate of young patients is similar with the rates of other patients with other primary diseases. However, dialysis treatment is much better than a transplant for the old patients considering complications of diabetes.

Kidney Failure Caused by Lupus Nephritis

Kidney transplant should be conducted when the lesions of other organs are controlled. As we know, the transplant number for lupus nephritis has increasingly grown year by year. The treatments for lupus are consistent with the applications of immunosuppressant after the transplant. The recurrence rate is not high, but the survival rate is lower than the primary glomerular disease.

Drug Poison

The transplant effect for kidney failure caused by drug poison is poor.

Oncosis

The primary tumor should be resected before metastasis.

3 The Treatments of ABO Blood Type Antibodies

We need to remove A and B antibodies as much as possible to avoid super acute rejection. Decreasing the titer of ABO antibodies, alleviating the rebound of antibodies due to B lymphocyte transformation, and regulating the coagulation function of the recipients are the three key points. There are three common methods to decrease the antibodies' titer such as plasma exchange (PE), plasma double filtration plasmapheresis (DFPP), and plasma immune adsorption (IA).

The specific clinical schemes for reducing antibodies include PE, DFPP, IA, PE + DFPP, PE + intravenous immunoglobulin (PE + IVIG), and PE/DFPP + CMVIg. All of the methods are to reduce and to prevent the rebound of antibodies.

3.1 The Plasma Treatments

3.1.1 Plasma Exchange (PE)

In ABOi kidney transplant, in order to remove A and B antibodies and reduce the risk of rejection, we use fresh frozen AB blood type plasma exchange to replace the patients' plasma or albumin replacement fluid though membrane plasma separation in vitro.

Characteristics

1. Small molecules, middle molecules, and macromolecules, especially the toxin combined with protein, all can be removed.
2. Plasma exchange has certain effects on correcting disorders of electrolyte acid-base balance in liver failure, but the effects are far less than hemodialysis and hemofiltration. The water overload cannot be improved by PE.
3. PE requires not only a large number of plasma to supplement essential protein and clotting factors but also brings about viral infections.
4. The replacement in PE is mainly fresh frozen plasma (FFP), with some substitute such as low molecular weight dextran and hydroxyethyl starch.

Complications

1. Complications caused by citrate hypocalcemia: Major symptoms are oral and distal limb skin numbness, and severe symptoms are muscle spasms and arrhythmia. Continuous intravenous injection of 10% calcium gluconate or calcium chloride 10–20 mL for more than 15 min can prevent and treat these

complications. Metabolic alkalosis usually occurs in the patients with kidney failure due to poor excretion of citrate.
2. Bleeding tendency: Albumin replacement fluid can expend clotting factors. Blood coagulation time (CT) extends to 130%, and activated partial thromboplastin time (APTT) extends to two times when a unit of plasma is replaced. These indexes are back to normal after 4 h. The exchange for many times in the short period may lead to the loss of blood clotting mechanism. Therefore, for patients with high risk of bleeding tendency such as pulmonary hemorrhage, the supplement of 1000–2000 mL FFP is necessary.
3. Virus infections: FFP can bring about the potential infections of hepatitis virus and human immunodeficiency virus (HIV). The replacement of 1 unit of plasma needs 10–15 units of FFP, and the infection risk should not be ignored. There is no effective prevention against infections, and we must control the application of FFP strictly. For patients who need a lot of FFP replacement, such as those with thrombotic thrombocytopenic purpura (TTP), hepatitis B vaccine may be beneficial to prevent hepatitis B virus infection.
4. Anaphylaxis: Anaphylaxis usually occurs during FFP infusion, and the major symptoms are chill, skin rashes, fever, and hypotension. Laryngeal edema and cardiorespiratory failure rarely occur. Before the plasma exchange, applications of anti-allergic drugs such as corticosteroids, promethazine, and adrenaline can reduce the incidence and severity. The anaphylaxis to disinfectant of membrane separator has been reported.
5. Hypokalemia: We should pay more attention to patients with low potassium because albumin solution doesn't contain potassium ions. The potassium concentration can decrease to 75% after each replacement of 1 unit of plasma. Adding 4 mmol calcium to per liter albumin will help prevent hypokalemia and its complications like cardiac arrhythmia.
6. Drugs elimination: Regular hemodialysis technology has less influence on the drugs with high protein-binding rate. However plasma exchange can decrease drug concentration in blood theoretically, such as cyclophosphamide [3].

3.1.2 Immunoadsorption (IA)

Immunoadsorption therapy is a technology of blood purification which has been developed in the recent 15 years. During the procedure of immunoadsorption, adsorbent column, combining specific antigens, antibodies, or affinity ligand with adsorption carriers, can selectively remove specific antibodies of the blood plasma in order to reduce postoperative rejection of transplant. Immunoadsorption therapy is very different from general nonspecific blood perfusion.

Immunoadsorption (IA) therapy, based on plasma exchange, provides for plasma antibodies with higher selective eliminations. At the same time, IA could cause less loss of useful components in plasma and avoid the side effects of plasma input. For the patients in hypersensitive immune status, IA can remove HLA antibodies before the transplant quickly and reduce the incidence of acute rejection.

IA is used once every other day to reduce the antibodies titer below the average level 1:8. Splenectomy should be conducted during the transplant surgery if necessary. Immunoadsorption for three times and large dose of gamma globulin, rituximab, ATG, anti-IL-2 antibodies, etc. should be used postoperatively when the immunosuppressive treatments are Tac+MMF+Pred (tacrolimus+mycophenolate mofetil+prednisone) and after transplant. Antibodies titer may increase after transplant, but it will be much lower than the preoperative level.

Compared with plasma exchange in the past, the immune adsorption has obvious advantages on the efficacy and safety. Due to the reinfusion of patients' own plasma without exogenous plasma and replacement fluid, IA can prevent infectious diseases and some complications of plasma exchange such as the citrate salt poisoning, abnormal blood clotting mechanism, allergic reactions, low blood pressure, and hypokalemia.

In addition, immune adsorption does not affect the metabolism of other drugs and costs less. The use of replacement fluid and anticoagulants in extracorporeal circulation during IA may bring about the complications like hypotension, hypocalcemia, arrhythmia, allergic reaction, infection, hemolysis, bleeding, or clotting disorders [4]. We should pay attention and attend to the complications effectively.

3.1.3 Double Filtration Plasmapheresis (DFPP)

After the second separation of the plasma, DFPP can transfuse patients' own plasma and other blood components without AB antibodies pathogenic substances. The membrane plasma separation was first presented by Millward et al. in 1978. Based on the technology, DFPP are created to separate the pathogenic substances whose molecular weight are between 15-3million daltons. Agishi et al. conducted DFPP for the first time in 1979. Today, DFPP has been widely used in the removal of antibodies and other therapies of clinical diseases, especially kidney disease. We should pay attention to the complications such as bleeding, hypotension, and hypoalbuminemia.

3.2 Applications of Immune Induction

The treatments of PE, IA, or DFPP will cause the rebound of antibodies. Conventional immunosuppressants and rituximab help to solve the problem by reducing the production of antibodies.

3.2.1 Rituximab

Rituximab, a chimeric monoclonal antibody of rat CD20, which can be combined with CD20 antigen in B lymphocyte to remove B lymphocyte, is used in the treatment of B-cell lymphoma initially. Recent reports say that rituximab can effectively prevent humoral rejection. Tyden et al. reported that in the 11 patients' cases of ABOi transplant, with the treatments of a dose of rituximab for 10 days before the surgery, conventional dose of MMF, FK506, prednisone, as well as immunoadsorption (IA), infections and failure of grafts never occur in all the patients. In addition, rituximab can replace splenectomy, and using rituximab 4 weeks before the transplant is recommended.

3.2.2 Immunosuppressive Therapy Before Transplant

Calmodulin neural protein inhibitor (CNI), glucocorticoid, and one kind of antiproliferative drugs are regarded as the primary immunosuppressive treatment for maintaining immunosuppression by many centers in China. Tacrolimus (FK506) are the first-line drugs of the CNI.

3.2.3 Other Immune Induction Agents

According to the guidelines, we should start using immunosuppressants before or during the transplant. IL-2 receptor antagonists are recommended as the first-line drugs of induction therapy. For patients with high risks, such as high panel reactive antibodies, retransplantation, delayed graft function, anti-thymocyte globulin (ATG), or IL-2 receptor, monoclonal antibody is extremely necessary for induction therapy.

4 Perioperative Management of Transplantation

4.1 Preoperative Managements of Transplantation

4.1.1 Preoperative Hemodialysis

Hemodialysis determines early recovery of graft function and long-term survival rate of the recipients during ABOi kidney transplant. The frequency, the treatment history, and the therapeutic effect of dialysis all have comprehensive influence on the recipients who are already under the treatment of hemodialysis before transplant. Preoperative dialysis can also affect the whole transplant for patients who has never taken the treatment of hemodialysis before.

The purposes of complete dialysis before the transplant are:

1. To eliminate water sodium retention: it must be ensured that there is no water overload before the transplant, because the overload will harm the suture or heal of incision and increase the risk of intraoperative rehydration and blood transfusion. However excessive ultrafiltration dehydration should be avoided considering intraoperative hypotension, insufficient perfusion of kidney, and even delayed graft function.
2. To remove toxins: uremic toxins can affect platelet function and cause surgical bleeding. What's more, uremic toxins increase the chance of postoperative infection and delay the healing of incision. Inadequate dialysis may cause pericarditis. Preoperative dialysis for 3–4 times should be conducted. Especially when urea nitrogen is more than 35.7/L, dialysis once a day for 3–5 days before the transplant are the best.
3. To regulate electrolyte and acid-base disorder: Potassium is the most important among electrolytes. Besides arrhythmia, high potassium produces side effects of neuromuscular blockers during anesthesia. Ideal serum potassium level before transplant is 4.0 mmol/L. For patients without residual kidney function, under the normal diet, serum potassium increased 1.0–1.5 mmol/L for 1 day. Serum potassium should be no more than 3.0 mmol/L after dialysis on the last day before transplant. For patients with cardiovascular disease, who can't tolerate low potassium, the dialysis fluid that contains potassium 3.0 L should be used. What's more, we can extend the dialysis time or conduct an additional dialysis without heparin 12 h before transplant.

   The PH disorders should be corrected. However, there is no need to correct the concentration of plasma strictly because the mild acidosis are safer, which could decrease the chance of arrhythmia caused by hyperventilation.

4. To correct anemia: when hematocrit (HCT) is under 20% preoperative, we should add the dose of erythropoietin or use the transfusion of deposited red blood cells to increase HCT to 20–35%. These treatments can not only improve the tolerance of surgery but also shorten the bleeding time.

In summary, regardless of the blood purification methods, complete dialysis, urea nitrogen below 11.6 mmol/L, creatinine below 353.6 μmol/L, hemoglobin over 80 g/L, hematocrit of red cells over 25%, serum potassium below 4.5 mmol/L, normal cardio-thoracic proportion, and dry weight without edema or other complications all contribute to the improvement of the patients' long-term survival rate and the reduction of long-term complications.

4.1.2 Routine Examinations Before Transplant and Monitoring of ABO Antibodies

Rituximab should be used 28 days before transplant. Mycophenolate mofetil (MMF) + tacrolimus (FK506) should be used 10–14 days before transplant. We conduct the plasma exchange and/or DFPP. Furthermore, we monitor the antibody levels and other indexes at different time points during plasma exchange, the surgery, and even the transplant matching. The antibodies include anti-A-IgG, anti-A-IgM, anti-B-IgG, and anti-B-IgM. The routine examinations include blood routine, liver and kidney function, graft glomerular filtration rate (GFR) and effective renal plasma flow (ERPF), blood coagulation function, the proportion of CD19, B lymphocytes in peripheral blood lymphocytes, the proportion of CD4+/CD8+T lymphocyte in peripheral blood, etc.

4.1.3 Preoperative Stem Cell Induction of Immune Tolerance

At the People's Hospital of Guangdong province China from 2008 to 2013, five cases of combined living kidney and hematopoietic stem cells transplant between relatives are conducted. These five cases are regarded as the study group (group A), and another five cases of living kidney transplant between relatives which are conducted at the same time are regarded as the control group (group B). After the follow-up studies for 5–50 months, the microchimerism positive rate is 10% in group A, and the rate is 60% in group B, which means the immunosuppression in group A is better. The combined living kidney and hematopoietic stem cell transplant between relatives provides us with a feasible method for inducing immune tolerance.

4.2 Managements in Operation

Other than general anesthesia, which are conducted for transplant by most kidney transplant centers abroad, continuous epidural anesthesia is the most common choice for kidney transplant domestically. Early studies showed that continuous epidural anesthesia accounted for 72%. In recent years the proportion of general anesthesia has increased. General anesthesia can provide the surgery with painless conditions, complete muscle relaxation, unobstructed respiratory tract, adequate oxygen, and stable hemodynamic. What's more, it can avoid the epidural hematoma and intraoperative agitation. From the beginning, general anesthesia is recommended for kidney transplant.

Preoperative prophylactic antibiotics are needed, and antibiotics should be used for 5 days after the surgery. Oral immunosuppressive drugs ought to be taken half an hour before surgery. Methylprednisolone 500 mg should be added to saline 250 mL for intravenous infusion, and the infusion must be finished before the opening of blood flow in transplanted kidney. Heparin is locally used in vascular anastomosis for anticoagulation. Human serum albumin 20 g should be intravenously dripped before arterial anastomosis considering that albumin helps the early recovery of renal function.

Five percent sodium bicarbonate can be intravenously dripped before the arteries are open to reduce the metabolic acidosis. Infusion of 5% mannitol 250 mL and cefuroxime Sammy 80 mg is needed after the vessels are open. Mannitol is the scavenger of free radical. Mannitol and osmotic diuretics can reduce the edema and ischemia-reperfusion injury of the transplant kidney. Electrolyte solution can expand blood volume and keep blood pressure a little higher than the normal level to ensure that renal allograft perfusion. Dopamine can be used if necessary. The kidney ought to be wrapped by special bag filled with brine ice cubes to stay cryostat. The drugs in different kidney transplant centers are different, and we could make a choice according to the experience. It is worth mentioning that the local use of low molecular weight heparin in vascular anastomosis is not recommended.

4.3 Early Postoperative Management of Kidney Transplant

4.3.1 Treatments of Catheter, Double J Tube, and Drainage Tube

According to some reports, the exact time to remove catheter after kidney transplant is not the same. If there is no obvious leak of the ureter-bladder anastomosis, the catheter is usually removed 10–14 days after the surgery. At the same time, we remove the double J tube by pulling out the silk sewed in bottom of the tube or through the cystoscope. The double J tube as ureteral stent can also be pulled out after 6–12 weeks because it can protect the reconstruction of urinary tract. The graft drainage tube can be removed when the drainage is less than 10 mL/day or when the drainage tube has been retained for 3 weeks, and the ultrasonic exam show that there is no obvious effusion around graft.

4.3.2 Treatments of Early Postoperative Complications

Oliguria or Anuria

Early oliguria or anuria after transplant can be caused by infection, acute rejection, urinary or vascular obstruction, toxicity of calcineurin inhibitor (CNI), delayed graft function and dehydration, etc. Infections and/or rejections can cause fever. The toxicity of calcineurin inhibitor (CNI) can cause fremitus. The quick determination of

CNI drugs' concentration in blood helps diagnosis. Careful physical examinations help find the primary infection. Graft kidney tenderness is a specific sign of rejection. Hydronephrosis, renal blood flow, and renal volume can be monitored through ultrasonic examination. Acute rejections usually increase renal blood flow impedance. Dehydration can be diagnosed by the rehydration test and central venous pressure measurement. Oliguria or anuria can often be corrected by appropriate treatments. Otherwise, kidney replacement therapies are in need as soon as possible.

Urinary Fistula

Urinary fistula is one of the most common complications after kidney transplant and the incidence is up to 3–5% before the wide use of ureteral stent. Urinary fistula can occur in the ureter, bladder, or kidney essence, and the most common cause is ischemic necrosis of the ureter. Retaining enough perirenal fat in "golden triangle" area during the repair of the kidney and the placing of the ureteral stent contribute to the prevention of postoperative urinary fistula. We can try to place the ureteral stent in graft kidney through the endoscope after the failure of conservative treatments for urinary fistula, but the success rate is low. If the ureteral length of transplanted kidney is enough, the reanastomosis of ureteral bladder or the reanastomosis of graft ureter and the original ureter is under consideration. Furthermore, we should pay attention to the urinary fistula caused by rejections.

Arterial Thrombosis

The incidence of arterial thrombosis in the first week after transplant is about 0.5%. The high-risk factors include atherosclerosis, unexplained desquamation of intima, poor vascular anastomosis, artery twist, multiple arteries, child donors, etc. When the primary graft dysfunction or acute anuria occurs, the arterial thrombosis should be taken into account. Ultrasound examinations and CT artery enhancement scanning can be used for the diagnosis. Once diagnosed, the surgery is essential. Percutaneous arteriography and thrombus removal in 12 h of disease time may be feasible. Considering the poor tolerance on warm ischemia, most graft kidneys are usually resected.

Venous Thrombosis

Venous thrombosis occurs rarely in kidney transplant. The total incidence is around 0.5%. Primary graft dysfunction, severe hematuria, or anuria may be the evidences of renal vein thrombosis. Once the thrombus is diagnosed, the success rate of thrombus removal is low, and graft nephrectomy is often conducted as the treatment.

Hematuria

Early hematuria after kidney transplant is often caused by urinary catheter, ureteral stent, or urinary tract reconstruction. If hematuria is still out of control after bladder douche, blood clot removal and coagulation hemostasis should be conducted through cystoscopy. If the above treatment fail, the surgery is in need.

4.4 The Monitoring of Graft Function

Changes in renal function after transplant are unpredictable. Diuresis, oliguria, or anuria may occur on each patient. We need to measure urine volume strictly every hour in 5–7 days after transplant. When renal function is back to normal, we can measure urine volume every day. Serum creatinine is measured once a day in early 3 days after the operation, 2–3 times in the next 2–4 weeks and once a week in the next 2–3 months. Ultrasound examination can monitor the urinary obstruction, perirenal hematoma, and kidney blood flow. Kidney biopsies are necessary for the diagnosis when serum creatinine keeps increasing unexplainably.

5 The Monitoring for Rejection

5.1 ABO Blood Group

Both preoperative and postoperative tests of ABO antibodies are needed, and the preoperative titer ought to be less than 1:8.

5.2 Other Blood Types

There is Rh blood type, etc.

5.3 HLA Antibodies

We use cross matching tests to find out whether there is HLA antibody to the donor in the recipient's serum, and HLA antibodies indicate the possibility of rejection.

5.4 Anti-Endothelial Cell Antibodies (AECA)

Endothelial cell itself is the antigen and can be damaged by anti-endothelial cell antibodies (AECA). AECA can be detected in many inflammation diseases such as Behcet's syndrome, Wegener's granulomatosis, systemic lupus erythematosus, systemic sclerosis, antiphospholipid syndrome, ulcerative colitis, and primary sclerosing cholangitis. The titer of AECA is closely related to the state of these diseases. Corresponding syndromes with AECA positive may indicate vasculitis or other rheumatic disease.

5.5 Cold Agglutinin Antibodies

Cold agglutinin is a cold, reactive, anti-erythrocyte IgM antibody, which is the most likely to be bound to red blood cell (RBC) membrane antigens in the temperature of 4 °C. Cold agglutinin exists in the common human's serum, and it isn't clinically significant when its titer is less than 1:32.

5.6 The Monitoring of Cellular Immune

5.6.1 Peripheral T-Cell Count

Monoclonal antibody immunofluorescence or flow cytometer are used for monitoring T-cell count in peripheral blood. T-cell total count and the CD4/CD8 ratio will increase in the early 1–5 days of acute rejection. The ratio will decrease because of cytomegalovirus (CMV) infections. According to some reports, acute rejections may occur when CD4/CD8 ratio is more than 1.2 (CD4/CD8 > 1.2), and the opportunity of infections may increase when the ratio is less than 1.08 (CD4/CD8 < 1.08). The dynamic monitoring of peripheral T-cell count help diagnose acute rejections and infections.

5.6.2 CD4/CD8 Ratio Measurement

CD4 count, as a specific index, can directly indicate the body's immune function. CD4 count fluctuates with different physiological conditions, but the CD4/CD8 ratio is relatively stable. Infections are closely related to the CD4 count and the CD4/CD8 ratio. The incidence of infections increase especially when the ratio is less than 0.20, as well as the opportunity of opportunistic infections. What's more, acute rejections are inclined to occur when CD4/CD8 ratio is more than 1.2.

5.6.3 The Activity of Killing Cells

We monitor the cytotoxic T cells (Tc) and natural killer cells (NK) to analyze the activity of killing cells. Dynamic monitoring is better. The acute rejection will increase the activity, and immunosuppressors can inhibit the activity. The donor's inactivated lymphocytes are regarded as stimulating cells, and the recipient's lymphocytes are regarded as reacting cells. Stimulating cells from the donor's inactivated lymphocytes and reacting cells from the recipient's lymphocytes are mixed in the mixed lymphocyte culture (MLC) to monitor the activity of NK and Tc.

5.6.4 Serum Cytokines

Acute rejection and infection can increase the titer of IL-2R in serum. The dynamic monitoring of IL-2R has great clinical significance. IL-2R can be released when the T cells are activated by acute rejections or infections, especially the CMV infection. However, IL-2R decreases obviously when cyclosporine A (CsA) causes renal function damage. The increase of serum creatinine together with the increase of IL-2R contributes to the diagnosis of acute rejections. In general, the levels of IL-2R are significantly different among different peoples, and there is no standard of diagnosis, which limits its clinical application. However, dynamic monitoring can overcome the shortcoming.

5.7 The Monitoring of Complements

In ABOi kidney transplant (ABOi-KT), there exist C4d sediments in the injured vascular endothelial cells of kidney graft, which means vascular endothelial cell injury is associated with C4d sediments. Both of them lead to rejections. As a result, the clinical monitoring of C4d is extremely important.

5.8 The Monitoring of Acute Phase Reactants

Transplant rejection is actually immune inflammation against the graft. Reactants in acute phase such as C-reactive protein (CRP) are related to the acute rejection.

5.9 Changes of ABO Antigens

Tatsu Tanab et al. noticed the changes of ABO antigens in the recipient after ABOi (A to B, B to A) kidney transplant by immunohistochemical examination of postoperative renal tissue. A or B antigens decreased to 91.8% in first 3 months after transplantation, 85.8% in early 5 years, 64.1% in 10 years, and about 57.6% after 10 years[5–7]. These changes of antigens may be associated with qualitative and quantitative changes in endothelial cells of the renal allograft. What's more, changes in endothelial cells may be associated with severe vascular rejections, which damage the transplanted renal vascular wall, and then stem cells from the recipients' blood circulation enter into the damaged blood vessels. After tissue repair, changes occur in endothelial cells [8, 9].

In ABOi kidney transplant (ABOi-KT), the vascular endothelium of grafts is always damaged to different degrees, and C4d sediment is the evidence, which can be found in the damaged endothelial cells of all ABOi-KT graft. However the kidney function is still normal. In summary, the immune response can damage the ABO antigen on the surface of the endothelial cells but doesn't cause renal function failure [10, 11]. What's more, severe damage of ABO antigen synthetase leads to the ABO antigens reduction in ABOi kidney transplant [12].

6 Comparison of ABOi-KT Protocols

6.1 European Managements

In Europe anti-CD20 monoclonal antibody (rituximab) and the immune adsorption column of AB antibodies without splenectomy are the primary treatments for ABOi transplant. According to the specific immune suppression scheme, a dose of rituximab (375 mg/m^2) should be used 2–4 weeks before immune adsorption. Traditional immune inhibitors including tacrolimus (FK506), mycophenolate mofetil, and prednisolone ought to be used 1 week before transplant. During the preoperative immune adsorption, glycosorb column, connecting A and B antigen to low molecular weight carbohydrate column of agarose gelmatrix, removes A and B antibodies. General speaking, ABO antibodies concentration could be less than 1:8 after four times adsorptions. After the last adsorption, intravenous immunoglobulin (0.5 g/kg) can avoid the postoperative rebound of antibodies. Immune adsorptions must be completed for more than three times in 9 days.

The specific scheme, which was created by Tydén et al. from Karolinska Institute, Sweden, achieved success in Sweden and Germany. According to the follow-up studies for 4 years, serum creatinine levels of the recipients are all normal, and there is no delayed creatinine abnormality. Gradually, the specific scheme get confirmed and applied widely in Europe [13, 14].

6.2 Japan Managements

As the largest ABOi-KT country, ABOi-KT accounts for almost 1/3 kidney transplantation in Japan [15, 16]. Takahashi et al. mainly used double filtration plasmapheresis (DFPP) to remove the blood type antibody [15].

They released the data from 494 cases of ABOi-KT from 1989 to 2001, during which a variety of immunosuppressive programs were used, including the use of immunosuppressants, in vitro antibody-removing strategies (preoperative antibody titer 1:8–1:16), anticoagulation, and splenectomy (98%). The transplantation scheme has been gradually improved. The original immunosuppressant were *anti-lymphocyte globulin* (ALG), *deoxidization fine guanidine rhizomorph*, and *cyclophosphamide*.

According to the review of living organ transplantation historical cases, the short-term prognosis of ABOi-KT was different to ABOc-KT, but there was no significant difference in the long-term prognosis. The recipients' survival rates, respectively, were 93% in 1 year, 89% in 3 years, 87% in 5 years, and 84% in 7 years. And the graft survival rates, respectively, were 84% in 1 year, 80% in 3 years, 71% in 5 years, and 65% in 7 years. There was no significant difference in various blood group combinations. Since 2001, the clinical application of new immunosuppressant *mycophenolate mofetil* and *basiliximab* (anti-CD25 monoclonal antibody) has, respectively, raised the rate of 1 year and 2 years to 96% and 94%. This data suggested that new immunosuppressive protocols have successfully improved the short-term graft survival rate of ABOi-KT. According to the registered cases, splenectomy is considered to be an important element of ABOi-KT, but it could not significantly improve the short-term and long-term curative effect. In 2004, it was replaced by desensitization protocols in 4 weeks before the operation, including DFPP, such as anti-CD20, *mycophenolate mofetil steroids*. These schemes required no additional postoperative antibody removal or intravenous immune globulin (IVIG) and have become the commonly used program of ABOi-KT in Japan [17].

6.3 US Managements

In America, Montgomery from John Hopkins University mainly used plasma exchange and high-dose intravenous immunoglobulins repeatedly to remove and neutralizing the blood type antibody. The first dose of *rituximab* was properly used before surgery on the basis of the patient's condition [2], and then *tacrolimus* and *mycophenolate mofetil* immunosuppression was applied, or steroids and *zenapax* was used after the transplantation operation. The postoperative treatment included three times of plasmapheresis. During the follow-up, the mean serum creatinine of the recipients was (1.3 + 0.1) mg/dL. Their initial experience did not show the use of rituximab could avoid the risk of splenectomy [17].

Though all roads lead to Rome, the three plasmaphereses have not much difference in the graft survival rate and the patient's long-term survival rate of postoperative [18].

7 Clinical Experience

Since the first ABOi-KT was performed in December 2006 in China, many centers have launched this operation. We have accumulated rich clinical experience in many aspects, such as the improvement of CD20 desensitization scheme, the prevention and control of thrombotic microangiopathy and consumptive clotting disorders, and the clinical application of immunosuppressor to adapt to the phenomenon and ABO/Rh blood group system incompatible kidney transplant. Some typical cases are summarized as follows: in order to guarantee authenticity and integrity, we had no change or modification on the inappropriate treatment measures and methods in this article. Informed consents from the patients for publication have been obtained.

7.1 The Prevention and Control of Thrombotic Microangiopathy and Consumptive Clotting Disorders

Case 1 [19]: Luo XX, male, 35 years old

He has received allograft renal transplantation in December 2002 due to chronic glomerulonephritis and chronic renal failure (uremia period). After the transplantation, he received immunosuppressive therapy, not discharged from the hospital until the renal function returned to normal. In November 2005, the patient restored blood dialysis treatment because of reduplicated herpes virus infection, *tacrolimus* (FK506) drug toxicity and overwork, which led to renal allograft failure after transplantation. In April 2006, the graft renal was removed. Up to the present day, the patient could not maintain hemodialysis due to the peripheral vascular badly damaged by repeated puncture, so he had to be hospitalized to undergo a relative renal transplantation again.

Physical examinations: T 37.5 °C, R 20 times/min, P 80 times/min, BP 130/98 mmHg, moderately nourished, chronic anemia features. In dwelling vein needle was visible on the left neck. The right neck shows a venous puncture scar. Bilateral upper extremity superficial repair puncture site was visible. Lungs are clear, having no rales. Normal soft abdomen; there was an "L"-shaped surgical scar on the right lower abdomen. No abdominal tenderness and rebounding pain. The liver and spleen did not touch under the rib, without knocking pain in the liver area. Abdominal shifting dullness was negative, with bowel sound normal. Double kidney can't be palpated, without renal percussive pain, double ureter-bladder region without tenderness, and bladder region without filling. The arms and legs were not edematous, and the superficial vein was punctured.

Laboratory examination after admission: Routine blood test, hemoglobin, 79 g/L, RBC 2.26 × 10^9/L; electrolyte, K^+ 5.31 mmol/L; renal function, Cr 1059.6 μmol/L, BUN 30.07 mmol/L; blood type, type O (Rh+); hepatitis complete set, HBs Ag (+), Hbe-Ab (+); other tests, stool routine, liver function, blood sugar, blood fat, blood coagulation function, CMV-DNA, sputum culture, swabs, HIV, and syphilis detection, were negative. For patients with anuria, routine urine and urine culture were not done.

Auxiliary examination after admission: Electrocardiogram (ECG), sinus tachycardia; ultrasound (abdominal viscera and double kidney), bilateral renal atrophy, without exception; color Doppler ultrasound (heart), ventricular septal and left ventricular posterior wall were thickening, decreased left ventricular diastolic function; X-ray, cardiopulmonary no exception.

The patient's father was willing to donate a kidney to him, but his blood type is type A, Rh (+). According to the relevant inspection, the donors and the recipient had the ABO blood group incompatibility, but the HLA had four matched sites. The population reactive antibody (PRA) level of the recipient respectively was 47.9% (class I antibody) and 27.3% (class II antibodies). Other aspects conformed to the requirements of the transplantation (details are shown in Table 12.1). Approved by the hospital ethics committee, ABOi-KT was planned.

The recipient received *FK506+ MMF+Pred* combined induction therapy 7 days before surgery. Double filtration plasmapheresis (DFPP) was carried out on the seventh day, fifth day, and third day preoperative, and plasma replacement (PE) was performed on the day before the operation to remove the recipient's anti-A and anti-B antibody in the blood plasma, the antibody titer falling to standard level before surgery. The recipient received continuous renal replacement therapy (CRRT) and intravenous drip anti-CD20 monoclonal antibody (*rituximab*). Intravenous drip freeze-dried fibrinogen to correct blood coagulation dysfunction 1 h before the transplantation.

Table 12.1 Tissue matching of donors and recipients

	Blood type	HLA-A	HLA-B	HLA-DR	PRAI (%)	PRAII (%)	CDC
Recipient	O	11/11	54 (22)/60 (40)	4/4	47.9	27.3	5%
Donor	A	11/–	13/60	4/17			

Table 12.2 Application of blood products in ABOi-KT recipients in early

	D	R	RBC (U)	Blood plasma (mL)	Cryoprecipitate (U)
LUO XX	A	O	26.0	12,000	32
ZHANG XX	B	A	20.5	1400	18.75
LI XX	A	O	18.5	3000	8.75
ZHANG XX	A	O	1.5	1400	10
P XX	B	O	2.0	1100	8

After the preoperative preparation, the patient received renal transplantation on December 14, 2006. It was visible in the operation that the left iliac blood vessels of the recipient are normal, no deformity or mutation. We anastomosed the donor renal vein with the left lateral iliac vein of the recipient end-to-side. The renal artery and the left iliac artery line anastomosed end to end. After opening the renal arteries and veins for 1 min, we could see pale yellow urine stream; the graft size, texture, color and luster, and beat of the transplanted kidney were normal. The donor kidney was placed inside the "J pipe" and took bladder countercurrent anastomosis. The whole operation was smooth. Unfortunately, a large amount of bleeding occurred in the postoperative incision because of incomplete correction of coagulation dysfunction caused by the three times' DFPP. The following blood products were used throughout the operation: PRBC 26 U, frozen plasma 12,000 mL, and cryoprecipitate 32 U (Table 12.2).

Immunosuppressive therapy was performed postoperatively. On the date of surgery, the patient received 7 mg/(kg day) intravenous injection of *methylprednisolone*, with a daily decline of 80 mg to 80 mg/day, and then changed to 40 mg oral prednisone, daily decrease 5 mg, maintaining 20 mg/day; *mycophenolate mofetil* (MMF) 2.0 g/day, intravenous infusion, 6 days after take orally 1.5 g/day instead; giving FK506, 4 mg/day (Fig. 12.1) after 2 days of the operation. At the same time, transfusing blood, plasma, albumin, and other support therapies and anticoagulant therapies was undergoing.

Postoperative renal function of the recipient had a good recovery, with no signs of rejection occurring. The patient smoothly resumed eating after the operation (Fig. 12.2 shows the recipient eating in the laminar flow ward). Twenty-five days after surgery, his serum creatinine fell to 132.8 μmol/L, and other biochemical indicators were normal. Plasma anti-A antibody titer: IgG was 1:16, and IgM was 1:8. Plasma anti-B antibody titer: IgG was 1:16, and IgM was 1:16 (Figs. 12.3 and 12.4). PRAI antibodies were 46.4%, Class II antibodies are 0 (Fig. 12.5). The patient was discharged from the hospital after a period of monitoring and treatment.

The continued follow-up after the discharge showed that the patient's physical condition is well within half a year, the serum creatinine being stable at 112 μmol/L, with the urea nitrogen tendency for 6.3 L, serum Na^+ being 138 mmol/L, K^+ being 3.60 mmol/L, Hb being 112 g/L, and other biochemical indication being normal. Plasma anti-A antibody titer: IgG was 1:32, and IgM was 1:16. Plasma anti-B antibody titer: IgG was 1:32, and IgM was 1:16. PRAI antibodies were 17.9%, and Class II antibodies were 3.6%. No infection, gastrointestinal bleeding,

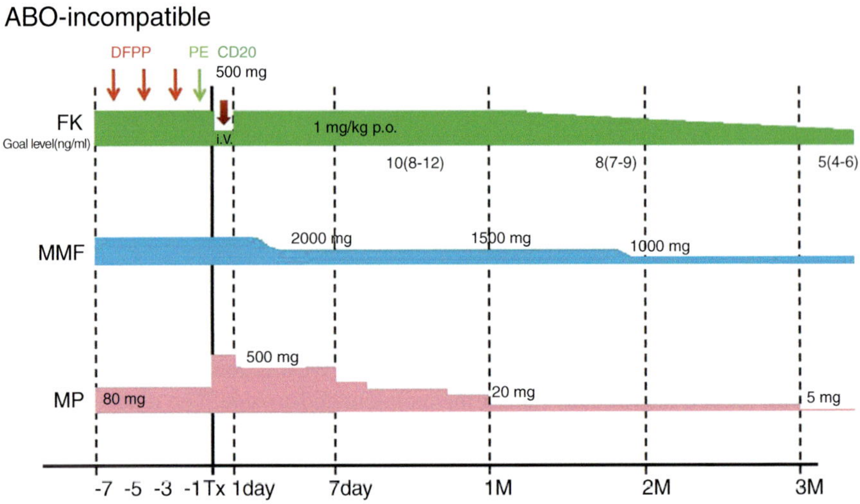

Fig. 12.1 Perioperatve immunosuppressive protocols

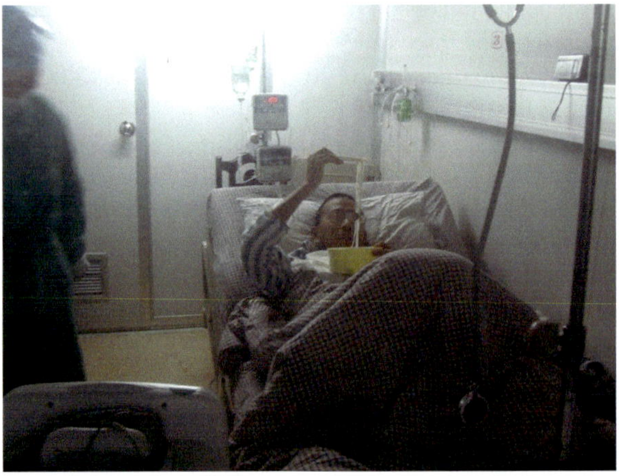

Fig. 12.2 Recipient eating in laminar flow ward 7 days after operation

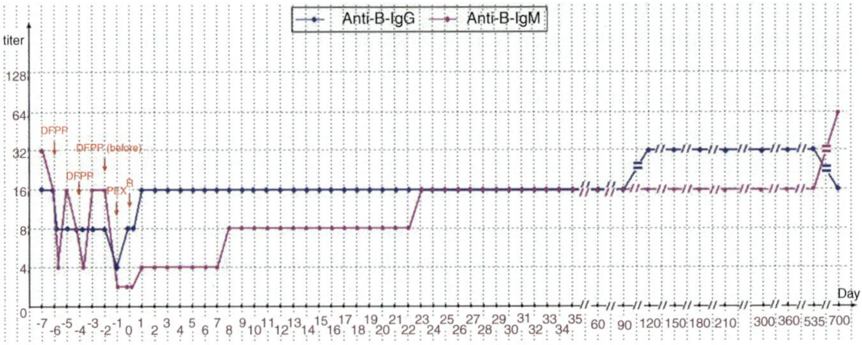

Fig. 12.3 Changes of anti-B antibodies titer

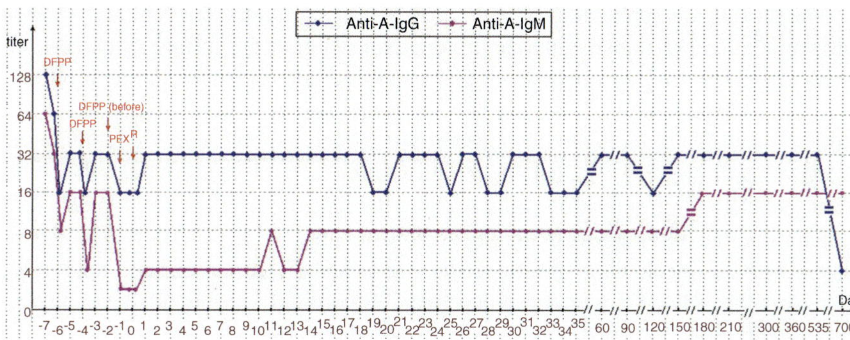

Fig. 12.4 Changes of anti-A antibodies titer

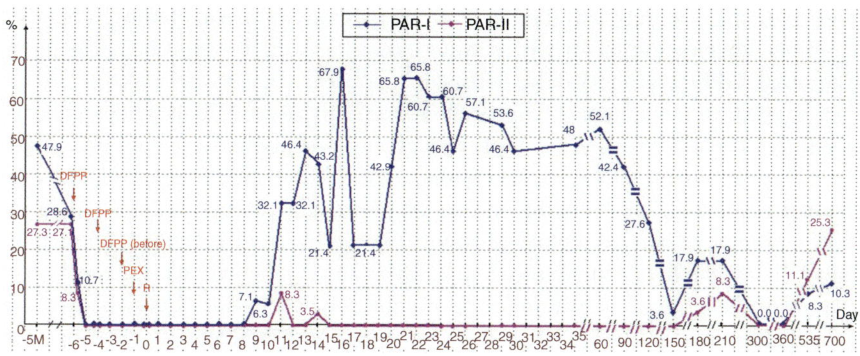

Fig. 12.5 Changes of HLA-I and HLA-II antibodies

hematoencephalic, erythronoclastic anemia, and other graft complications occurred. The recipient can engage in the general social work.

Subsequently, the patient was followed up outside the hospital, and the graft renal survived well.

This was the first case of ABO-KT in mainland China [17]. Up to December 14, 2016, the patient had survived 10 years with the graft renal. In this successful ABOi-KT case, we have gained the following experiences.

Firstly, immunosuppressive therapy plays a critical role in the transplantation. A multicenter randomized controlled study showed that the immunosuppression of *tacrolimus* had significant effect on the maintenance of the graft renal function, and mycophenolate might inhibit the blood type antibody in ABOi-KT. Therefore, the two schemes were combined as a basic immunosuppressive program.

Secondly, although using plasma double filtration (DFPP) to remove the blood group antibody will lead to hyperlipidemia and low-protein coagulation disorders, DFPP is a reliable way to remove the prestored plasma anti-A and anti-B antibody. Moreover, DFPP can also clean out the anti-HLA antibodies for those patients who have group-reactive antibody positive.

The third is the application of anti-CD20 *rituximab* monoclonal antibody. CD20 antigen is a kind of transmembrane protein expression in the surface of pre-B lymphocyte and mature B lymphocyte. It plays an important role in regulating proliferation and differentiation of B lymphocyte. *Rituximab* is a kind of human-mouse chimeric anti-CD20 monoclonal antibody. Rituximab may be acting by eliminating B cells. B cells are very efficient antigen-presenting cells, particularly after they have been activated. Such activation could occur at the time of rejection. The rapidity with which rituximab eliminates circulating and presumably tissue CD20+ B cells is consistent with this mechanism of action. *Rituximab* can be used for immunosuppressive therapy in the ABOi-KT without splenectomy. Accordingly, we did not have splenectomy in this case, but *rituximab* was administered to patients before surgery.

At last, postoperative hemostasis is critical. In early ABOi-KT cases, we have mainly drawn lessons from Tokyo Women's Medical University who made a scheme based on DFPP. The Asahi EC-20w filter used for DFPP has a 0.01 μm small hollow fiber aperture. Not only was the blood group antibody in plasma removed but also the blood coagulation factor with similar molecular weight would be cleaned out. Therefore, DFPP has a risk of hemorrhagic tendency.

Coagulation and anticoagulation system keep a dynamic balance under a normal condition. Once the balance is broken, bleeding or thrombosis would occur. The liver plays an important role in the regulation of this dynamic balance: (1) the liver synthesizes almost all of the blood coagulation factor (except factor IV); (2) the liver can remove activated clotting factor; (3) the liver is the production of plasminogen; (4) the liver can produce antiplasmin; and (5) the liver has the function of removing the original activation cycle of fibrinolytic enzyme. Lacking of blood coagulation and (or) fibrin is prone to have bleeding tendency or bleeding. The blood coagulation disorders are mainly because (1) coagulation factors are filtered out and reduced in circulation and (2) clotting factor increased consumption leading to DIC. Therefore, early hemostasis based on coagulation function is very important.

It can be seen from Table 12.2 that in the early ABOi-KT practice, postoperative bleeding often occurs due to the shallow understanding of secondary coagulation dysfunction and the perioperative influence triggered by DFPP. In order to treat the bleeding, we had to use large amounts of concentrated red blood cells, plasma, and cold deposits. With the further understanding of coagulation dysfunction caused by DFPP, we put the blood coagulation function adjustment in an important place of preoperative work. So, the use of blood products was also similarly reduced to the need in ABOc-KT.

But we should attach great importance to the subsequent prevention against thrombotic microangiopathy and the resulting systemic consumptive coagulation dysfunction.

Case 2: Zhu XX, male

The main complaints are "Found the serum creatinine increased for more than 7 years, regular hemodialysis for six months, had a nasal congestion and runny nose for 1 day." The patient had been hospitalized due to fatigue and lack of appetite in

May 2008. The biochemical examination showed serum creatinine was 340 μmol/L. The treatment of renal preservation combination of traditional Chinese and Western medicine didn't produce satisfactory effect. Since then, the level of serum creatinine has been continuously increasing, and the renal function has deteriorated gradually. In August 2015, the patient revisited the hospital because of aggravating symptoms of fatigue and lack of appetite. Assay of serum creatinine was 760 μmol/L, given hemodialysis treatment up to now, after put a femoral vein double lumen tube. One day before, the patient got a nasal congestion, runny nose again, and treated himself with oral amoxicillin, but the effect was poor.

This time, the patient wanted a relative ABOi-KT. After admission, the patient had good mental state, diet, and sleep, with 24-h urine 1000 mL, and normal stool.

History of past illness: Examination in 2000 found that the urine protein is positive (2+), treated as chronic nephritis (unspecified), no further consultation. In September 2015, left forearm arteriovenous fistula angioplasty was performed. The history of hepatitis, tuberculosis, and other infectious diseases was denied, and there was no history of trauma, no history of gastrointestinal bleeding and hemorrhoids or other bleeding history, no history of blood transfusion, and no food allergy. The history of vaccination is unspecified.

Physical examinations: T 36.5 °C, R 20 times/min, P 95 times/min, BP 136/85 mmHg; wt: 81 kg, moderately nourished, chronic anemia features. Double lung breath sounded coarse, having no rales. The heart rate was 95 beats per minute, with regular rhythm. Without pathological murmur in valve auscultation area; normal soft abdomen; no abdominal tenderness and rebounding pain. The liver and spleen did not touch under the rib, without knocking pain in the liver area. Abdominal shifting dullness was negative, bowel sound being normal. The left arteriovenous fistula had wind-like vascular murmur. No edema of lower limbs; no abnormalities were detected in the nervous system.

Laboratories and auxiliary examination: routine blood test, routine clotting function test, and liver function are all normal. Renal function, serum creatinine 360.00 μmol/L; urea nitrogen, 12.10 mmol/L; lithic acid, 142.00 μmol/L; serum carbonate, 28.70 mmol/L; K^+, 4.25 mmol/L; Na^+, 145.00 mmol/L; CL^-, 97.90 mmol/L; Ca^{2+}, 2.11 mmol/L; inorganic phosphorus, 0.84 mmol/L. Virological examination, HIV, and syphilis detection were negative. Electrocardiogram (ECG), sinus rhythm and abnormal t waves; X-ray, no abnormalities; abdominal B ultrasound, double atrophy of kidney; the liver, spleen, and pancreas were normal; no abnormal bilateral iliac vessels. Ultrasonic cardiogram: aortic broadening; left atrial enlargement, aortic broadening; left atrial enlargement. The left ventricular diastolic function decreased and the systolic function was normal.

Donor: Zhu XX, male, 62 years old, the recipient's father. The relevant examination showed no contraindication. With a history of mild hypertension (taking a single antihypertensive drug, blood pressure can be controlled at about 120/80 mmHg). No infectious diseases and chronic disease; no surgical trauma history; no blood transfusion and drug allergy experience; the vaccination was unspecified. Blood type B, RhD-positive, creatinine 59.00 μmol/L; urea nitrogen 4.50/L; lithic acid 152.00 μmol/L, serum carbonate 21.40 mmol/L; serum creatinine clearance rate 123.13 mL/min.

Coagulation and urine, liver function, electrolyte, blood lipid, and blood glucose were all normal. No positive results were found in infectious disease tests.

Chest X-ray showed double lung markings. ECG was normal. B ultrasound prompts hepatobiliary spleen, and the pancreas and kidney showed no abnormalities. Ultrasonic cardiogram: aortic broadening, left atrial expansion; left ventricular wall thickness. Left ventricular diastolic function is reduced, and left ventricular systolic function is normal. Normal lung ventilation function. ECT: double renal perfusion machine function was normal. Glomerular filtration rate: 95.6 mL/min; the left side was 46.1 mL/min, and the right side was 49.5 mL/min. Urinary 64 CT: bilateral renal artery calcification; the rest had no obvious abnormalities. Bilateral renal vein showed no abnormalities. Multiple calcifications of abdominal aorta wall. No obvious abnormalities were found in the bilateral renal pelvis, ureter, and bladder. The tissue matching of donor and recipient is shown in Table 12.3.

In this case, we used the latest perioperative treatment plan (Fig. 12.6). *Rituximab* was administered 28 days before surgery with a dose of 200 mg. Before the operation, the patient's blood type antibody titer was low to 1:2 level (Fig. 12.7). Immunosuppression induction and the treatment were the same as before. The patient recovered well postoperatively. Ten days after then operation, the patient's serum creatinine has been reduced to 100 μmol/L and maintained its stability. After a long period of time (currently monitored for 34 days after surgery), the serum antibody titer of recipients was still maintained at a low level (Fig. 12.7).

Table 12.3 The tissue matching of donor and recipient

	Blood type	HLA-A	HLA-B	HLA-DR	PRAI/II (%)	CDC
Donor	O	31/24	52/4	10/14		5%
Recipient	B	31/–	51/4	16/14	-/-	

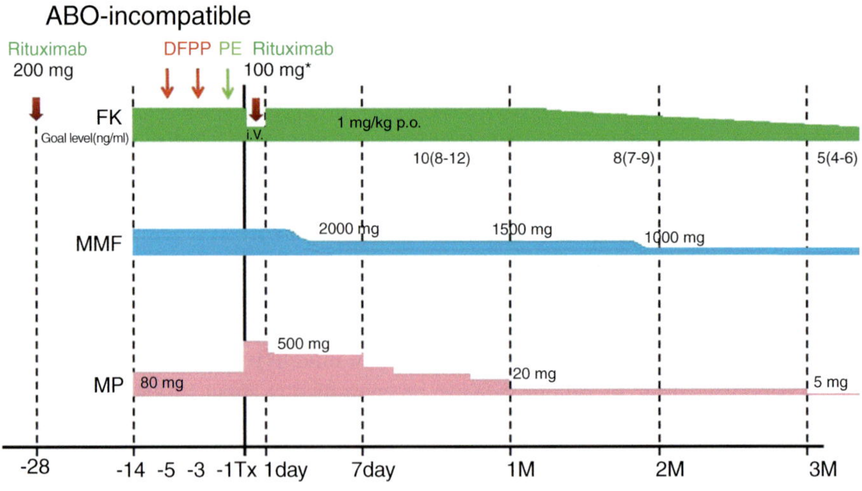

Fig. 12.6 New perioperative treatment scheme

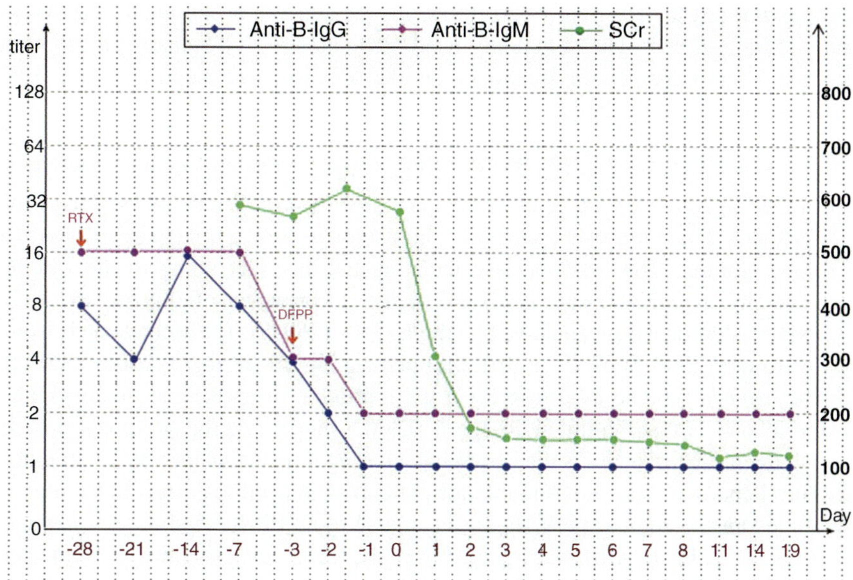

Fig. 12.7 Changes of anti-B antibodies and creatinine in perioperative recipients

After the use of a new perioperative protocol, thrombotic microvascular disease has become the most common complication instead of bleeding. In this way, effective anticoagulant therapy was more important. Because the ABO blood type was not compatible between the donor and the recipient, blood group antigens expressed on the surface of graft renal vascular endothelial cells and renal tubular epithelial cells can be combined with the blood type antibody in the recipient leading to plasma coagulation cascade and microvascular thrombosis in graft renal vascular. Anticoagulation is an important therapeutic measure to prevent the graft renal vascular of micro thrombosis.

There are many types of commonly used anticoagulants. In Chinese market there were unfractionated heparin, low molecular weight *heparin*, and natrium citricum. The former two are more frequently used in the ABOi-KT, while the latter one is used more in the centrifugal plasma separation (For example, the anticoagulant of fresh frozen plasma in blood bank is natrium citricum).

Heparin is a commonly used anticoagulant agent. The molecular weight is 6000–25,000 Da. Intravenous *heparin* anticoagulant has quick effect. It mainly plays an anticoagulant role through the combination and activation of *antithrombin* (AT-III). Specifically, the activation of AT-III can inactivate some factors, such as thrombin, activation factor XII, activation factor IX, and activation factor X, inhibit the fibrinogen changing to fibrin, and thereby inhibit the blood coagulation process. Heparin's half-life is about 1 h, which is inactivated in the liver and excreted by the kidneys. We have to add *heparin* to maintain the efficacy when the treatment time is more than 1 h. When we use heparin, the routine monitor of coagulation function is activated clotting time (ACT) and the Lee-White clotting time (LWCT). Activated clotting time (ACT) is normally 120–150 s, and the Lee-White clotting time (LWCT) tends to be 5–8 min. The commonly used methods are vivo heparinization, vitro heparinization, edge heparin treatment, and heparin-free treatment. Here is a brief description of these methods.

1. Vivo heparinization: It is suitable for patients without bleeding tendency. It can be injected directly into the veins of the body, and *heparin* can be added during the treatment. There are two options for the use of *heparin* on people with normal blood clotting. The first one is calculating the dose according to the weight. Generally, the initial dosage is 0.5–1.0 mg/kg (1 U *heparin* = 0.008 mg) (62.5 U), and the additional dose could be 6–8 mg/h (750–1250 U). The second one is using 16–40 mg (2000–5000 U) at first and then adding 20–28 mg/h (2500–3500 U). The *heparin* scheme used to prevent the formation of graft renal microvascular thrombosis is that the initial dosage is 0.3–0.5 mg/kg and the additional dose is 6–8 mg/h. The standard is the Lee-White clotting time maintained at 20–30 min.
2. Vitro heparinization: It is suitable for patients who need to correct the tendency of bleeding as soon as possible. In the course of DFPP, the first dose of *heparin* is not given, but *heparin* was injected from the artery, and protamine was injected from the vein to maintain basically the constancy of the clotting time of body. The dose of *heparin* injection was 0.375* blood flow *60. The amount of protamine can be determined referring to the instructions, normally 1:1 usage.
3. Edge heparinization: It is suitable for the patients with mild bleeding tendency. The standards is the Lee-White clotting time maintained at 9–16 min. The dose of *heparin* depends on ACT. If the patient's ACT exceeds the normal value of 40%, there is no need to use the first dose of heparin; directly add *heparin* 600 U/h. If not, the first dose is 750 U (equivalent to 6 mg heparin), and then maintain the additional dose of 1200 U/h, and monitor the ACT; reduce to 600 U/h when the ACT maintain at the standard value. If the patient's LWCT is more than 20 min, the first dose of *heparin* is not given. Just check it every half an hour during the treatment to determine whether to add heparin. *Heparin* was given as 6 mg/h (750 U) when it was added.

Low molecular weight *heparin* is a low molecular weight anticoagulant drug isolated from heparin. Its average molecular weight is 4000–6000 Da. It plays an anticoagulant role mainly by inhibiting the activation of *antithrombin* III. At the same time, it can maintain the anti-X an activity, thus weakening the effect of thrombin inhibition, enhance the antithrombotic effect, and reduce the risk of bleeding. In the course of treatment, a single dose of low molecular weight *heparin* 5000–6000 U can maintain for 4 h. However, its half-life is 2 h, so it can reduce the added dose. The dose of 6000 IU, H, bid is also suitable.

No matter which scheme is used, once the patient is in hypercoagulable or normal coagulation state, anticoagulant drugs should be used as soon as possible after operation to ensure the relatively low coagulation state, so as to prevent the patient from thrombotic microvascular disease.

7.2 Immune Adaptation Phenomenon

Case 3: Li XX, male, 48 years old

He was admitted to the hospital because of nausea and vomiting and oliguria for 5 months. He has a history of chronic glomerulonephritis. Physical examination: BP 150/90 mmHg, chronic anemia features. Biochemical examination, urine occult blood (+) and urine protein (+); blood routine test, Hb 76 g/L; renal function, Cr 592 μmol/L, BUN 23.52 mmol/L, UA 384 mmol/L. The other examinations showed no obvious abnormality. Admission diagnosis: (1) chronic glomerular nephritis, chronic renal failure (uremia period); (2) renal hypertension; (3) renal anemia. On June 11, 2008, the patient accepted ABOi-KT. The postoperative recovery was smooth. The current renal function: Cr 163 μmol/L, BUN 20 mmol/L, UA 208 mmol/L.

The healthy donor was Tang XX (uncle), male, 60 years old, from Dongan County, Hunan Province, who got admission for his voluntary donation to one kidney. Previous physical rehabilitation, the history of hepatitis, tuberculosis, and other infectious diseases was denied; there was no history of trauma, no history of blood transfusion, and no food allergy; the history of vaccination is unspecified. No obvious abnormal signs were found in the hospitalized patients. Biochemical examination: Blood routine, urine routine, and stool routine are normal; coagulation function, biochemical complete set, hepatitis A, and other auxiliary examinations were normal.

Physical examination: No obvious abnormal signs. The following were checked: the three conventional, blood coagulation function, biochemical full set, such as hepatitis, a full range of auxiliary examination for all the normality. The match detail refers to Table 12.4.

As can be seen from the above two figures, we have reduced the recipient's titer of anti-donor blood group antibodies. Anti-B IgG and IgM have been below 1:4 (Fig. 12.8), anti-A IgG and IgM have been below 1:8 before the operation, but from the eighth day after surgery, this value will increase at a rate of one to two orders per day. Despite being given DFPP treatment, it was still elevated. Especially on the 13th and 17th day, anti-A IgM increased to a high level of 1:512, which is four orders of magnitude exceeding the base titer. However, the level of serum creatinine was not changed (Fig. 12.9). There occurred no thrombotic microvascular disease and no serum creatinine increase until discharge. This kind of ABOi-KT recipients showed increased antibody to donor blood group, but there was no rejection, which was called immune adaptation.

Table 12.4 Tissue matching donor and recipient

	Blood type	HLA-A	HLA-B	HLA-DR	PRAI (%)	PRAII (%)	CDC
Recipient	O	11/–	13/60	12/–	0	0	
Donor	A	11/–	54/60	4/12			10%

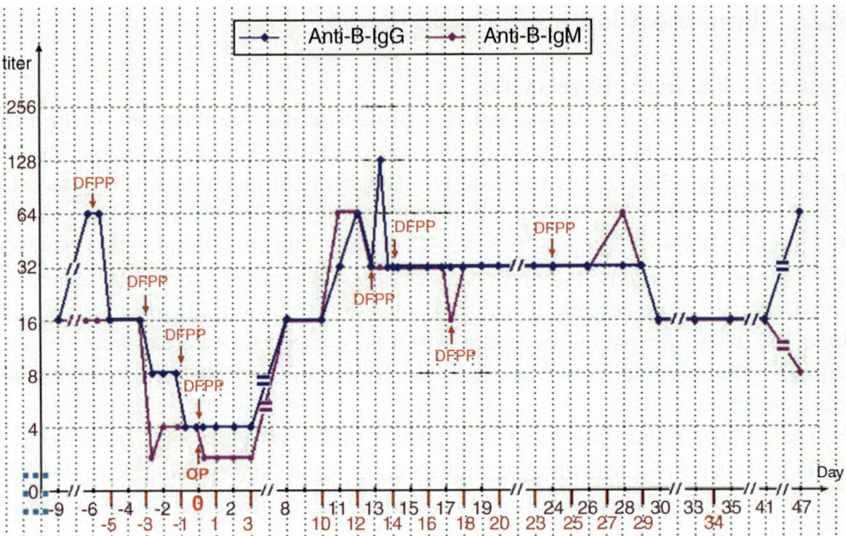

Fig. 12.8 Changes of anti-B antibody titer during perioperative period of Li XX

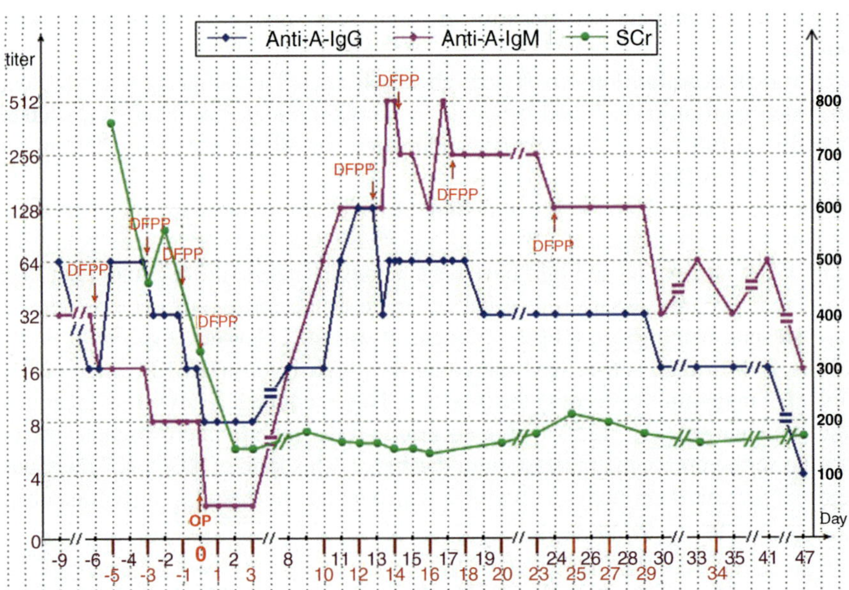

Fig. 12.9 Changes in the titer of anti-A antibody and serum creatinine of Li XX during perioperative period

7.3 ABO-Incompatible Renal Transplantation/Rh Double Blood Type System

Case 4: Hou XX, male, 28 years old

He was admitted to the hospital because of repeated systemic fatigue, loss of appetite, shortness of breath after activity lasing 3 years, skin itching, oliguria for half a year still June 24, 2010.

Three years ago, the patient began to have unexplained fatigue, lack of appetite, shortness of breath after activity, slightly relieved after the break. No cold, fever, no cough, expectoration, no facial edema, etc. During the visit in local hospital, the serum creatinine was 180 μmol/L and urine protein (+++). There was no obvious relief of symptoms after drug treatment (specifically unknown). In December 2009, the patient's symptoms gradually increased and began to have itching, and urine volume decreased. Assay of serum creatinine was 700 μmol/L. Irregular hemodialysis began in the local hospital. But the effect was poor. The patient had the highest creatinine level of 1131.1 μmol/L and urea nitrogen 36.49 mmol/L. So far, the patient's urine volume has been reduced to 100 mL/day. This time, the patient was hospitalized to receive a living relative donor ABOi-KT.

Past medical history: Facial paralysis in 2006; a history of mild hypertension (irregular taking of antihypertensive drug); no infectious diseases and chronic disease; no surgical trauma history; having a blood transfusion history; no drug allergy experience. The vaccination was unspecified.

Physical examinations: T 37.3 °C, R 20 times/min, P 96 times/min, BP 160/95 mmHg; wt: 58 kg, moderately nourished, chronic anemia features. Double lung breathe sound clear, having no rales. Heart sound blunt, with regular rhythm. There was no tenderness and percussion pain in both kidney areas, no tenderness in the bilateral ureter areas, and no swelling in the suprapubic bladder area. There was edema of lower extremities (±).

Laboratories and auxiliary examination: Blood type O Rh (−), routine blood test: RBC 2.65×10^{12}/L, PLT 158×10^{9}/L, Hb 78 g/L, LC 0.3×10^{9}/L, LYM 9.28%, NE 86.80%, and routine clotting function test; liver function is normal. Routine urine test: glucose in urine1+, BLD1+, urine protein3+; Renal function: serum creatinine, 866.00 μmol/L; urea nitrogen, 21.5 mmol/L; 24-h creatinine clearance rate 0.1 mL/min; 24-h urine protein quantification 48.4 mg; ESR 18 mm/h; Virological examination: HIV and syphilis detection were negative. Anti-"O," tumor markers, and thyroid function were not significantly abnormal. CMV-IgG, 113.9; CMV-IgM, 0; anti-B-IgG 1:64, anti-B-IgM 1:64. HLA: A (2/24), B (51/62), Bw (4/6), DR (9/15), and DRw (51/53). PRA class I and class II are 0%. Chest X-ray, bilateral pleural effusion; double lower lung infection is not excluded; enlargement of the heart shadow; abdominal B ultrasound, double kidney ultrasound changes, double kidney diffuse lesions, and double renal atrophy were considered. Ultrasonic cardiogram: left atrium, left ventricular mass, ventricular wall thickness, left ventricular diastolic and systolic function, pericardial effusion, and ventricular wall motion were reduced. Lung function showed severe mixed pulmonary ventilation dysfunction, severe restrictive pulmonary ventilation dysfunction, and severe obstructive pulmonary ventilation dysfunction. Heart rate variability report, low heart rate variability; 24-h dynamic electrocardiogram, paroxysmal two-degree type, two sinoatrial block, incidental two-degree, two atrioventricular block, paroxysmal ST-T change. Bilateral iliac vascular color Doppler ultrasound: no obvious abnormalities.

At 19:58, August 2, 2010, routine blood test showed that WBC decreased to 2.66×10^9/L, RBC 2.19×10^{12}/L, Hb 61 g/L, and PLT 43×10^9/L. The blood routine check at 21:57 showed WBC 3.16×10^9/L, RBC 2.6×10^{12}/L, Hb 73 g/L, and PLT 57×10^9/L; according to these results, bone marrow suppression was considered. The operation was discontinued, and the antirejection drugs such as *mycophenolate mofetil* and *tacrolimus* were discontinued. The line of bone marrow puncture on August 4, 2010, showed that the proliferation of bone marrow granulocytes was active, the proportion of young and middle-aged granulocytes increased, the red cell proliferation was active, the proportion of late red blood cells increased, the production plate of megakaryocyte decreased, the platelets scattered into small piles, and the proportion of neutrophils in blood increased.

Hou XX, a healthy donor, male, 54 years, was admitted for his voluntary kidney donation to his son.

Past medical history: No infectious diseases and chronic disease; no surgical trauma history; having a blood transfusion history; no drug allergy experience. The vaccination was unspecified.

Physical examinations: T 36.5 °C, R 20 times/min, P 80 times/min, BP 94/64 mmHg; wt: 65 kg, conscious, automatic body position. No positive signs of the heart, lung, and abdomen. There was no tenderness and percussion pain in both kidney areas, no tenderness in the bilateral ureter areas, and no swelling in the suprapubic bladder area. There was edema of lower extremities (±).

Laboratories and auxiliary examination: Blood type B Rh (+), EB virus antibody positive; renal function: serum creatinine, 103.1 μmol/L; urea nitrogen, 5.66 mmol/L; 24-h creatinine clearance rate 58.0 mL/min; 24-h urine protein quantification 87 mg; thyroid-stimulating hormone 5.6 μIU/ml (mIU/L) and cardiac troponin 0.43 ng/mL; ESR 9 mm/h; nephrogram (GFR, 64.8 mL/min; L, 35.5 mL/min; R 29.3 mL/min), right renal blood flow perfusion slightly decreased, and glomerular filtration function was slightly impaired; left renal blood flow and glomerular filtration function was not abnormal. Abdominal X-ray and intravenous urography showed (1) left renal pelvis and upper group of renal arc curve between the left and right kidney a cyst. Lumbar degeneration. Pulmonary function showed mild obstructive pulmonary ventilation dysfunction. The 24-h dynamic electrocardiogram showed occasional atrial premature contractions and sparse ventricular premature beats. CMV-IgG is 29.5; CMV-IgM is 0; CMV-DNA is negative. Virological examination showed HIV and syphilis detections were negative. The other examinations including blood routine, urine routine, stool routine, liver function, blood

Table 12.5 Tissue matching of donor and recipient

	ABO	Rh	HLA-A	HLA-B	HLA-DR	PRAI (%)	PRAII (%)
Donor	O	–	2/24	51/62	9/15	-	-
Recipient	A	+	24/–	54/62	4/15		

electrolyte, blood coagulation function, HBV-DNA, TB-IgG, TB-DNA, chest X-ray, cardiac ultrasound, abdominal B ultrasound, and double renal artery CTA showed no obvious abnormalities.

Tissue matching of donors and recipients is shown in Table 12.5.

After two hospital consultations on July 21, 2010, and August 31, 2010, regular treatment was administered such as hemodialysis, antivirus, anti-infection, blood pressure control, heart protection, diuresis, CRRT (CVVH), and DFPP treatment to reduce the anti-titer, and the patient's condition was improved. We applied to the health authorities for approval, and after having assessed the patient's general condition, we believed that the patient could tolerate the surgery, and then both ABO- and Rh-blood-type-incompatible renal allografts were performed under general anesthesia on September 1, 2010.

Intraoperative situation: we, respectively, performed end-to-side anastomosis to left renal vein of the donor with right external iliac vein of the recipient, and left renal artery of the donor with right external iliac artery of the recipient; we gave intravenous methylprednisolone (MP) 350 mg; leak detection experiments showed that anastomotic had no bleeding. Intravenous administration of furosemide 100 mg and inosine 1.0 g. Opening the renal vein and the renal artery blood flow, after 5 s, there was urine out flowing from the ureteral stump of donor kidney. There was no obvious bleeding and oozing on the graft kidney, and the tension, pulsation, and temperature of the graft kidney were normal. Hydropathic compressing graft kidney by hot saline wet was to promote renal blood supply. The intraoperative blood loss was about 250 mL. Three hundred milliliters AB Rh (+) plasma, 3.5 U O Rh (−) CRBC, human albumin 50 mL × 2 bottles, and prothrombin complex 200 U were transfused during the operation.

Postoperative condition: On September 2, B ultrasound showed that there was a small amount of effusion in the perirenal and right iliac fossa and a mass of unknown property, which was considered as the possibility of hematoma. Hemostatic agents such as cold precipitation, fresh frozen plasma, platelet, and other coagulation agents were used to stop bleeding. From September 2, 10:00 pm, the patient began to have difficulty breathing, feeling obvious shortness of breath even after slight activities, and cardiogram monitor showed oxygen saturation is low. On September 4, the chest and abdomen CT indicated pulmonary field and heart shadow change and pericardial and pleural effusion, which was considered as the possibility of heart failure pulmonary edema. Pulmonary infection is not excluded either; right pneumothorax. Normal change of right graft kidney. Accumulation of blood in renal bed; abdominal dropsy. After anti-infection, anti-immune rejection, blood transfusion, acid suppression, stomach protection, diuresis, and other symptomatic supportive treatment, the patient's condition improved. On September 13, the renal allograft drainage tube was removed, and the catheter was removed on September 15. Later, the patient was in overall good condition with stable vital signs and good abdominal wound healing and was transferred to the general ward on September 20.

Such case with rare ABO- and Rh-blood-type-incompatible renal transplantation has very low clinical probability, but the complex perioperative management still has a high clinical reference value.

The Rh blood group is the most significant blood type found after the discovery of ABO blood group, and it is also one of the most complex blood group systems. Rh-incompatible blood transfusion can endanger the patient's life. The proportion of Rh-negative blood in Chinese Han people ranged from 0.2 to 0.5%. However, the rate of Rh-negative blood recipients and pregnant women stimulated by Rh-positive antigen was as high as 99.6–99.8%. After an Rh-positive blood transfusion, more than 50% of the Rh-negative patients would produce anti-Rh antibodies. Since the Rh blood group antibody is a kind of immune antibody, if the Rh-positive blood reentered, the blood transfusion reaction is likely to occur; Rh blood test is equally important to ABO blood type. It should be noted that Rh-negative recipients must undergo Rh blood group identification, and it must be checked whether they have immune anti-Rh antibodies, so we can prevent the transfusion hemolytic disease caused by blood group incompatibility. It is feasible for Rh-negative recipients to receive Rh-positive donors in the absence of organ shortage. The Rh antigen only expresses on the surface of red blood cells, and vascular endothelial cells do not express the antigen. There are only a few red blood cells transfused from the donor's kidney into the recipients' circulatory system. Therefore, the proportion of anti-Rh antibodies produced by the Rh-negative recipient after receiving the Rh-positive donor's kidney was low. But we need to pay attention to the transfusion of blood products to recipients in the following aspects: (1) in emergency transfusion, Rh-negative blood can be transferred to Rh-positive recipient who has compatible A, B, and O blood type. (2) Rh-negative plasma can be transfused to Rh-positive patients if the blood is successfully crossed with the recipient's red blood cells. (3) Rh antigen does not exist on the surface of platelets. It is advisable to use products containing red blood cells below 0.4 mL. (4) Every recipient will undergo antibody screening tests before transfusion. For each patient, with anti-D antibodies test before red blood cell transfusion, only about 1 in 300,000 patients, Rh-negative-concentrated red blood cell transfusion is preferable. But in emergency cases, infusion of Rh-positive red blood cells is also feasible.

A group of foreign data display that incompatibility in the Rh blood group does not affect the short-term survival rate of renal transplant recipients. Therefore, we suggest that Rh blood type incompatibility is not a major obstacle to renal transplantation. If the donor and recipient are well matched, the kidneys have adequate lavage, and the appropriate immunosuppressive agents are used, the Rh-negative patients can still receive donor kidneys to Rh-positive recipients. But we should pay attention to improving the long-term survival rate.

Nowadays, in many European countries, especially in Sweden and Germany, *rituximab* has been used in different immunosuppressive protocols of ABOi-KT and has become a common method of blood group antibodies purge. Tyden et al.

reported the first case of using immune sorbent and *rituximab* instead of splenectomy to complete ABOi-KT. The immunosuppressive protocols commonly used in Europe and other countries are as follows: a single dose of *rituximab* (375 mg/m^2) was administered for 2–4 weeks before immunization, and the conventional protocols combined *tacrolimus*, *mycophenolate mofetil*, and prednisone which were used 1 week before immunization. The blood group antibody was removed by immune adsorption before operation, and the concentration of antibody was less than 1:8. Finally, IVIG 0.5 g/kg. In order to avoid the rebound of antibody concentration, immune adsorption therapy was applied on the ninth day after operation. During the follow-up, serum creatinine levels remained normal, and no incidence of blood type antibody occurred. The program has successfully treated 60 patients in Germany and Sweden within 5 years.

In ABOi-KT, plasmapheresis, CMV-IgG, and anti-VD20 can be used instead of splenectomy. The treatment scheme is as follows. The recipients received four to five times plasmapheresis to remove the blood group antibodies preoperatively and to ensure that the serum antibody titer was less than 1:16. 1–2 days before transplantation, a single dose of *rituximab* (375 mg/kg) was used. After transplantation, *tacrolimus* and *mycophenolate mofetil* were used, followed by steroids. The postoperative treatment also included intravenous immunoglobulin and plasmapheresis on the first day, third day, and fifth day after operation. The mean serum creatinine level was 1.2–1.4 mg/dL, and renal function is stable after the implementation of this scheme (Fig. 12.10). The patient's blood group antibody returned to the preoperative level (Fig. 12.11), but no humoral rejection occurred.

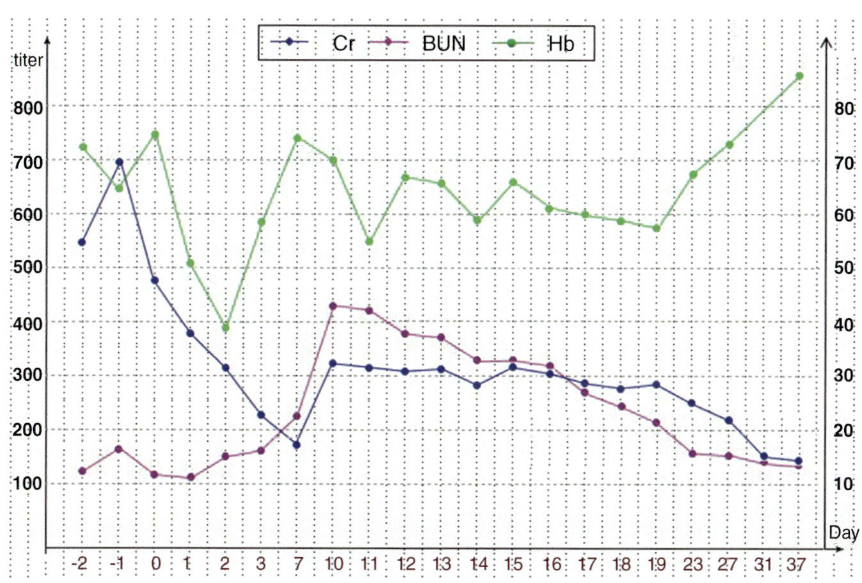

Fig. 12.10 Postoperative changes of hemoglobin and renal function

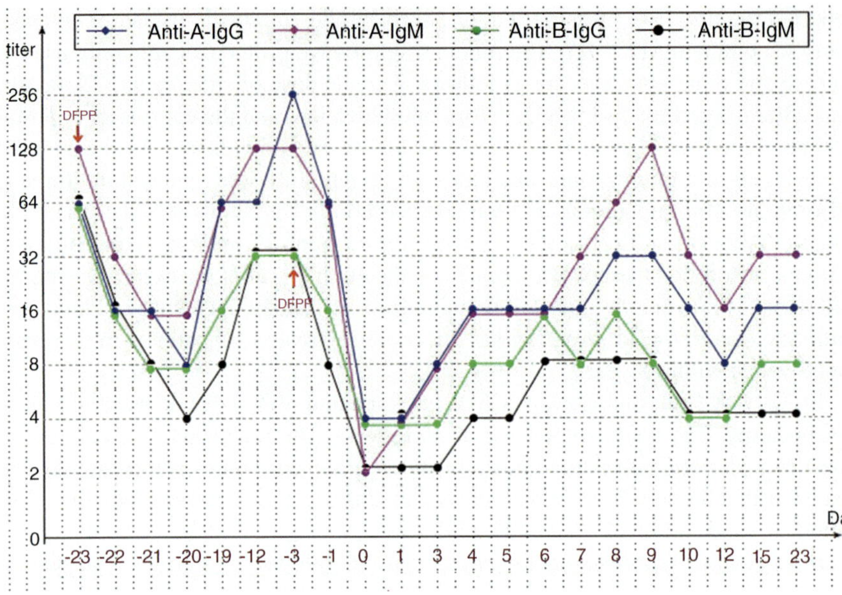

Fig. 12.11 Changes of blood group antibodies after surgery

Japan has the leading position in the world in ABOi-KT area. During 1989–2001, Japan had tried various immunosuppressive protocols, including an in vitro antibody removal program to make the recipient's preoperative titer less than 1:16. There are also drug immunosuppression, anticoagulation, and splenectomy (98% recipients received splenectomy). The immunosuppressive triple regimen is based on calcium-dependent phosphatase inhibitors, steroids, and antibody metabolites. After transplantation, antibody clearance therapy is not routinely required. Review of the past Japanese cases shows that the short-term prognosis of ABOi-KT is not as good as that of ABOc-KT, but the long-term prognosis is almost the same. The survival rates of ABOi-KT recipients after 1, 3, 5, 7, and 9 years, respectively, were 93%, 89%, 87%, 85%, and 84%, the graft renal survival rates, respectively, were 84%, 80%, 71%, 65%, and 59%. After 2001, with the use of new immunosuppressive protocols, MMF, and anti-CD25 molecular antibodies, the survival rates of graft survival rates increased to 96% and 94%. Since 2004, splenectomy has been replaced by DFFP, *rituximab*, MMF, and steroids because it has failed to improve short-term prognosis. Studies in other centers, including Tokyo Women's Medical University and John Hopkins University, have reported no significant differences in the 5-year survival rate and 5-year graft survival rate between ABOi-KT and ABOc-KT.

7.4 An Early Japanese Report

Case 5: A 24-year-old patient with nephrotic syndrome, male, blood type A
The patient was diagnosed with end-stage renal disease at the age of 3, continuous ambulatory peritoneal dialysis (CAPD) was first used, but peritonitis occurred. In April of the same year, it was changed to hemodialysis (HD). In 1986, when the patient was 9 years old, the patient underwent ABOc-KT. The donor was the patient's mother (blood type A1, HLA-A, B, DR: ALL, –, B54, –, DR4, DR8). Unfortunately, the patient had to accept HD because of the CAN occurrence in 1999 when the recipient was 22 years old.

In March 2001, the patient required a second kidney transplantation. The kidney donor was his father, who was blood type B. The cross matching and typing from donor lymphocytes was strong positive, and thus MP 4 mg/dL, MMF 50 mg/day, and CYA 50–100 mg/day were given to ensure the titer of the T-cell antibodies is close to preoperative standard. In October, the cross matching turned to negative, but the recipient is highly immune responder, so continued to immunosuppressive therapy. The donor and recipient tissue matching are shown in Table 12.6.

In March 2002, the patient had only one preoperative DFPP because of the low titer of anti-B blood type antibodies (IgM = 1:8; IgG = 0). ABOi-KT was performed on April 3, 2002, when the preoperative antibody titer was decreased (IgM = 1:2; IgG was 0), and the result of cross matching test was negative.

After surgery, the recipients received immunosuppressive therapy with CyA, MP, MMF, and infliximab. The graft renal function was stable. The serum creatinine was 5.2 mg/dL on the second day and 0.6 mg/dL on the fifth day. On the ninth day after operation, the titer of anti-B-cell IgM antibody increased to 1:32, which was immediately treated with DFPP. Although no clinical symptoms were found, MP shock treatment was still performed for the patient. We switched the calcineurin inhibitor from CyA to FK506 to prevent acute rejection. On the 12th day after operation, the patient received the second DFFP treatment because the titer of anti-B-cell antibody increased again (IgM = 1:64). On the same day, the recipient began to demonstrate cytomegalovirus viremia, granulocytopenia, and thrombocytopenia. Thus we reduced the dose of MMF to 50 mg/day and gave high titer gamma protein of ganciclovir and CMV.

Although the titer of anti-B-cell antibody IgM maintained at 1:32–1:64 for a period of time, yet in order to reduce the risk of infection, they still did not give strong immune suppression and just kept an eye on the situation of recipient. After

Table 12.6 Tissue matching of donor and recipient

	Blood type	HLA-A	HLA-B	HLA-DR	PRAI (%)	PRAII (%)
Recipient	A	11/24	54/56	4/–	0	0
Donor	B	24/–	52/54	8/–		

a period of time, the titer of anti-B-cell antibody began to decline. The serum creatinine level was maintained at 0.6–0.8 mg/dL, and the graft renal function was well.

A few months later after transplantation, FK506 2.5 mg/dL, MP 8 mg/day, and MMF 500 mg/day were administered. After 1 year, the immunosuppressive protocols were adjusted to FK506 2 mg/dL, MP 4 mg/day, and MMF 500 mg/day. The renal function of the recipient recovered well.

According to incomplete statistics, the 1-year survival rate of adult renal transplant recipients in our country is above 90%, or even 95% in some centers. But only about 50% of the patients survived for 10 years or more. According to the statistics of American kidney information system, the 5-year survival rate and 10-year survival rate of living donor kidney transplantation were respectively 88% and 76%. The 5-year survival rate and 10-year survival rate of cadaveric renal transplantation were respectively 76% and 54%. Pediatric living donor kidney transplantation mainly refers to recipients under 18 years old. More than 50% of pediatric kidney transplant recipients in North America are living kidney transplantation. The 5-year survival rate of living kidney transplantation in children was over 96%, the survival rate of donor kidney in 1 year was more than 95%, and the rejection rate was lower than 25%. The reason for the decrease of rejection rate may be related to the substitution of FK506 for CSA, MMF, and Rapa instead of Aza. Methylprednisone is generally not used or discontinued.

In addition, laparoscopic nephrectomy results in more DGF and rejection than open nephrectomy, and the 1-year and 2-year survival rates are also slightly lower. This effect is more obvious in younger patients.

References

1. Shishido S, Hyodo YY, Aoki Y, et al. Outcomes of pediatric abo-incompatible kidney transplantations are equivalent to abo-compatible controls. Transplant Proc. 2012;44:214–6.
2. Warren DS, Montgomery RA. Incompatible kidney transplantation: lessons from a decade of desensitization and paired kidney exchange. Immunol Res. 2010;47:257–64.
3. Beimler J, Zeier M. Abo-incompatible transplantation—a safe way to perform renal transplantation? Nephrol Dial Transplant. 2007;22:25–7.
4. Kobayashi T, Liu D, Ogawa H, et al. Removal of blood group a/b antigen in organs by ex vivo and in vivo administration of endo-beta-galactosidase (abase) for abo-incompatible transplantation. Transpl Immunol. 2009;20:132–8.
5. Montgomery JR, Berger JC, Warren DS, et al. Outcomes of abo-incompatible kidney transplantation in the United States. Transplantation. 2012;93:603–9.
6. Toki D, Ishida H, Setoguchi K, et al. Acute antibody-mediated rejection in living abo-incompatible kidney transplantation: long-term impact and risk factors. Am J Transplant. 2009;9:567–77.
7. Tanabe T, Ishida H, Horita S, et al. Decrease of blood type antigenicity over the long-term after abo-incompatible kidney transplantation. Transpl Immunol. 2011;25:1–6.
8. Rienstra H, Boersema M, Onuta G, et al. Donor and recipient origin of mesenchymal and endothelial cells in chronic renal allograft remodeling. Am J Transplant. 2009;9:463–72.
9. Kwon O, Miller S, Li N, et al. Bone marrow-derived endothelial progenitor cells and endothelial cells may contribute to endothelial repair in the kidney immediately after ischemia-reperfusion. J Histochem Cytochem. 2010;58:687–94.

10. Taylor RP, Lindorfer MA. Impact of low-dose rituximab on splenic B cells: evidence for the shaving reaction. Transpl Int. 2010;23:116–7.
11. Li Y, Williams ME, Cousar JB, et al. Rituximab-CD20 complexes are shaved from Z138 mantle cell lymphoma cells in intravenous and subcutaneous SCID mouse models. J Immunol. 2007;179:4263–71.
12. Tasaki M, Nakajima T, Imai N, et al. Detection of allogeneic blood group a and b enzyme activities in patients with abo incompatible kidney transplantation. Glycobiology. 2010;20:1251–8.
13. Genberg H, Kumlien G, Wennberg L, et al. Isoagglutinin adsorption in abo-incompatible transplantation. Transfus Apher Sci. 2010;43:231–5.
14. Silvestre C, Furian L, Marson P, et al. Desensitization with plasmapheresis and anti-CD20 for abo incompatible kidney transplantation from living donor: experience of a single center in Italy. Transplant Proc. 2014;46:2209–13.
15. Takahashi K, Saito K. Abo-incompatible kidney transplantation. Transplant Rev (Orlando). 2013;27:1–8.
16. Tasaki M, Saito K, Nakagawa Y, et al. 20-year analysis of kidney transplantation: a single center in Japan. Transplant Proc. 2014;46:437–41.
17. Oettl T, Halter J, Bachmann A, et al. Abo blood group-incompatible living donor kidney transplantation: a prospective, single-centre analysis including serial protocol biopsies. Nephrol Dial Transplant. 2009;24:298–303.
18. Zschiedrich S, Kramer-Zucker A, Janigen B, et al. An update on abo-incompatible kidney transplantation. Transpl Int. 2015;28:387–97.
19. Yi Wang, Zhi Gang Luo, Peigen Gui, et al. A case report of living relative ABO incompatible kidney transplantation which had preserved the spleen of recipients. Chinese J Organ Transplant. 2007;28:694–5.

Experience with ABO-Incompatible Lung Transplantation

13

Bo Wu, Li Fan, and Hang Yang

Abstract

In this chapter, we focused on introducing the experience with ABO-incompatible lung transplantation, including the selection of patients and donors, the indications for lung transplantation, the perioperative treatment of ABO-incompatible lung transplantation, and the treatment of postoperative complications. In the end, we showed two case reports of ABO-incompatible lung transplantation.

Keywords

ABO-incompatible · Lung transplantation · Selection of donors · Selection of recipients · Indications · Complications · Immunosuppression · Rejection Bronchiolitis obliterans syndrome

Nowadays, there are many treatments for early respiratory diseases with preserved lung function, but the treatment of end-stage lung disease is not enough. Allograft lung transplantation is the only feasible method for the treatment of end-stage lung disease on the basis of successful experiments, which makes more and more patients with end-stage lung disease get the hope of life. In 1963, Dr. Hardy tried the first lung transplant in humans, and the patient survived for 18 days after the operation. Since then, 40 lung transplants had been reported in the world in about 20 years, but only one patient lived for about 10 months. In the early 1980s of the last century, the new highly effective immunosuppressive drug, cyclosporine A, was put into clinical practice and made lung transplantation, like other solid organ transplantations, enter a new period of vigorous development. Three main operations,

B. Wu (✉) · L. Fan · H. Yang
Department of Pulmonary and Critical Care Medicine, Lung Transplant Center, Wuxi People's Hospital, Nanjing Medical University, Wuxi, Jiangsu, China
e-mail: 15852759830@126.com; manutdfl123@126.com; yanghang-0000@163.com

Y. Wang (ed.), *ABO-incompatible Organ Transplantation*,
https://doi.org/10.1007/978-981-13-3399-6_13

including single- and double-lung transplantation and heart-lung transplantation, have been successively successful. So far, around 60,107 cases of single- and double-lung transplantation have been completed worldwide, and the rate of about 4000 cases has increased each year. Lung transplantation in mainland China dates back to 1979. In the Beijing Institute of Tuberculosis, Professor Xin Yuling tried to perform a lung transplant for two patients with tuberculosis. From January 1994 to January 1998, a total of about 20 cases of lung transplantation were carried out in Beijing, Guangzhou, and other places. However, because of the complications and the low survival rate of the patients, the clinical lung transplantation in our country has stagnated for 5 years. Until September 2002, Professor Chen Jingyu of Wuxi People's Hospital successfully carried out lung transplantation for emphysema for the first time in our country, which started the work of lung transplantation in our country again. In 2010, the National Health and Family Planning Commission of PRC commissioned the Wuxi People's Hospital to establish the data center of lung transplantation in China, which is responsible for the daily management, operation, maintenance, and data verification of the data centers for lung transplantation. At present, including Wuxi People's Hospital, China-Japan Friendship Hospital of Beijing, and The First Hospital Affiliated of Guangzhou Medical College, a total of 31 transplant units have been registered. According to the data from the China lung transplantation data center, 18 hospitals have carried out lung transplants in the country since 2005 to the end of 2016. Since 2002 to the end of 2016, 918 cases of lung transplantation have been completed.

The lungs are respiratory organs, communicating with the atmosphere, affecting by the environment, more exposure to pathogens, and the respiratory tracts of patients after transplantation have poor self-clearance ability, and the transplanted lung has more severe ischemia reperfusion injury than other transplanted solid organ. In addition, lung transplantation requires higher surgical skills and better lung donors, and the postoperative patients have more severe rejections and complications. Therefore, lung transplantation has the most difficult level in human solid organ transplantations. Lung transplantation has been in China for many years, but with the increasing number of patients with end-stage lung diseases, the biggest obstacle facing clinicians is not the medical technology itself. In developed countries, patients begin to consider lung transplant in waiting list and prepare for lung transplant when the expected life is less than 2 years. But in China, many patients won't think about lung transplant until the last few months of their lives, and they die without time to wait for the optimum lung donor. To patients suffering from end-stage lung diseases, medical treatment is often difficult to be effective, relying on the ventilator, ECMO and other auxiliary device to relieve the symptoms and prolong life, but even so, the survival time of patients often can't keep long. An excellent lung transplant team should include the technical elites in department of thoracic surgery, respiratory medicine, ICU, anesthesia, central laboratory, professional nursing, and other related disciplines. Transplant surgeons should not only have the technical skill on the operating table, but also become experts in organ acquisition, anesthesia, operating cooperation, postoperative anti-rejection, anti-infection treatment, rehabilitation and follow-up management. At present, the lung preservation technique requires cold ischemia time within 4~6 h; the excessive prolongation of time will lead to the increase of rejection and organ ischemia injury. Therefore, the entire operation time generally required is within 6 h; otherwise the risk of surgery may increase and even lead to failure of lung transplantation. So, from the moment the lung is taken out of the donor, the lung transplant is a race against time.

1 Selection of Donors and Patients

1.1 Selection of Donors

Due to the severe shortage of donors, 2000 patients in the United States are waiting for lungs each year, and only 10–20% of the available donors are standard donors. In order to maximize the use of donors, based on in vitro evaluation of lungs, many research centers use expanded standard donor and marginal donor as important supplements to donor sources, especially use of lungs without heartbeat. Loyola University reported 18 cases of lung transplant recipients with heavier illness that could not wait for standard lungs and accepted no heartbeat lungs, the average thermal ischemia time was 36 min (19~93 min), and the average cold ischemia time was 349 min (221~480 min). As a result, 88.8% of the recipients were discharged (16/18), with a 1 year survival rate of 88.5% (14/16) and a maximum survival of 3410 days (9 years and 4 months), reaching a similar effect with heartbeat lung transplantation [1].

1.1.1 Donor Inclusion Criteria

1. Inclusion criteria for brain-dead donor — "Chinese criteria for brain death (exposure draft)". 2. In line with medical ethics standards. 3. Cardiopulmonary death donor inclusion criteria: three objective indicators (no spontaneous breathing, no spontaneous heartbeat, dilated and fixed pupils without light reflex), cardiopulmonary resuscitation for 30 min and invalid.

1.1.2 Lung Selection Criteria

1. Lung transplantation donor age <60 years and heart-lung transplantation donor age <55 years.
2. No history of primary heart disease (heart donor) and lung disease (lung donor).
3. No history of smoking and no history of heart and lung surgery.
4. No severe chest trauma, no extensive pulmonary contusion, and no aspiration pneumonia/abscess; clear and normal chest X-ray plain film.
5. When $FiO_2 = 1.0$, PEEP = 6.65 kPa, PaO_2 >40 kPa (300 mmHg).
6. Lung compliance is normal (tidal volume = 15 mL/kg, peak pressure <39.9 kPa).
7. Bronchoscopy shows normal finding, with no evidence of aspiration or inflammation; if the bronchoscopy does not find signs of airway mucosal inflammation, the G (+) bacteria and purulent secretion can be ignored.
8. ABO blood type and size match with recipients.

9. Malignant diseases (except for primary intracranial tumors), HIV, and hepatitis virus screening are negative. Those who meet this standard are "ideal donors."
10. Due to the severe lack of donors and the increasing number of patients, many transplant centers will relax the selection criteria for the lungs, and other countries in the world are relaxing the selection criteria.

Potential lung donors who fail to meet these criteria are still classified as lung donors and are called "marginal donors"; criteria such as donor age, smoking history, Gram stain (+), etc. can be moderately relaxed; so far, incompatible ABO blood type lung transplantation also has progressed abroad [2].

1.2 Selection of Recipients

1.2.1 Recipient Exclusion Criteria

1. Malignant tumors which happened within 2 years (except for skin squamous cell carcinoma and basal cell carcinoma); but a few centers take bronchioloalveolar carcinoma as an indication, which is still controversial.
2. Organ dysfunction in another system that cannot be cured.
3. Chronic extrapulmonary infection that cannot be cured and severe thoracic or spinal deformity.
4. Poor compliance to treatment or follow-up and psychological or mental illness that cannot be cured.
5. Lack of solid and reliable social support [3].

1.2.2 General Condition of Recipients

To select a lung transplant recipient, the patient's age, heart, kidney, liver, nutrition, immunity, and mental state should be evaluated.

Age: Hosenpud concluded that the prognosis of older recipients was poorer than younger recipients according to the data registered in the International Society for Heart and Lung Transplantation, thus making the following recommendations: (1) heart-lung transplantation ≤55 years old, (2) sequential bilateral lung transplantation ≤60 years old, and (3) single-lung transplantation ≤65 years old. But the actual clinical work should depend on specific circumstances.

Renal function: Normal renal function is generally required to potential recipients of lung transplantation because the renal toxicity of the immunosuppressive agents such as cyclosporine A and tacrolimus (FK506), which are used after lung transplantation, will accelerate the deterioration of renal function in patients with renal dysfunction.

Liver function: Liver function is generally required to be normal, without portal hypertension, for lung transplantation to be feasible. Patients with hepatitis B history, hepatitis B virus DNA-positive patients and hepatitis C patients suffering from serious liver injury are not suitable for lung transplantation. Postoperative high-dose steroid medication will cause hepatitis B and hepatitis C virus to activate again, to speed up replication, and to induce the recurrence of hepatitis.

Cardiac function: patients with coronary heart disease are generally not suitable for lung transplantation. Surgery has the risk of inducing myocardial infarction, which is consistent with foreign perspectives; a patient with severe left ventricular systolic and diastolic dysfunction cannot be a lung transplant recipient but can be a heart-lung transplant recipient. A patient with chronic hypoxia, pulmonary hypertension, right heart enlargement, and abnormal right heart function still can be a lung transplant recipient. Because hemodynamics will change after single or bilateral lung transplantation, right heart function and volume can be improved significantly. However, severe heart disease (especially heart failure) is still a relative contraindication of lung transplantation, and about 9% of patients who die within 90 days after lung transplantation die of perioperative heart failure, and such patients may consider heart-lung transplantation.

The nutrition state of recipients is closely related to postoperative rehabilitation, reduction of infection, and accelerated wound healing, so the weight is desirable to be in the range of 70–130% of the ideal weight.

The volume of donor lung and recipient lung is required to match; a too large donor lung will cause pulmonary tamponade after closing the chest, which will affect venous return, causing cough and weakness in clearing secretions, and there will be atelectasis and infection problems as well. If the donor lung is too small, there will be a cavity left in the chest, which is susceptible to have pyothorax, especially to recipients with inflammatory lung diseases.

Donor lung procurement: all donor lungs adopt raffinose low-potassium dextran solution (R-LPD) as organ-preserving solution. The specific parameters of perfusion and preservation are shown in Table 13.1 [4].

Synchronous procurement of the heart, lungs, liver, and kidneys: multiple donor organ procurement requires close cooperation of cardiac surgery, thoracic surgery, and other departments. Clear preoperative division is needed. Generally, heart-lung transplantation group completes intubation of aorta and pulmonary artery before abdominal surgery group completes hepatorenal intubation. After the two groups complete intubation, perfusion is carried out, respectively, at the same time. The thoracic group should consider the needs of the liver and the heart when cutting the inferior vena cava. Generally, the inferior vena cava is cut at 0.5 cm above the diaphragm. The heart and lung transplant doctors carry out the separation together after

Table 13.1 Lung perfusion and preservation plan recommended by Toronto Lung Transplantation Group in 2004

Index	Range
Antegrade perfusion volume of R-LPD solution	50–60 mL/kg
Retrograde perfusion volume	250 mL/pulmonary vein
Pulmonary arterial pressure of antegrade perfusion	10–15 mmHg
Temperature of perfusate	4–8 °C
Mechanical ventilation	VT 10 mL/kg, PEEP 5 cm H_2O
Oxygen concentration/oxygen ratio	≤50%
Tracheal blocking pressure	15–20 cm H_2O
Storage temperature	4–8 °C

the whole of the heart and lung is acquired, ensuring the integrity of the left atrial sleeve of the donor lung as far as possible. Close cooperation is required in transplant teams.

Separation and clipping of the heart and lung: move the heart and lung to another operating table. Heart and lung transplant doctors carry out the separation together. Separate the aorta and pulmonary artery at 3 cm above the aortic ring and 1 cm above the pulmonary arterial ring. Cut off the left atrium at the proximal atrial wall 0.5 cm away from the opening of upper and lower pulmonary vein, and complete the separation of the heart and lung. Move the two lungs to another operating table, and perform the retrograde perfusion of donor lungs again.

Separation of the left and right donor lung: dissociate the distal part of the pulmonary trunk of the donor lung in the operating room, and divide the left and right pulmonary arteries from the middle of the initial segment. Cut the back wall of the left atrium open in the middle of the left and right pulmonary veins. Clip under direct vision. Left superior and inferior pulmonary veins and part of the back wall of the left atrium formed the left part of left atrial sleeve. Right superior and inferior pulmonary veins and part of the back wall of the left atrium formed the right part of left atrial sleeve. Cut off the left main bronchus near the carina using a cutting stapling device, and separate the left and right donor lungs. Dissociate left and right pulmonary arteries to their first branches, and ligate the bronchial artery. Retain the connective tissue around the bronchus as much as possible. Cut off the left and right main bronchus about two cartilage rings above the opening of bilateral superior lobar bronchus. Use a large cotton pad saturated with R-LPD solution to cover and protect the donor lungs when the clipping is completed, and wait for the recipients [5].

1.2.3 Indications for Transplantation of Recipients

End-stage benign pulmonary diseases with lung function severely damaged, medicine and routine surgery invalid, daily activities severely restricted, life expectancy only 1–2 years, no dysfunction of other important organs. Chronic obstructive pulmonary disease (COPD), idiopathic pulmonary fibrosis (IPF), pulmonary cystic fibrosis, α-1 antitrypsin deficiency, and idiopathic pulmonary hypertension account for 85% of the whole lung transplantation spectrum of diseases. The remaining 15% is composed of relatively rare diseases such as sarcoidosis and pulmonary lymphatic leiomyomatosis. When selecting lung transplant recipients, the life expectancy of patients doing or not doing lung transplantation and the improvement of patients' quality of life after lung transplantation should be comprehensively measured, to determine whether to include the patients in the transplant waiting list (see Table 13.2). The International Society for Heart and Lung Transplantation registered more than 51,400 cases of adult lung transplant recipients in more than 155 transplant centers worldwide. According to the registration in 2015, the median survival time of adult lung transplant recipients is about 5.6 years, and the median survival time of bilateral lung transplantation is longer than single-lung transplantation (6.6 years vs. 4.6 years).

Table 13.2 Indications for inclusion in the lung transplant list

Diseases	Lung function	Arterial blood gases	Others
Emphysema	FEV1 <25% of expectation	PCO_2 >55 mm Hg and PO_2 <60 mmHg	Pulmonary hypertension
Pulmonary cystic fibrosis	FEV1 <25% of expectation	PCO_2 >55 mmHg and PO_2 <60 mmHg	Frequent hospitalization
Idiopathic pulmonary fibrosis	FVC <60% of expectation DLCO <39% of expectation FVC or DLCO decrease over 10% in the follow-up of past 6 months	Hypoxia after activity	Ineffective medical treatments
Pulmonary hypertension			III–IV grade pulmonary hypertension after using medicine

Table 13.3 Evaluation of lung function

	Before transplantation		After single-lung transplantation		After bilateral lung transplantation
	COPD	Pulmonary interstitial fibrosis	COPD	Pulmonary interstitial fibrosis	
FEV1%	40–50%	About 20%	63.2%	51.2%	87.9%
PaO_2	≤50 mmHg		84–92 mmHg		98.8 mmHg
$PaCO_2$	≥50 mmHg		34–48 mmHg		
6-min walk test	≤300 m(with oxygen)		Over 600–700 m (without oxygen)		
Ventilation			Ventilation of transplanted lung is 37%, while autologous lung is 63%	Ventilation of transplanted lung is 60%, while autologous lung is 40%	
Blood flow			Blood flow of transplanted lung is 80%, while autologous lung is 20%	Blood flow of transplanted lung is 82%, while autologous lung is 18%	

Preoperative Evaluation of Lung Function (Table 13.3)

There are a few differences between obstructive lung diseases and interstitial lung diseases. When VC is about 20–50%, FEV1% of the former is 40–50%, FEV1% of the latter is around 20%, over half of the patients need oxygen therapy. In that condition, almost all the patients show PaO_2 ≤50 mmHg and $PaCO_2$ ≥50 mmHg and can only walk 300 m in the 6-min walk test.

1.3 Therapeutic Regimen

1.3.1 Immunosuppression

Standard triple immunosuppressive therapy (CNI, antiproliferatives, and corticosteroids) can be used in ABO-incompatible lung transplantation, which can reduce rejection reaction after transplantation.

Inductive Treatment

Rabbit antithymocyte globulin (RATG) can be used in inductive treatment. MMF can directly inhibit B cells and reduce the production of B cells [6]. There are some antibodies in RATG that can directly kill B cells, therefore increasing the efficiency of immunosuppression early after the operation.

Furthermore, RATG is likely to control antibody response. If there is unstable hemodynamics or moderate to severe reperfusion injury, RATG treatment can be delayed to the second or third day after operation. If there is severe bronchospasm or dysfunction in hemodynamics, OKT3 can be used instead of RATG treatment after acute adverse reaction is relieved.

Maintenance Treatment

Cyclosporin A, steroid, MMF used as maintenance immunosuppressive treatment instead of azathioprine in some improved immunosuppressive therapies.

1.3.2 Intraoperative Treatment

ABO-incompatible lung transplantation can take advantage of extracorporeal circulation to do plasmapheresis during operation, wiping off donor-specific alloantibody of blood cell, with no need of immunosuppressive treatment or splenectomy.

1.3.3 Transfusion of Blood Products

Children who accepted ABO-incompatible lung transplantation cannot transfuse whole blood. It must be informed to the family members and be reminded to medical workers when accepting emergency treatment or surgery in the future. Type O red blood cell and type AB plasma are safe to be transfused to all blood types. If the recipient needs to transfuse red blood cell, the type of red blood cell should match with the ABO blood type of the recipient. If the recipient needs to transfuse platelet or plasma, the type of blood products should match with the ABO blood type of the donor.

1.3.4 Intravenous Immunoglobulin(IVIG)

The purposes of using IVIG:

1. Supplement immunoglobulin depleted by nonspecific immunoadsorption to reduce the risk of infection
2. Regulate and treat a series of autoimmune diseases and antibody-mediated rejection of HLA-sensitized patients after transplantation [7]

1.3.5 Other Treatments

Other treatments such as ventilation, etc. are not different from other ABOi organ transplantations, so we don't go into details here.

2 Diagnosis and Treatment of Postoperative Complications

2.1 Monitoring of Rejection

2.1.1 Imaging

Reperfusion Pulmonary Edema

The image findings are pulmonary cloudy shadows; the lesions usually appear in the entire transplanted lung, especially the basal segment of lower lobe; hilar shadow is not enlarged, lung volume doesn't shrink; and the shadow of exudation generally absorbs and disappears spontaneously within 3 days.

Acute Rejection

Chest X-ray shows slight grid-form shadow of the pulmonary interstitium, consolidation of the pulmonary segment, and pulmonary mass around the hilus. In addition, it's reported that the interlobular septal thickening and the aggressive or new pleural effusion suggested the diagnosis of acute rejection, the sensitivity was 68%, and the specificity was 90%. The manifestation of high-resolution CT (HRCT) includes ground glass opacity (GGO), pulmonary segment consolidation, interlobular septal thickening, pleural effusion, and lung volume reduction. Among them, GGO is characteristic, which is related to alveolar interstitial inflammation and alveolar inflammatory cell infiltration, indicating that acute rejection is similar to alveolitis.

2.1.2 Sputum Cytology

Chronic graft rejection is the main prognostic factor. Previous techniques for monitoring rejection were invasive and might harm the patients. Induced sputum test is a noninvasive and safe method for monitoring inflammation of lower respiratory tract in lung transplant patients. It was found that neutrophils in sputum reflected the major inflammatory processes related to pathogenesis, inflammation stimulation, tissue damage, and airway wall changes of chronic rejection. These findings were consistent with the results of bronchoalveolar lavage and tissue biopsy studies. According to the researchers, neutrophils increased significantly in bronchoalveolar lavage fluid or lung tissue during chronic rejection. Therefore, a series of studies will furtherly assess the sensitivity and the predictive value of induced sputum test in chronic rejection of lung transplantation. The possible mechanism of neutrophils on chronic rejection elucidates that the targeted new anti-inflammatory drugs (e.g., leukotriene B4 antagonists or selective phosphodiesterase inhibitor) may be an effective treatment for chronic rejection [8].

2.1.3 Pulmonary Perfusion Imaging

Good perfusion of transplanted lung postoperatively measured by radionuclide pulmonary perfusion imaging is one of the objective signs of successful operation and demonstrates the transplanted lung survival and function. In general, the vascular resistance of the transplanted lung is significantly lower than that of the lateral lung; thus more blood flows to the transplanted lung.

The blood perfusion of the transplanted lung should be measured in time. Perfusion of the transplanted lung usually varies a lot and mainly depends on the original pulmonary resistance of the recipient. For instance, the original pulmonary resistance of a COPD patient was normal; perfusion of unilateral transplanted lung will account for 50–60% immediately after lung transplantation and increase to some degree several months after surgery. By contrary, if a pulmonary hypertension patient undergoes lung transplantation, perfusion of unilateral transplanted lung will account for 90–95% immediately after surgery and decrease gradually after months. Dynamic pulmonary perfusion imaging can monitor the functional status of the transplanted lung and predict the possibility of rejection. It indicates the rejection, and corresponding treatment measures should be taken when the perfusion of transplanted lung decreases by 5% [9].

2.1.4 Pulmonary Function Test

Acute rejection often results in fever, cough, and dyspnea. Physical examination shows pleural effusion and pulmonary rale. Pulmonary function test shows deterioration of the lung function and hypoxemia, but the sensitivity and specificity are not high. More than 10% decrease of the baseline in FVC or FEV1 and over 10–15% decline of the baseline in FEF 25–75% may indicate acute rejection, infection, or other graft complications. Although rejection and infection can't be distinguished, the specificity of the diagnosis of graft complications is still 84% by pulmonary function test [10].

2.1.5 Transbronchial Lung Biopsy (TBLB)

TBLB is the primary means of identifying rejection and infection. The sensitivity of diagnosing acute rejection was 70–95%, and the specificity was 90–100% as reported. Four to six biopsies are usually done. The main morphologic change of acute rejection is perivascular lymphocyte infiltration. The infiltrating cells could affect alveolar septum, and lymphocytes infiltrate in the airway in the later period.

It is controversial whether routine TBLB should be performed in asymptomatic patients. A survey of 50 transplant centers showed 69% of the centers maintained routine TBLB to monitor rejection [11].

2.2 Pathological Histology of Rejection in Early and Late Transplantation

2.2.1 Hyperacute Rejection

Hyperacute rejection usually occurs 24–48 h postoperatively, the diagnosis based on clinical, serological, histological, and immunofluorescent findings. If the following manifestations occur, hyperacute rejection should be suspected: severe pulmonary congestion and edema and massive bloody foamy sputum in the bronchus of the transplanted lung. Obvious pulmonary edema, alveolar hemorrhage, intravascular platelet and fibrin thrombus, capillary congestion, interstitial infiltration of neutrophils, and injury of endothelial and epithelial cells are observed under light microscopy. The histological examination is the only method to make a definite diagnosis. Immunofluorescence shows that IgG deposits in the endothelium distribute along the wall of blood vessels and alveoli. IgG mediated lymphocytotoxicity is strongly positive in cross match of T and/or B lymphocytes between donor and recipient. If the patient could survive, diffuse alveolar damage will form.

2.2.2 Acute Rejection

Acute rejection is characterized by perivascular and interstitial mononuclear cell infiltration and respiratory tract inflammation. Differentiation between acute and chronic rejection is whether the irreversible vascular or airway eosinophilic hyaline change exists. However, there is no conclusion whether preventive TBLB should be performed to monitor rejection. Burns et al. [12] compared TBLB with surgical biopsy for the diagnosis of rejection and found the diagnosis rate had increased by 33% through surgical biopsy; 15 of 41 patients switched treatments based on the change of diagnosis. Thus surgical biopsy has a certain value. The biopsy specimens are pathologically classified into four types:

1. Lymphocytic infiltration around the pulmonary small arteries and veins can confirm acute rejection.
2. Acute rejection is suspected when lymphocytic infiltration is observed.
3. Unexplained diffuse alveolar destruction and interstitial inflammation, biopsy specimens are nonspecific.
4. Normal.

The biopsy specimens which are confirmed as acute rejection are classified into A0–A4 grade according to the region and severity of mononuclear cell infiltration histologically.

- Grade A0: no acute rejection, no pulmonary parenchymal mononuclear cell infiltration, hemorrhage, or necrosis.
- Grade A1: scattered mononuclear cell infiltration in the outer membrane of the small pulmonary vein.
- Grade A2: obvious mononuclear cell infiltration around the small pulmonary vein, accompanied by infiltration of the endothelium and inflammation of the airways, but no infiltration of the alveolar septum.
- Grade A3: significant mononuclear cell infiltration around the pulmonary vessel and into the adjacent alveolar septum, accompanied with lymphocytic bronchiolitis.
- Grade A4: significant mononuclear cell infiltration around the vessel, bronchus, and alveolar septum; macrophages, hemorrhages, fibrous tissue and hyaline membrane can be found in the alveolus.

In addition, lung rejection study group (LRSG) classified acute rejection with airway inflammation as class B and divided it into B0–B4 grades according to the severity of the inflammatory reaction. Acute rejection often accompanies by airway inflammation, and imaging is difficult to differentiate. Bronchoscopic lung biopsy can determine acute rejection and whether it is associated with airway inflammation, but sometimes bronchoscopic biopsy can't obtain the lesion due to material restrictions. Chest X-ray or CT has important reference value to judge whether there is pulmonary lesion, guide the localization for bronchoscopic biopsy and increase the accuracy of the biopsy.

The clinical manifestations of acute rejection include discomfort, fatigue, fever, chest tightness, shortness of breath, chest pain, and infiltrates or pleural fluid in chest X-ray. White blood cells increasing moderately, decrease of arterial partial pressure of oxygen (PaO_2), and decrease of forced expiratory volume in 1 second (FEV1) can be observed in typical patients. There is no specific manifestation in chest CT, which has limited effect on diagnosing acute rejection. The sensitivity is 35% and the accuracy rate is 53%. Sometimes abnormal chest X-ray appears earlier than symptoms and abnormal lung function; interstitial infiltration of pulmonary hilum is common in X-ray. It was reported that GGO was 65% sensitive to the diagnosis of rejection, and GGO was best suited for guidance of the timing and localization of TBLB.

Bronchoscopic bronchoalveolar lavage (BAL) and TBLB play an important role in diagnosis of rejection and infection. Cytological diagnosis of BAL shows an increase in the absolute number of lymphocytes and an increase in the number of persistent polymorphonuclear cells during acute rejection. However, other lung pathological changes, such as replantation, pneumonia, and atelectasis, can lead to the same lavage fluid findings, making it difficult to distinguish between rejection and infection through cell counts. TBLB is the gold standard for the diagnosis of acute rejection, and the sensitivity and specificity are more than 90%. A large crocodile forceps should be used to obtain the best quality and quantity of tissue. Biopsy needs to be performed in at least two locations and usually requires at least five lung parenchyma specimens, including the bronchial wall. Hopkins et al. reported that 10~12 specimens should be taken in order to improve the positive rate of TBLB. The disadvantage of TBLB is that it can cause pneumothorax, pulmonary infection, and bronchial hemorrhage. Although thoracoscopic biopsy or small incision open lung biopsy (OLB) can obtain more tissue compared with TBLB, the Toronto Lung Transplant Group considered that OLB had little significance when performed immediately after operation. Instead, OLB showed more meaningful results when performed more than 45 days after operation, where patients can receive timely diagnosis and treatment and avoid empirical therapy. Weill et al. suggested timely OLB in patients with worsening or undiagnosed conditions [12]. Methylprednisolone is commonly used in the treatment of acute rejection. For patients who have failed to respond to methylprednisolone and have poor prognosis, anti-T cell immunoglobulin (ATG) or OKT3 should be attempted.

2.2.3 Chronic Rejection: Bronchiolitis Obliterans Syndrome (BOS)

The main clinical manifestation of chronic rejection is progressive decline in FEV1, even before dyspnea appears. Some patients develop acute fever with dyspnea and wheezing. The imaging findings include diffuse, bilateral reticular lesions, alveolar lesions, and patchy pneumonia. Manual measurements of FEV1 daily with spirometry during the follow-up period after transplantation are suggested. Although chronic rejection continues to develop, chest radiograph and CT scan may be normal. The pathological feature of chronic rejection is bronchiolitis obliterans (BO). BO is an inflammatory response of the terminal bronchiolus and alveolar duct. Diagnostic pathological changes are specific, with inflammatory exudate and connective tissue regularly arranged and evenly distributed in the terminal bronchioles, respiratory bronchioles, alveolar ducts, and alveoli and the lesions in different organizing stages. Some areas are mainly composed of inflammatory cells and protein exudates, while others are mainly composed of loose, myxoid connective tissue or dense collagen fibers with no obvious inflammation. Alveoli near the affected airways contain foamy macrophages, inflammatory cells, and cell debris and sometimes cholesterol crystals. This inflammatory response, which is confined to the alveolar lumen, is a clue to the BO. The alveolar septum has different degrees of chronic interstitial inflammation and alveolar collapse. Evenly-distributed nodule, connective tissue plug, organized connective tissue and inflammatory obstruction showed by low power lens in the terminal respiratory tract are predictive for the diagnosis of BO. It can also show epithelial cell desquamation, the bronchial wall gradually replaced by fibrous tissue, eventually complete fibrous obstruction, and excessive expansion of the alveoli.

BOS is used to describe functional decline after transplantation, which is not a mechanical obstruction due to acute rejection, infection, or complications of bronchial anastomosis. BOS is characterized by chronic inflammation, thickening of the fibers, and narrowing of the lumen of the terminal or respiratory bronchioles. Lesions can cause partial or complete obliteration of the lumen. Scar tissue may be concentric or eccentric, accompanied by destruction of the smooth muscle wall usually. In addition, it often results in decreased mucus secretion or obstructive pneumonia. Pathological morphology is divided into active stage and quiescent stage.

1. Active stage. It is characterized by a large number of fibrous scars accompanied by infiltration of mononuclear cells in and around the bronchiolar lumen. In the early stage, there are mononuclear cell infiltration in the bronchioles, walls, smooth muscles, and mucous membranes (with lymph cell mainly). The mucosal epithelial cells are necrotic, exfoliated, and proliferated, and some of them develop flat cell metaplasia. With persistent inflammation, epithelial cell hyperplasia, macrophages, and fibroblasts appear, gradually form mucosal subepithelial fibrosis tissue. Microscopically, the inner membrane of bronchioles shows concentric circles fibrous tissue hyperplasia and fibrotic proliferation and the bronchiolar lumen partially or completely occluded. Polyp-like tissue can also be formed in the bronchioles of acute rejection, containing lymphocytes, neutrophils, macrophages, hemosiderin, and foamy tissue cell. Furtherly proliferation

of fibroblasts and the polypoid structure of the connective tissue block the lumen. The fibrous tissue in the lumen may extend outward into the thoracic diaphragm in a bar-like manner, accompanied by dilation of the proximal airway.

2. Quiescent stage. It is characterized by a large number of fibrous scars, not accompanied by infiltration of inflammatory cell in and around the bronchiolar lumen.

3 Other Complications

3.1 Immunosuppressive therapy related complications

3.1.1 The Posttransplant Lymphoproliferative Diseases (PTLD)

PTLD refers to a series of abnormal B cell proliferation responses, from benign hyperplasia of polyclonal to malignant lymphoma. In malignant tumor after SOT, the incidence of malignant PTLD is slightly less than non-melanoma skin cancer. Epstein Barr virus has been identified as a B cell proliferation stimulating factor. Due to the immunosuppression state of the cytotoxic T cells in the host, cell proliferation is usually in an uncontrolled situation. The incidence of PTLD is usually highest in the first year after transplant. Early onset of PTLD (≤1 year) can involve the transplanted lung, the typical manifestation is single or multiple nodules, usually associated with enlarged mediastinal lymph nodes. Late-onset PTLD (>a year) is often scattered in the abdomen.

3.1.2 Other Malignant Tumors

Skin malignancy after transplantation includes squamous cell carcinoma, basal cell carcinoma, mixed carcinoma (squamous cell carcinoma and basal cell carcinoma), etc. Patients with bronchioloalveolar carcinoma are in high risk of recurrence after lung transplantation. Lung cancer may rapidly progress in lung transplant recipients because of the lack of host antitumor immune monitoring mechanism in immunosuppressive therapy or special effects of CSA on promoting the growth of tumor [13].

3.2 Bleeding and Other Complications Related to the Operation

Because the lungs removed in lung transplantation belong to end-stage lung diseases, sometimes the lungs have lots of adhesions and are prone to hemorrhage in the surgery. Postoperative hemorrhage is also common. The incision of bilateral lung transplantation is larger than ordinary lung surgeries. It is prone to hemorrhage when extracorporeal circulation is used in the surgery. Other surgical complications include the stenosis, distortion, and obstruction of the pulmonary artery and left atrial sleeve after anastomosis; the injury of recurrent laryngeal nerves, phrenic nerves, and vagus nerves; etc. The injury of phrenic nerves in a proportion of patients will recover in 3 to 12 months after the operation, but the function of respiration and cough will be influenced early after the operation, so phrenic nerves should be protected in the surgery.

3.3 Infection After Transplantation

A variety of reasons such as termination of virus prevention, long-term use of immunosuppressive drugs and broad spectrum antibiotics make the long-term infection post lung transplantation present different characteristics. Infection is one of the major causes of death in the later period after lung transplantation and can also promote the occurrence and development of various complications such as BOS and PTLD. EB virus infection is closely related to lymphatic hyperplastic diseases which include Hodgkin's disease, non-Hodgkin's lymphoma, and lymphatic hyperplastic diseases post bone marrow transplantation and solid organ transplantation.

Bacteria are the most common pathogen of infection after ABOi lung transplantation. The main pathogenic bacteria were *Pseudomonas aeruginosa*. The clinical manifestation of *Pseudomonas aeruginosa* infection varies. Pulmonary *Pseudomonas aeruginosa* infection can be characterized by purulent bronchitis, pneumonia, bronchiectasis, etc. The systemic infection with *Pseudomonas aeruginosa* can also occur. Isolated infections such as strep discs of *Streptococcus pneumoniae* and *Pseudomonas aeruginosa* endophthalmitis caused by colonization of pathogens in the lung are rare in extrapulmonary tissues or organs. Mycobacterium infection is uncommon after lung transplantation. It can cause infection in the lung and empyema and soft tissue infection.

CMV infection is the most common viral infection after lung transplantation. The vast majority of CMV infections occur within 1 year, especially within 1–3 months after operation. The patients with repeated CMV infection are at a higher risk of developing BOS. The clinical manifestation of CMV infection is usually subclinical and not specific. It is difficult to make a definite diagnosis because of the low sensitivity of current detection methods for CMV. Because of the different diagnostic criteria, CMV prevention strategies are different in type and prevention time. It is reported that D+/R− patients are at high risk of CMV infection. CMV infection is a common cause of death within 31 days–1 year after lung transplantation and the mortality decreased rapidly 1 year later. In addition, CMV can increase the risk of bacterial and fungal infection and also contribute to the formation of BOS. Ganciclovir is the main drug in the treatment of CMV infection. In recent years, the incidence of resistance for ganciclovir has been over 6%, especially in patients with D+/R−. The use of antilymphocyte antibodies or daclizumab may be a risk factor. Community-acquired respiratory virus infections (respiratory syncytial virus, parainfluenza virus, influenza virus, adenovirus, etc.) also have higher morbidity and mortality rates due to limited efficacy of antiviral drugs. Invasive aspergillosis is still the most common opportunistic fungal infection. The etiology and location of fungal infections are diverse because of the changes for antifungal strategy and immunosuppressive agents. Protozoan infections are rare in ABOi lung transplantation.

4 Case Reports

At present, ABO-incompatible lung transplantation has made great progress, and its short-term and long-term survival rate has also been significantly improved. Many patients with end-stage lung disease can survive by transplantation. However, compared with ABO-compatible solid organ transplantation, there is still some deficiency.

ABO-incompatible organ transplants are considered only when the recipient is critically ill and does not have a ABO-compatible donor. The success of ABO-incompatible organ transplants is associated with many factors, such as the recipient age, the preoperative patient status, and so on. Although there are many ways to inhibit hyperacute rejection, acute rejection, and other complications in ABO-incompatible organ transplantation, most of the drugs produce various adverse reactions [14]. Tacrolimus and cyclosporine are nephrotoxic and neurotoxic and may cause diabetes, hyperkalemia, metabolic acidosis, hypertension, and hyperlipidemia. MMF can inhibit bone marrow hyperplasia and cause gastrointestinal adverse reactions, viral infections (such as CMV and HSV), and spontaneous abortion. Corticosteroids can cause diabetes, hypertension, obesity, osteoporosis, ischemic necrosis, growth retardation, Cushing syndrome, mental problems, wound healing, adrenal hyperfunction, and cataract. Over-immunosuppressive therapy before and after transplantation can lead to various infections. Transplants can be performed only after controlling for infection. Infection should also be prevented after transplantation. The long-term survival rate of many solid organ transplants is still unsatisfactory, and the mechanism of long-term chronic rejection is not particularly clear. In addition, the protocol adopted by each organ transplantation center is not the same; it is difficult to reach a unified standard. On the pretransplant antibody level, the transplant centers also have different opinions. Due to technical limitations, the monitoring of antibody levels after transplantation is difficult for each transplant center to unify.

Case 1 [14]

In 2008, one ABO-incompatible lung transplantation was performed at the Hannover Medical School in Germany. The patient was a 21-year-old female with cystic fibrosis. She was considered to survive less than 6–10 weeks despite the efforts of all departments of the hospital. The only treatment for her is lung transplantation. On the fifth day after the urgent application, an AB donor was successfully paired. The donor HLA was A11, A26, B7, B39, DR7, and DR15, and the recipient was A11, B35, B44, DR13, and DR15. Eight hours before surgery, the patient underwent a plasmapheresis followed by infusion of 500 mg rituximab and 1000 mg methylprednisolone. During the extracorporeal circulation intraoperative, the plasma filtration was performed with infusion of 2 g/kg IVIG at the same time to maintain lower antibody titer. Triple transplantation immunosuppressive therapy (methylprednisolone, mycophenolate mofetil, tacrolimus) was used postoperatively. One week after surgery, infusion of rituximab and plasmapheresis was continued to maintain the titer of blood group antibody below 1:16. A week later, the titer of blood group antibody in the patient rebounded; the doctors immediately used anti-A and anti-B immune adsorption column to reduce the production of antibodies. The method was shown to be effective, and the antibody titer of the patient remained less than 1:16. The antibody titer did not rebound again. Thirty-seven days after operation, the pulmonary function of the patient was FEV1 for 0.9L and VC for 0.9L. Fifty-four days after the operation, the patient recovered well and was discharged. After discharge, the patient's pulmonary function further improved (116 days after surgery, FEV1 1.56L and VC 1.68L; after 265 days, FEV1 2.20L and VC 1.99L).

Case 2 [15]

A case of ABO-incompatible lung transplantation was performed at the Toronto Children's Hospital in 2012. The patient was aged 38 weeks, with a weight of 3720 g, and was diagnosed with congenital pulmonary surfactant protein deficiency. After 5 days of waiting, a DCD donor matching succeeded. But the donor's blood type was B, and the recipient's was type A. Preoperative and intraoperative preparation and treatment were the same as ABO-incompatible cardiac transplantation. Postoperative immunosuppressive therapy was basiliximab, methylprednisolone, mycophenolate mofetil, and tacrolimus. Supraventricular tachycardia occurred in the patient 8 days after surgery and improved after taking propranolol. The grafts were well functioning 15 days after surgery. There was no rejection in 7 weeks, 3 months, 6months after surgery by transbronchial lung biopsy.

References

1. Cypel M, Yeung JC, Liu M, et al. Normothermic ex vivo lung perfusion in clinical lung transplantation. N Engl J Med. 2011;364:1431–40.
2. Snell GI, Westall GP. Selection and management of the lung donor. Clin Chest Med. 2011;32:223–32.
3. Flint SM, Walker RG, Hogan C, et al. Successful ABO-incompatible kidney transplantation with antibody removal and standard immunosuppression. Am J Transplant. 2011;11:1016–24.
4. Ishida H, Miyamoto N, Shirakawa H, et al. Evaluation of immunosuppressive regimens in ABO-incompatible living kidney transplantation: single center analysis. Am J Transplant. 2007;7:825–31.
5. Pierson RN, Loyd JE, Goodwin A, et al. Successful management of an ABO-mismatched lung allograft using antigen-specific immunoadsorption, complement inhibition, and immunomodulatory therapy. Transplantation. 2002;74:79–84.
6. Solomon M, Grasemann H, Keshavjee S. Pediatric lung transplantation. Pediatr Clin North Am. 2010;57:375–91.

7. Dipchand AI, Pollock BarZiv SM, Manlhiot C, West LJ, VanderVliet M, McCrindle BW. Equivalent outcomes for pediatric heart transplantation recipients: ABO-blood group incompatible versus ABO compatible. Am J Transplant. 2010;10:389–97.
8. Everitt MD, Donaldson AE, Casper TC, et al. Effect of ABO incompatible listing on infant heart transplant waitlist outcomes: analysis of the United Network for Organ Sharing (UNOS) database. J Heart Lung Transplant. 2009;28:1254–60.
9. Fischer S, Hoeper MM, Tomaszek S, et al. Bridge to lung transplantation with the extracorporeal membrane ventilator NovaLung in the veno-venous mode: the initial Hannover experience. ASAIO J. 2007;53:168–70.
10. Banner NR, Rose ML, Cummins D, et al. Management of an ABO incompatible lung transplant. Am J Transplant. 2004;4:1192–6.
11. Levine SM. A survey of clinical practice of lung transplantation in North America. Chest. 2004;125(4):1224–38.
12. Burns KE, Johnson BA, Iacono AT. Diagnostic properties of transbronchial biopsy in lung transplant recipients who require mechanical ventilation. J Heart Lung Transplant. 2003;22(3):267–75.
13. Collins J, Kazerooni EA, Lacomis J, et al. Bronchogenic carcinoma after lung transplantation: frequency, clinical characteristics, and imaging findings. Radiology. 2002;224(1):131–8.
14. Strüber M, Warnecke G, Hafer C, Goudeva L, Fegbeutel C, Fischer S, Gottlieb J, Avsar M, Simon A, Haverich A. Intentional ABO-incompatible lung transplantation. Am J Transplant. 2008;8(11):2476–8.
15. Grasema H, de Perrot M, Bendiak GN, et al. ABO-incompatible lung transplantation in an infant. Am J Transplant. 2012;12:779–81.

14 The Animal Model in ABO-Incompatible Organ Transplantation

Gang Chen and Song Chen

Abstract

To better understand the mechanisms of such antibody-mediated rejection and explore novel strategies for clinical application, it is important to establish an animal research model of humoral rejection in ABO-incompatible organ transplantation. In this chapter, we will discuss the following issues: the ABO tissue groups and blood groups in nonhuman primates, natural anti-blood group antibody levels in sera of nonhuman primates, outcomes of ABO-incompatible organ transplantation in nonhuman primates, and establishment of humoral rejection models in ABO-incompatible organ transplantation in nonhuman primates.

Keywords

Animal model · Nonhuman primates · Humoral rejection models

G. Chen (✉)
Institute of Organ Transplantation, Tongji Hospital, Huazhong University of Science and Technology, Wuhan, China

Key Laboratory of Organ Transplantation, Ministry of Education/Ministry of Public Health, Wuhan, China

Tongji Hospital, Tongji Medical College of Huazhong University of Science and Technology, Wuhan, China
e-mail: gchen@tjh.tjmu.edu.cn

S. Chen
Institute of Organ Transplantation, Tongji Hospital, Huazhong University of Science and Technology, Wuhan, China

Key Laboratory of Organ Transplantation, Ministry of Education/Ministry of Public Health, Wuhan, China

Y. Wang (ed.), *ABO-incompatible Organ Transplantation*,
https://doi.org/10.1007/978-981-13-3399-6_14

Since more and more living-related kidney transplants have been performed these years due to the severe shortage of organ donors, it is no doubt that renal donor resource can be broadened in certain degree if the ABO barrier could be overcome. However, most ABO-incompatible renal allografts will develop irreversible hyperacute or acute antibody-mediated rejection without special pretreatment. To better understand the mechanisms of such antibody-mediated rejection and explore novel strategies for clinical application, it is important to establish an animal research model of humoral rejection in ABO-incompatible organ transplantation. Nonhuman primate animals can have blood type A and/or B antigens expressed on vascular endothelial cells in their organs and can contain natural anti-blood group A and/or B antibodies in their sera; therefore, the ABO-incompatible allografts may develop hyperacute or acute antibody-mediated rejection in the early period after organ transplantation. In this chapter, we will introduce the ABO tissue groups and serum preformed anti-blood group antibody levels in different species of experimental nonhuman primates, as well as the reported animal models of organ transplantation across the ABO barrier.

1 ABO Tissue Groups and Blood Groups in Nonhuman Primates

Like humans, nonhuman primates (including anthropoid apes, New- and Old-World monkeys) also express the ABH specificities of the ABO histo-blood group system on vascular endothelium, epithelial cells, and exocrine secretions. However, these ABH antigens are absent or only weakly expressed on the erythrocytes of Old- and New-World monkeys (Table 14.1) [1, 2].

The baboon and macaque (including rhesus monkey and cynomolgus monkey), two typical representative of Old-World monkeys, are frequently used in experimental transplantation research because of their physical traits and availability. As reported by Busch et al. in 2006 [2], blood groups A, B, and AB were represented, respectively, in 14%, 36%, and 50% of the 14 baboons they typed. Blood group O was not found among the 14 baboons [2]. In one of our studies, we found that blood groups B and AB were expressed, respectively, in 74% and 16% of the 38 rhesus monkeys we typed, and blood groups A (3%) and O (7%) were both rare [3]. In 98 cynomolgus monkeys we reported in total, there was a relatively equal representation of blood types A and AB (26% and 31%, respectively). Blood type B was represented by 42%, and blood type O was found in only one of these monkeys (approximately 1%) [3, 4] (Table 14.2).

Table 14.1 Known ABO blood types of the baboon and monkey [2]

Species	Known ABO blood types
Baboon	A, B, AB, O[a]
Monkey	A, B, AB, O[a]

[a]Blood type O is rare

Table 14.2 Blood group distribution in experimental baboons and monkeys [2–4]

Species	ABO group types
Baboon (n = 14)	AB (50%) > B (36%) > A (14%) > O (0%)
Rhesus monkey (n = 38)	B (74%) > AB (16%) > O (7%) > A (3%)
Cynomolgus monkey (n = 98)	B (42%) > AB (31%) > A (26%) > O (1%)

2 Natural Anti-Blood Group Antibody Levels in Sera of Nonhuman Primates

Nonhuman primate animals can regularly generate natural anti-A and/or anti-B antibodies directed against antigen(s) absent from the animal's body secretions [1]. The natural anti-A or anti-B antibody titers in baboons appear to be similar to that in humans, which has been reported to be mainly in the range of 1:32–1:128 [5]. Cooper et al. determined anti-A or anti-B antibody titers in 18 baboons using the direct saline agglutination assay [6] in 1993 [7]. The strength of the agglutination was measured by the American of Blood Banks grading system [8]. They reported that anti-A (n = 16) and anti-B (n = 2) antibody titers ranged from 1:4 to 1:256 (four titers were 1:32 or less, four titers were 1:64, and ten titers were 1:128 or 1:256). Increasing the antibody titer to 1:512 or above in the majority of cases through a "hyperimmunization program" clearly exposed the donor heart to a severe hyperacute rejection in their study [7].

Using a novel-modified flow cytometry method with human red blood cells as target cells [9, 10], we reported that the levels of anti-A and anti-B IgM antibodies in monkey sera were lower than that in human sera. More concretely, in 20 rhesus monkeys, anti-A (n = 14) and anti-B (n = 6) antibody titers ranged from 1:64 to 1:2048 (5 titers were 1:128 or less, 10 titers were 1:256 or 1:512, and 5 titers were 1:1024 or 1:2048). Similar results were observed in 20 cynomolgus monkeys: anti-A (n = 12) and anti-B (n = 8) antibody titers ranged from 1:64 to 1:2048 (5 titers were 1:128 or less, 9 titers were 1:256 or 1:512, and 6 titers were 1:1024 or 1:2048). However, the levels of anti-A/B IgM antibody in 32 human serum samples we tested were higher significantly. Anti-A (n = 16) and anti-B (n = 16) antibody titers ranged from 1:512 to 1:8192 (13 titers were 1:512 or 1:1024, 15 titers were 1:2048 or 1:4096, and 4 titers were 1:8192) [10].

3 Outcomes of ABO-Incompatible Organ Transplantation in Nonhuman Primates

As the sera of nonhuman primate animals regularly contain natural anti-blood group A and/or B antibodies directed against antigen(s) absent from the animal's body secretions [3, 4, 11], the A and/or B antigens expressed on vascular endothelial cells in organs can be a target for the host immune system and may result in hyperacute rejection (HAR) or acute antibody-mediated rejection (AAMR). In fact, however, ABO-incompatible organ transplantation in nonhuman primates does not always develop HAR or AAMR. An early study on cardiac allotransplantation across the ABO barrier in baboons had shown that only one-third of the allografts developed early antibody-mediated HAR, whereas the remaining 66% of the allografts developed acute cellular rejection as similar as what was seen in ABO-compatible cardiac allotransplantation [12]. In a kidney transplantation study we just completed in cynomolgus monkeys, ABO-incompatible renal allografts did not develop either HAR or AAMR as expected, and the allografts could survive more than 30 days with the treatment of cyclosporine (CsA) and mycophenolate mofetida (MMF) (unpublished data). These results indicate that humoral rejection models are not easy to be established in the situation of ABO-incompatible organ transplantation in nonhuman primates without specific presensitization. Relatively low levels of natural anti-blood group antibodies in the sera of experimental nonhuman primate animals may represent the main cause.

4 Establishment of Humoral Rejection Models in ABO-Incompatible Organ Transplantation in Nonhuman Primates

To ensure the occurrence of HAR or AAMR after ABO-incompatible organ transplantation in nonhuman primate animals, the anti-blood group antibody levels should be significantly elevated in circulation of the recipients before transplantation. This could be achieved by subcutaneous injection of the coupled compounds, A-KLH (blood group A antigen keyhole limpet hemocyanin) or B-KLH, emulsified in complete Freund's adjuvant [7]. Such hyperimmunization program resulted in a very potent stimulus to the immune system and significantly raised anti-A or anti-B IgM titers in all tested baboons (n = 18). When three of these animals were randomly selected as recipients to perform ABO-incompatible cardiac transplantation, all allografts developed HAR within 30 min [7]. In a study we just completed, 20 cynomolgus monkeys with tissue group B received a subcutaneously injection of A-KLH, resulting in significant raised titers of serum anti-A antibodies after 14 days in 70% of these animals. Four of them were randomly selected as recipients to receive a renal allograft from donor monkeys with tissue group A, and all allografts were hyperacutelly rejected (unpublished data). These results indicate that HAR models can be successfully established in ABO-incompatible organ transplantation in nonhuman primates with the use of hyperimmunization program. To date, no AAMR model in ABO-incompatible organ transplantation has been reported yet in nonhuman primates, possibly because the induced antibody responses against blood group antigens in the early period after organ transplantation are pretty weak in experimental baboons or monkeys. To reduce the degree of blood group antigen-induced hyperimmunization in recipients before transplantation or inhibit complement activation after transplantation may help to establish an animal model of AAMR in ABO-incompatible organ transplantation.

References

1. Socha WW, Marboe CC, Michler RE, Rose EA, Moor-Jankowski J. Primate animal model for the study of ABO incompatibility in organ transplantation. Transplant Proc. 1987;19(6):4448–55.
2. Busch J, Specht S, Ezzelarab M, Cooper DK. Buccal mucosal cell immunohistochemistry: a simple method of determining the ABH phenotype of baboons, monkeys, and pigs. Xenotransplantation. 2006;13(1):63–8.
3. Chen S, Wei Q, Li J, Xiang Y, Guo H, Ichim TE, et al. A simple and reliable method to blood type monkeys using serum samples. Transpl Int. 2009;22(10):999–1004.
4. Wang X, Chen S, Chen G. ABO typing in experimental cynomolgus monkeys using non-invasive methods. Sci Rep. 2017;7:41274.
5. Mollison PL. Blood transfusion in clinical medicine. Oxford: Blackwell Scientific; 1990. p. 555.
6. Walker RH. The technical manual. Arlington: American Association of Blood Banks; 1990. p. 567.
7. Cooper DK, Ye Y, Niekrasz M, Kehoe M, Martin M, Neethling FA, et al. Specific intravenous carbohydrate therapy. A new concept in inhibiting antibody-mediated rejection—experience with ABO-incompatible cardiac allografting in the baboon. Transplantation. 1993;56(4):769–77.
8. Marsh WL. Scoring of hemagglutination reactions. Transfusion. 1972;12(5):352–3.
9. Stussi G, Huggel K, Lutz HU, Schanz U, Rieben R, Seebach JD. Isotype-specific detection of ABO blood group antibodies using a novel flow cytometric method. Br J Haematol. 2005;130(6):954–63.
10. Zhang C, Wang XX, Wang L, Xiang Y, Wei Q, Wang WY, et al. Application of flow cytometry to detect ABO blood group antibody levels in rhesus monkeys and cynomolgus monkeys. Zool Res. 2011;32(1):56–61.
11. Oriol R, Cooper JE, Davies DR, Keeling PW. ABH antigens in vascular endothelium and some epithelial tissues of baboons. Lab Invest. 1984;50(5):514–8.
12. Cooper DK, Lexer G, Rose AG, Keraan M, Rees J, Du Toit E, et al. Cardiac allotransplantation across major blood group barriers in the baboon. J Med Primatol. 1988;17(6):333–46.

Mechanism Development of Accommodation and Tolerance in Transplant

15

Jina Wang and Ruiming Rong

Abstract

Administration of immunosuppressants in transplanted recipients promotes the allograft acceptance but also leads to serious side effects. Aiming at solving this issue in allotransplantation, researchers have paid attention to manipulate the immune response so as to induce an allograft tolerance (in which the immune response to foreign antigen or an allograft is selectively abolished due to generalized non-responsiveness or loss of the antigenic target) without immunosuppressants rather than unspecific immunosuppression. It is interesting to observe that until anti-blood group antibodies went back to normal levels in recipients several days after ABO-incompatible (ABOi) renal transplantation, there was still no allograft rejection in most of the recipients. The survival of ABOi-transplanted organs in coexistence with anti-allograft antibodies and complement which originally results in graft rejection was described as accommodation. Is this successful engraftment of ABOi allografts (accommodation) a certain level or type of allograft tolerance, or does it just reflect some other biological condition of allografts? Thus, the mechanism investigation of accommodation and tolerance could be significant for conquering humoral barriers to allotransplantation and promoting long-term survival of allografts.

Keywords

Organ transplantation · ABO incompatible · Accommodation · Tolerance Antibody · Immune response

J. Wang · R. Rong (✉)
Department of Urology, Zhongshan Hospital, Fudan University, Shanghai, China

Shanghai Key Laboratory of Organ Transplantation, Shanghai, China
e-mail: wang.jina@zs-hospital.sh.cn; rong.ruiming@zs-hospital.sh.cn

Y. Wang (ed.), *ABO-incompatible Organ Transplantation*,
https://doi.org/10.1007/978-981-13-3399-6_15

Tolerance is a status of the immune system unresponsiveness to substances or tissue that is capable of eliciting an immune response in a given organism, in contrast with traditional immune-mediated elimination of foreign antigens. It contains the spectrum of physiological mechanisms by which the organism decreases or eliminates an immune response to particular agents. And it is also used to depict the phenomenon underlying distinction between self and nonself, repressing allergic responses, permitting chronic infection instead of rejection or elimination, and averting maternal immune system from attacking fetuses. Immune tolerance does not usually mean immunosuppression artificially induced by lymphotoxic chemotherapy agents, immunosuppressant, sublethal irradiation, and so on. Nor does it mean to be other nonreactivity types, such as immunological deficiency. In the latter two cases, the host's physiology is mutilated but not fundamentally changed.

Accommodation is a unique immunologic condition that is different from immune tolerance. It is defined operationally as a state in which the transplanted organ works normally under the existence of antibodies in the recipient specifically targeting the allograft. The state of immune accommodation was initially observed in ABO-incompatible (ABOi) renal transplants. It was discovered that if anti-blood group A/B antibodies (anti-A/B antibodies) directed at attacking allogeneic blood groups are eliminated or controlled below a certain threshold at the time of ABOi renal transplantation and during the first 14 days of posttransplantation temporarily, renal allografts might survive and work for months or years without obvious injury even after anti-A/B antibodies go back to the circulation. The term "accommodation" was initially used to organ xenografts, like ABOi organ allografts, which appeared to resist acute and hyperacute vascular rejection. The resistance to injury lasted even after xenoreactive antibodies in experimental xenotransplantation or anti-A/B antibodies in human renal transplant recipients went back to recipients' circulation. Most astonishingly, biopsies of regular-working healthy grafts revealed persistent existence of ABO antigens locating on endothelial surfaces. It seems to be contradictory that there was coexistence of antibody and target antigen without obvious rejection or graft injury, which emboldened the concept that there might be a novel type of graft-recipient interaction. Though it is poorly understood, ABOi graft accommodation may provide clues to investigate the mechanism of alloimmune response, especially the antibody-mediated humoral alloimmune response and the complement-mediated destruction of allografts.

1 Mechanisms of Immune Tolerance of Transplant

1.1 Immune Tolerance Formation

The phenomenon of immune tolerance was initially depicted by Ray D. Owens in 1945, who observed that dizygotic twin cattle not only shared a common placenta but also shared a stable mixture of each other's erythrocytes and retained that mixture throughout life. Besides this, his study showed that one of the twin cattle could accept the skin graft from another twin cattle without rejection but would still reject skin grafts from other cattle. Furthermore Rupert E. Billingham and Peter Medawar validated this observation experimentally in 1953. At that time, Frank McFarlane Burnet assumed that in embryonic period and immediately after birth, cells gradually obtain the capability to discriminate between their own tissue substances and unwanted cells and foreign material. Sir Peter Medawar's team injected cells from young mouse into another fetal or neonatal mouse of different strains; afterward skin grafting from that of the original strain was performed when the mouse grew into adult, and no skin graft rejection was observed. However, the recipient mouse can still reject the tissue from the mouse of unrelated strains. It revealed that the mouse had tolerated the foreign tissue which would be rejected normally. Their experimental proof of Burnet's assumption was named "actively acquired tolerance." Burnet and Medawar were finally honored by "the discovery of acquired immune tolerance" and won the Nobel Prize in Physiology or Medicine in 1960.

Further mechanism investigation in immune tolerance induction found that several factors appear to be associated with the formation of immune tolerance.

Genetic Background. It is easier to induce immune tolerance in animals with relatively simple immune system (such as rats and mice). However, it is tough to induce a state of immune tolerance in animal models with complex immune system (such as rabbits and primates) after birth, especially in an adult. There are also differences in the induction of immune tolerance among different individuals in the same strain. For example, some individuals have a poor response to hepatitis B vaccine and produce no antibody or low-titer antibody, which may be related to the MHC polymorphism of individuals.

Body Age and Immune System Maturation. Exposure to a foreign antigen during embryonic period produces immune tolerance. It is prone to induce immune tolerance during the early neonatal period. Mother-to-child transmission of HIV and hepatitis B virus in the embryonic period usually leads to infection tolerance, whereas the infection during infancy can produce an immune response but not immune clearance against these infections.

Body Immune Status. It is hard to produce immune tolerance induced by foreign antigen stimulation in immune-mature individuals. However, it is possible to induce immune tolerance with the help of some immunosuppressive strategies, such as immunosuppressants and irradiation. Before the clinical application of effective immunosuppressants (such as cyclosporine A, tacrolimus), most of the allografts were rejected in transplant recipients with normal immunity. Induction of immune tolerance by transplantation and immunosuppressive agents is an effective way to achieve the goal of long-term graft survival.

Antigen Types and Characteristics. Monomer protein is easy to tolerate because it is not easy to be taken up and presented by the antigen-presenting cells (APCs). However, due to the high molecular weight and strong antigenicity, polymer is prone to induce immune response, and the use of immune adjuvants (such as BCG, lipopolysaccharide, etc.) can enhance the immune response. Some protein fragments can induce immune tolerance, such as orally *taken* type II collagen. Further studies have shown that 260–270 amino acid residues of the protein may be the epitope which is responsible for the induction of immune tolerance. The antigen epitope that can induce immune tolerance is called the tolerogenic epitope.

Antigen Dose. High-dose and low-dose antigen can induce immune tolerance, while appropriate dose of antigen causes the immune response. In 1964, Avrion Mitchison found that mice can't produce specific antibodies when injected with high dose (10^{-5} mol/L) and low dose (10^{-8} mol/L) of bovine serum albumin (BSA), while the strong immune response could be caused by an appropriate concentration (10^{-7} mol/L) of BSA. The tolerances induced by too high and too low dose of antigen are called low-zone tolerance and high-zone tolerance, respectively. It is also found that T cells and B cells have different doses of antigen to produce immune tolerance. T cells that produced tolerance need much lower dose of antigen than that in B cells and with a faster onset time and longer duration.

Antigen Administration Approach and Duration. It is easier to produce immune tolerance using oral administration of well-soluble and easy digestive protein by which the generation of antigen-specific suppressor T cells is easy to be induced. Lymphocytes with continuous antigen stimulation and lack of costimulatory signal are apt to undergo apoptosis and induce tolerance, such as the negative selection of T cells in the thymus.

1.2 Fundamental Mechanism of Immune Tolerance

The underlying mechanism of immune tolerance is complex and still unclear. Tolerance can be classified into peripheral tolerance and central tolerance depending on where the state is originally induced in other tissues and in lymph nodes (peripheral) or in the thymus and bone marrow (central). The mechanisms of how to establish these two forms tolerance are distinct, but the final effect is similar, while almost all of the allograft tolerance is induced through the peripheral tolerance way among organ transplantations.

1.2.1 Central Tolerance

Central tolerance is such a type of tolerance established by eliminating autoreactive lymphocyte clones before they grow into fully immunocompetent cells. The occurrence of central tolerance is in the thymus and bone marrow, thus allowing the elimination of a major percentage of autoreactive T and B lymphocytes before they develop into fully immunocompetent cells. The thymus, the major region of T-cell maturation, is composed of the thymic medulla and cortex. The medulla and the cortex are places where the process of negative selection and positive selection occurs separately, in which maturing lymphocytes are exposed to self-antigens presented by thymic dendritic cells (DCs) and medullary thymic epithelial cells or bone marrow cells. Self-antigens are submitted owing to endogenous expression and importation of antigen from peripheral sites through circulation blood and, in the case of thymic stromal cells, expression of other non-thymic tissues' proteins by the action of the transcription factor AIRE.

Those lymphocytes recognizing self-antigens with high avidity will be eliminated by induction of the autoreactive cell apoptosis or by induction of anergy.

Weakly autoreactive B cells still stay in an immunological ignorance state where they simply do not respond to their B-cell receptor stimulation. Some weakly self-recognizing T cells are selectively developed into natural regulatory T cells (nTregs), which act as guards in the periphery to calm down potential T-cell autoreactivity instances.

Central tolerance is the primary way by which the immune system learns to distinguish self from nonself. This negative selection process ensures that T and B cells initiating a potent immune response to the host's own tissues are cleared up while conserving the capability of recognizing foreign antigens. It is the step of lymphocyte education which is determined for avoiding autoimmunity. In virtue of negative and positive selection, lymphocytes leaving the thymus and bone marrow are self-antigens restricted and tolerant to most of self-antigens.

1.2.2 Peripheral Tolerance

Peripheral tolerance establishes after mature T and B cells entering the lymph nodes and peripheral tissues. Although central tolerance mechanisms are effective in eliminating the self-reactive lymphocyte clones by recognizing self-antigens in high affinity, some autoreactive T cells escaping intrathymic negative selection enter the lymph nodes and the peripheral tissues. Owing to the existence of escaping self-reactive T-cell clones in the periphery, there is still a regular risk of latent autoimmune responses in the recipient. However these potentially harmful self-reactive cells can be controlled by peripheral tolerance mechanisms effectively, which consist of the elimination of activated effector T cells, active regulation of effector T cells, clonal exhaustion, and anergy induction. Regulatory T cells (Tregs) modulate active regulation of the immune response avoiding inflammatory and autoimmune diseases and restricting responses to various foreign pathogen infections. Appropriate response to certain antigens can also be subsided by inducted tolerance after exposure in a certain context or repeated exposure. In these cases, there are induced Tregs (iTregs) differentiated from naïve $CD4^{+}$ helper T cells in the nearby lymphoid tissue or peripheral tissue.

Not only Tregs regulate peripheral tolerance. DCs also act a pivotal role in developing peripheral tolerance. Immature DCs (iDCs) can internalize self-antigens present in apoptotic cells and induce tolerance mechanisms such as the amplification of iTregs which control effector responses and prevent tissues from injury during pathogenic autoimmune response. Some DCs can alter indoleamine 2,3-dioxygenase (IDO) that eliminates the amino acid tryptophan required by T-cell proliferation and thus attenuate responsiveness. DCs are also able to induce anergy directly in T cells that recognize high-level expression of antigen and thus presented in a steady state by DCs.

B cells also produce CD22, a non-specific inhibitor receptor that restrains B-cell receptor activation, and there are also a subset of B regulatory cells (Bregs) expressing IL-10 and TGF-β. Peripheral tolerance is crucial to avoiding hyper-reactivity of the immune system to multifarious environmental entities.

1.3 Induction of Immune Tolerance

Based on a knowledge of the mechanisms that may facilitate the generation of immune tolerance, various protolerogenic regimens have been advanced. Although a number of these regimens have succeeded consistently in rodent transplant models, none comparable success has been observed in nonhuman primates or humans. Despite the shortness of direct application from rodent models to humans, some approaches have been general components of clinical regimens aiming at inducing tolerance or at least lessening immunosuppression in clinical transplantation. We will summarize the tolerance induction strategies that have progressed to the stage of testing in nonhuman primate transplant systems and clinical setting.

1.3.1 T-Cell Depletion Strategies

Profound depletion of T/B cells with monoclonal antibodies (such as anti-CD3, anti-CD4, anti-CD8 monoclonal antibodies) decreases the quantity of T cells competent of reacting to allografts and eliminating the quantity of alloreactive T cells under the threshold essential for the occurrence of allograft rejection. It is theorized that T cells appearing in the existence of allografts may go through some forms of selection so that those recognizing allografts are depicted less functional or even eliminated. Beside these, at the time of T-cell repletion, the "danger" signals present perioperatively (such as surgical trauma, allograft ischemia-reperfusion injury) are absent, and alloimmune stimulation in this more quiescent immunologic milieu would be more tolerogenic.

Despite the theoretical function of eliminating donor-reactive T cells, it is explicit that T-cell elimination strategy alone is scanty to avoid allograft rejection or permit tolerance induction.

1.3.2 Costimulatory Pathway Blockade

Costimulatory blockade is an immunosuppression strategy that blocks the vital costimulating signals required for complete sensitization of alloreactive T cells. Treatment of murine transplant recipients with antibodies that ablate these costimulatory pathways (such as the CD40-CD154 or CD28-CD80/86 pathways) results in significantly prolonged allograft survival. However, it did not work when this strategy was applied into primate transplant models. Combined use of anti-CD86 and anti-CD80 antibodies did lengthen rhesus renal allograft survival but without tolerance. Belatacept (CTLA-4-Ig; it is CD28 antagonists) and anti-CD40 monoclonal antibodies (ch5D12 and Chi220 antibodies) could prolong renal allograft survival of rhesus, but it did not induce tolerance as well. Given the risk of serious thrombotic complications when using anti-CD154 monoclonal antibodies, it was brought to an abrupt halt. Coupling blockade of the CD40-CD154 and CD28-CD80/86 pathways (anti-CD40 and anti-CD86 antibody, belatacept and anti-CD40) substantially prolonged allograft survival but also did not permit tolerance induction.

These data indicate that with increasing knowledge of the alloimmune response, it may still be capable of inducing long-term, immunosuppressive medicine-free survival of allografts employing the strategy of costimulatory pathway blockage.

1.3.3 Mixed Chimerism Approaches

One of the most prospective methods of inducing transplant tolerance is infusion of the donor's hematopoietic cells meanwhile of the organ transplantation so as to get transient induction of hematopoietic chimerism compound. This chimerism allows the generation of central immune tolerance, as the engrafted donor hematopoietic cells traffic to the thymus, enabling elimination of donor-specific T cells. Mixed chimerism enables long-range allograft survival in murine, and it has been proven to be effective in allowing allograft survival without further immunosuppression in a variety of nonhuman primate transplant systems. Success in these primate studies led to several clinical trials of mixed chimerism induction in human transplant recipients. The Stanford group, the Northwestern University group, and Massachusetts General Hospital group have applied this technique in renal transplant recipients and demonstrated that durable renal allograft survival without immunosuppression was achieved in some recipients.

1.3.4 Cellular Therapies

To induce peripheral tolerance, some researchers have focused on adoptive transfer of regulatory cell populations. Regulatory cell populations may also have great effect on maintaining transplant tolerance. The candidates involve iDCs, regulatory macrophages, Tregs, Bregs, and mesenchymal stromal/stem cells owing to their ability of inducing tolerance in antigen-specific way.

Dendritic Cells and Regulatory Macrophages. The potential to induce tolerance is straight related to DC maturation state, in which T-cell tolerance is induced by iDCs expressing low surface levels of costimulatory molecules and MHC class II. Immature DCs are also applied in the development of mixed chimerism, which is a method to induce transplant tolerance. Regulatory macrophages are activated (M2-polarized) macrophages that can produce IL-10, favor Th2-polarized T-cell responses, and have T-cell-suppressive properties. The applications of regulatory macrophages in clinical renal transplantation have allowed to diminish the dosage of immunosuppressants to induce operational tolerance to allografts.

Regulatory T Cells (Tregs). Given the significant effect of Tregs on inducing/maintaining immune tolerance and the unambiguous immunoregulatory mechanisms, their application has been advanced as a strategy of inducing specific immune tolerance. Adoptive transfer of recipient Tregs expanded ex vivo was used in rhesus transplant recipients and got interesting results. In that study, half of the treated rhesus recipients showed long-term survival of renal allografts while demonstrating donor-specific unresponsiveness in mixed lymphocyte reactions and donor-specific acceptance of skin grafts, both of which indicate achievement of a tolerant state. Although specific adoptive transfer of Tregs has not been used yet in primate solid organ transplant models, one study showed that ex vivo expanded Tregs derived from rhesus macaques could suppress allo-immune response. Besides the transferring of "recipient"-derived Tregs, certain "donor"-derived cells were also used to promote recipient Tregs expansion and resulting in donor-specific hyporesponsiveness. The results showed that 1-ethyl-3-(3′-dimethylaminopropyl)-carbodiimide (EDCI)-treated donor splenocytes can be adoptively transferred into cynomolgus monkey recipients of islet allografts to promote donor-specific Tregs expansion and promote prolonged islet allograft acceptance.

Despite the extended experimental research approving a role for Tregs in transplant tolerance, astonishingly there is few data approving their role in clinical transplant tolerance. In fact, most of the studies addressing the function of Tregs in transplant animal model suggest they arise in response to immune response so as to limit the graft injury, rather than arising de novo as a means of establishing immune tolerance.

B Cells. B cells are regarded a central part of the adaptive immune response to alloantigens, acting through several mechanisms to modulate allograft injury. However, there is a developing perception that B cells may also be related to the development and maintenance of tolerance after organ transplantation. The role of Bregs has been best established in the tolerance induction of experimental animal models, but the existence of comparable B-cell populations in humans remains undiscovered. Currently, the most unambiguous character identifying Bregs is their expression of IL-10, which is also regarded vital for their modulatory function. It is recently reported that IL-10-expressing B cells may have effect mechanistically on an operationally tolerant status after renal transplantation. The relationship between specific type of B cells and allograft tolerance is just based on the observation of long-term tolerant recipients rather than the prospective research of tolerance induction. Thus, it is not certain whether B cells take part in the development of tolerance or are simply an epiphenomenon of tolerant state.

Many tolerance induction strategies can work well in rodents but are unsuccessful in nonhuman primates and, in turn, may not be applicable in humans. However, many of the induction strategies as mentioned above have been translated to preclinical nonhuman primate models and even to clinical trials. Currently, limitations in understanding the immune tolerance mechanisms of humans, the lack of reliable assays/biomarkers which can accurately forecast the development of tolerance, and the absence of the ideal animal model restrict the more widespread development of tolerance in clinical setting. However, the future for transplant immune tolerance induction remains promising; some new and novel tolerance strategies are coming up, the most promising of which may be extended to translational nonhuman primate transplant models and clinical setting.

2 Mechanisms of Immune Accommodation of Transplant

Hyperacute rejection is mainly referring to the binding of preexisting and/or de novo anti-graft antibodies to endothelium and subsequent complement pathway activation, leading to allograft endothelial cell activation, which in turn brings about vigorous allograft rejection. Ordinarily, ABOi renal transplantation is precluded by the presence of antibodies against blood group antigen A or B (or both in patients with blood type O)—resulting in acute antibody-mediated rejection (ABMR) of allografts. The concept of accommodation is based on the discovery in the 1980s by researchers who successfully performed renal transplantation between ABOi recipients. The ABOi allografts were grafted under immunosuppression in addition with multiple plasmapheresis that were administered before transplantation, so that the allografts can survive without hyperacute rejection in the existence of low-level anti-graft antibodies. It was also viewed that at the time the anti-blood group antibodies went back to normal levels after transplantation, the allografts can still function well for months or years without the evidence of rejection.

Anti-HLA antibodies are commonly regarded destructive for allografts, and the existence of these antibodies in a transplant recipient indicates hyperacute rejection. Accommodation is also considered to occur in allografts surviving in patients with anti-HLA antibodies when antibodies go back to circulation after termination of plasmapheresis, though it appears less prevalent. It is shown that immune accommodation is also crucial to successful engraftment in ABO-compatible but HLA-incompatible (the crossmatch-positive) allograft transplant.

The mechanisms of immune accommodation are still not completely illuminated. It is generally thought that immune accommodation is mainly correlated with previous elimination of anti-graft antibodies, Th2 immune response, inhibition of complement, and expression of protection genes in grafts. It is a complicated process to induce immune accommodation, which involves the synergy of multiple factors that participate in recipients and in grafts.

2.1 Animal Models of Immune Accommodation Investigation

Graft accommodation was originally elucidated in the context of human ABOi renal transplants where graft rejection did not develop despite the existence of antibodies specific against donor blood groups. Although accommodation is also considered to occur in allografts surviving in recipients with anti-HLA antibodies when antibodies go back to circulation after termination of plasmapheresis, it is not prevalent in clinical setting. Until now, we know little about the exact mechanism of accommodation in human organ transplantation. An appropriate animal model established of ABOi organ transplantation would give diplomatic recognition of researching elaborate mechanisms of accommodation that is impossible to investigate in humans.

The first animal model that was used for investigating graft accommodation was baboon cardiac transplantation. The baboon can express A and/or B blood group antigens on its vascular endothelial cells. Anti-A and/or anti-B antibodies are directed against these antigens, the epitopes of which are carbohydrate structures. Cardiac allografting across the ABO barrier in the baboon can lead to hyperacute ABMR. The recipient baboon was over immunized against the incompatible A/B antigen before heterotopic allografting of ABOi donor hearts. The continuous intravenous infusion of the specific synthetic A/B trisaccharide and addition of triple pharmacologic immunosuppressive significantly prolonged allograft survival without ABMR after discontinuation of carbohydrate therapy. Baboon transplant model is the most suitable model for mimicking the human immune response after ABOi organ transplantation. However, due to the big body size and high cost of the baboon, it is hard to be a widespread application in the immune accommodation investigation.

The second allograft accommodation model was built in concordant cardiac xenotransplantation, such as rat-to-mouse and hamster-to-rat combinations. In this model, T-cell activation was suppressed by cyclosporine A (CsA), and complement was blocked by cobra venom factor (CVF). With the administration of the complement inhibitor CVF and T-cell immunosuppressant CsA posttransplantation in recipients, xenograft accommodation was induced. Xenograft accommodation was also achieved by repeated i.v. injections of low-dose anti-α-Gal IgG1 to Rag/galactosyltransferase (Rag/GT)-defective recipient mice that received rat hearts. Due to the hyperacute rejection caused by preexisting xenoreactive natural antibodies, accommodation has not been observed in discordant xenotransplantation models, such as from pig to primate. However, many strategies have been proposed to reduce complement-mediated xenograft EC injury. Besides the blood group antigens and HLA antigens, there are also other protein antigens that exist in the xenotransplantation, which makes the investigation of immune accommodation more complicated.

The third accommodation model has been built in the α1,3 galactosyltransferase knockout (KO) animal model. In mice, there is a structure of α-gal epitope which is tightly related to blood group A/B antigens in human. Beside this, the anti-Gal antibody contains the majority of human anti-B antibodies and of the induced anti-A/B antibodies in ABOi renal allografts. The KO mice lack α-gal epitopes owing to the disruption of their α1,3 galactosyltransferase gene, while the wild-type (WT) mice expressing α-gal epitopes are not able to produce anti-Gal, even though they are widely immunized with tissues or cells that express α-gal epitopes. Therefore, there may be analogous immunological mechanism between the KO mice transplanted with organs from WT mice and individuals with blood group O transplanted with ABOi allografts. It is shown that being exposed of anti-Gal B cells to α-gal epitopes lasting 7 days without the presence of T cells leads to allograft accommodation. In addition, Griesemer who transplanted WT (wild-type) swine kidneys into α1-3 Gal-deletion swine demonstrated experimentally inducible accommodation. Spontaneous accommodation was discovered in renal allografts in juvenile animals, indicating that there is a low level of antibody rather than decrease in antibody or B-cell levels, which allows the following engraftment and accommodation.

2.2 Mechanisms of Immune Accommodation

The immune accommodation state was first observed in human ABOi renal transplants in the 1980s. Figuring out how accommodation develops and by what mechanism it is established is of great significance in both clinical transplantation and transplant immunology. Due to the absence of appropriate experimental animal model that can mimic the human immune system, the exact mechanism of accommodation in human is still far from clear. However, investigations in pursuit of the state of accommodation over the last two decades have developed an important understanding of the mechanisms involved.

It was originally proposed that three changes may contribute to the establishment of accommodation: a change in antigens on the graft, a change in the allograft, and a change in antibodies in recipients. It is also thought that induction of graft accommodation requires complement depletion, the upregulation of complement regulatory components, and the induction of anti-apoptotic and cytoprotective genes/proteins.

2.2.1 Endothelial Cell Surface Antigens

In ABOi transplant recipients, allografts can still survive and function without ABMR occurring even after the anti-ABO antibody returned in the circulation. The first speculation is that accommodation may involve a change of the allograft endothelial cells' antigenic profile. The change of antigen epitopes on the graft during the transplantation results in no longer binding of antibodies to these antigens. Koestner et al. published a case report about the change of ABO blood antigen in a recipient after the ABOi heart transplantation. The case is that the patient of blood type O neglectfully received a cardiac allograft from donor with blood type B. The expression of ABO-type antigens on the vascular endothelial cells of the cardiac allograft was monitored by the researchers for 44 months. The alteration of the antigenic profile of the allograft endothelial cells from B to H is progressive and complete. There was also a case report of B to O cardiac transplantation in which the researchers also found that the level of B antigen staining on endothelial cells was less than that observed in control heart tissue.

However, no antigenic profile change of the graft endothelium was observed in ABOi cardiac transplants in infant who had achieved accommodation in the presence of anti-donor antibodies. Tasaki et al. measured the α1,3 galactosyltransferase and α1,3-*N*-acetylgalactosaminyltransferase, which was related to the synthesis of blood group A/B antigen (A/B enzymes), in the sera and allografts of ABOi renal transplant recipients. No obvious alteration in the distribution or strength of A/B antigens in the ABOi allograft was observed in the period of the study.

In summary, the change of antigen profiles on allograft endothelium does not seem to act as a pivotal role in accommodation, considering that accommodated organs are still capable of binding antibody to the same degree as those at basal line.

2.2.2 Blood Type Antibody/Alloantibody

Low blood type antibody/alloantibody titer or subsaturating amount of these antibodies may prior induce graft accommodation. Reduction and maintenance of anti-A/B antibodies during the first 2 weeks after transplantation below a threshold that is considered to be safe for ABOi organ transplantation. Accommodation requires a low titer of anti-graft antibodies state before transplantation and a gradual slow-paced return of the anti-graft antibodies to the circulation after transplantation. However, it is shown that accommodation does not appear when all anti-donor Ab expressions are inhibited. Total elimination of IgM antibodies increases the hardness of inducing accommodation, which was observed in some xenotransplantation models. For example, porcine ECs preincubated with human sera xenoreactive natural antibodies are capable of inducing resistance to complement-mediated injury, while the elimination of IgM antibodies from the preincubation sera weakened the protecting effect of ECs from injury. Ding et al. showed that gradual injection of low-dose anti-graft antibody (anti-α-Gal IgG1) alone could also induce immune accommodation. Thus, the antibodies' absolute levels count, in that the time required for antibody induction postoperatively may offer grafts the chance to engage accommodation.

Complement fixation (C4d deposition) in accommodated grafts indicates that the antibody binding is complete, while the less cytotoxicity involves some form of modulatory pathway as the foundation of graft survival in accommodation. Heslan et al. viewed the infiltration of B cells in accommodated grafts and thought the local restriction of grafts in situ alloantibody expression should have great significance for the accommodation state. Some studies suggest that low levels of alloantibodies may be advantageous for graft survival by upregulating anti-apoptotic genes/proteins in grafts and promoting the state of accommodation. Dalmasso et al. observed that antibodies against ECs are capable of inducing protective responses in ECs, just as the responses viewed in ECs of xenograft accommodation. Delikouras et al. confirmed that porcine EC cultured with polyclonal human IgG could induce the expression of "survival genes," including hemoxygenase 1 (HO-1) and Bcl family members on ECs. Jindra et al. showed that low concentrations of anti-donor HLA antibodies can upregulate the expression of anti-apoptotic proteins in grafts, confer endothelial cell resistance to injury, and facilitate a state of graft accommodation.

Accommodation may be relevant to antibody subclass modifications and a progressive and slow-paced of these antibodies going back to circulation. Yu et al. found that human IgG2, which is specific for Galα1-3Gal, can block the bind of IgM and prevent complement activation in cells producing Galα1-3Gal antigen. They further determined that the heavy chain repertoire of human anti-Galα1-3Gal antibodies can be altered by sensitization with xenogeneic tissues. Besides, accommodating mice showed an accumulation in the anti-Gal IgG2b subclass, while a change in IgG subclass to IgG2 could attenuate the injury resulting from humoral immunity in human.

Smith et al. suggested that without the existence of immunosuppression, anti-HLA alloantibodies may not be related to steady accommodation compared to carbohydrate antigen/ABOi, which may bring about more steady accommodation. The role of antibody in immune accommodation needs further investigation; the only thing that is certain is that the antibody is involved in the induction of immune accommodation.

2.2.3 Expression of Cytoprotective Genes and Molecules

It is observed that some protective and anti-apoptotic genes/molecules are upregulated in accommodated grafts. The vasculature of accommodated mouse heart grafts shows overexpression of the gene HO-1. This gene is undoubtedly needed for accommodation, firmly elucidated by xenotransplant model from HO-1-deficient mice-to-rat recipients with which Soares et al. authenticated that heart grafts from HO-1 WT mice acquired accommodation, while those from HO-1-deficient mice did not. HO-1 acts a pivotal role in regulating decay-catalyzing factor expression by endothelium and ameliorating the damage caused by ischemia-reperfusion innate to all transplanted organs. NF-κB activation can improve the HO-1 cytoprotective effect in ECs, since H-ferritin may be such a gene among the NF-κB-dependent genes targeted by HO-1. The expression HO-1 in ECs is capable of downregulating some proinflammatory gene expression which is related to EC activation. HO-1 is also up-modulated in the period of AMR, thus making it not a biomarker of accommodation state, but it should be considered as permission for accommodation.

Other cytoprotective genes, including A20, Bcl-2, Bcl-XL, nitric oxide synthase, and indoleamine 2,3-dioxygenase, are also upregulated in accommodated grafts. There is a large amount of evidence indicating that these genes are induced in endothelial cells in low (rather than high)-concentration Abs against multiple epitopes by a nitric oxide-dependent process taking part in signaling via adenosine A2 receptors and PI3K/AKT pathway. For instance, Bcl-XL expression by glomerular and peritubular capillaries has been depicted as a specific biomarker of accommodation.

It is found that cytoprotective genes are expressed both in accommodated grafts and in grafts suffering from rejection. Other investigators have found that these genes are not overexpressed in accommodated ABO-incompatible allografts. Although the functional significance of these genes in vivo has not been built, they are hypothesized to restrict the vascular response to inflammation, by depressing NF-κB stimulation. Alternatively, diverse protective genes may offer different types of protection from injury.

Other cytoprotective molecules have been authenticated in accommodated porcine graft models and human ABOi renal allografts, including syndecan-4-phosphate, heparan sulfate, Muc-1, and members of the tyrosine kinase receptor family.

2.2.4 The Complement System

Evidence indicates that complement acts a pivotal role in ABMR. The mechanism of graft accommodation might refer to heightened regulation of complement or heightened resistance to complement.

Attenuation of complement by internalization and shedding of complement complexes and up-modulation of decay-accelerating membrane cofactor protein or CD59 have been advanced as mechanisms contributing to accommodation which was observed after ABOi renal transplantation in human. Dalmasso et al. observed that xenoreactive antibodies induce CD59 expression which regulates the membrane attack complex of complement, and this alteration results in heightened resistance to complement-regulated cell lysis. Furthermore, Dorling et al. found that resistance of porcine endothelial cell lysis was induced by xenoreactive IgG. However, xenograft expression of CD59 which is regarded as a product of a transgene does not avoid rejection. In fact, complement inhibitors alone and jointly have failed by themselves to bring about long-term survival of xenografts only if xenoreactive antibodies or antigens they distinguish were also manipulated.

Tang et al. found that hepatocytes naturally resist complement-regulated lysis resulting from heightened regulation of complement independent of the concentration of expression of complement modulatory proteins but demanding function of the AKT/PI3K pathways. Ding et al. used the rat-to-mouse xenotransplant model and found that upregulation of complement modulatory proteins may abolish complement-regulated rejection and allow xenograft accommodation.

2.2.5 Other Factors

Other factors inducing protective gene expression in ECs are anti-inflammatory cytokines (including IL-4, IL-6, IL-10, and IL-13), which are related to Th2 immune responses. Furthermore, the increasing of IL-4 and IL-10 secreting by Th2 cells has been observed in the peripheral blood and spleen of rats with accommodated xenografts.

2.3 Relationship Between Accommodation and Immune Tolerance

Induction of immune tolerance to allograft induction is always being considered the holy grail in organ transplant immunology. The clinical use of new and potent immunosuppressants reduces the occurrence proportion of acute allograft rejection rather than lengthening the long-term survival of allografts obviously. The development of chronic rejection is the main cause of terminal allograft failure. The immunological mechanisms, the foundation of chronic rejection, are not fully understood but seem to be related to continuous production of anti-donor/anti-allograft antibodies. Both alloantibodies and chronic rejection are pivotal problems in tolerance induction procedures. Interestingly, accommodation is indeed a state where the allograft functions regularly with the existence of anti-graft antibodies in the recipient.

Tolerance and accommodation together can explain avoidance of allograft rejection by the alloimmune response more completely than by each one of them. Tolerance mainly focuses on alterations of the recipient's immune system, while accommodation is involved in the changes of the target allograft. Tolerance endows allografts with immune privilege, which means that recipients' immune system shows "specific non-responsiveness" to allografts even without immunosuppression. Accommodation permits allografts to endure active alloimmune responses but at a biological expense. Besides these, in condition of accommodation, the recipient preserves the ability of rejecting other allografts from the same donor, but the satisfactory observation is that accommodated allograft is still being protected even if re-transplanted to a new recipient. However, in condition of tolerance, the recipient could accept other allografts from the same donor, but tolerant allograft can still be rejected if re-transplanted into a new recipient.

The orchestrated combination of tolerance and accommodation will embody the mechanism to explain why alloimmunity does not damage allografts. Further mechanism investigating both accommodation and tolerance and the relationship between these two statuses can coordinate recipient's immune defense with avoidance of immune response to allografts.

Bibliography

1. Hourmant M, Cesbron-Gautier A, Terasaki PI, et al. Frequency and clinical implications of development of donor-specific and non-donor-specific HLA antibodies after kidney transplantation. J Am Soc Nephrol. 2005;16:2804–12.
2. Zhang Q, Liang LW, Gjertson DW, et al. Development of posttransplant antidonor HLA antibodies is associated with acute humoral rejection and early graft dysfunction. Transplantation. 2005;79:591–8.
3. Lefaucheur C, Nochy D, Hill GS, et al. Determinants of poor graft outcome in patients with antibody-mediated acute rejection. Am J Transplant. 2007;7:832–41.
4. Piazza A, Poggi E, Ozzella G, et al. Post-transplant donor-specific antibody production and graft outcome in kidney transplantation: results of sixteen-year monitoring by flow cytometry. Clin Transpl. 2006:323–36.
5. Bach FH, Ferran C, Hechenleitner P, et al. Accommodation of vascularized xenografts: expression of "protective genes" by donor endothelial cells in a host Th2 cytokine environment. Nat Med. 1997;3:196–204.
6. Haas M, Segev DL, Racusen LC, et al. C4d deposition without rejection correlates with reduced early scarring in ABO-incompatible renal allografts. J Am Soc Nephrol. 2009;20:197–204.
7. Galili U. Xenotransplantation and ABO incompatible transplantation: the similarities they share. Transfus Apher Sci. 2006;35:45–58.
8. Griesemer AD, Okumi M, Shimizu A, et al. Upregulation of cd59: potential mechanism of accommodation in a large animal model. Transplantation. 2009;87:1308–17.
9. Koestner SC, Kappeler A, Schaffner T, et al. Histo-blood group type change of the graft from B to O after ABO mismatched heart transplantation. Lancet. 2004;363:1523–5.
10. Lee PS, Poh KK. Endothelial progenitor cells in cardiovascular diseases. World J Stem Cells. 2014;6:355–66.
11. Quaini F, Urbanek K, Beltrami AP, et al. Chimerism of the transplanted heart. N Engl J Med. 2002;346:5–15.
12. Lagaaij EL, Cramer-Knijnenburg GF, van Kemenade FJ, et al. Endothelial cell chimerism after renal transplantation and vascular rejection. Lancet. 2001;357:33–7.
13. Tasaki M, Nakajima T, Imai N, et al. Detection of allogeneic blood group A and B enzyme activities in patients with abo incompatible kidney transplantation. Glycobiology. 2010;20:1251–8.
14. Dehoux JP, Hori S, Talpe S, et al. Specific depletion of preformed IgM natural antibodies by administration of anti-mu monoclonal antibody suppresses hyperacute rejection of pig to baboon renal xenografts. Transplantation. 2000;70:935–46.
15. Ding JW, Zhou T, Ma L, et al. Expression of complement regulatory proteins in accommodated xenografts induced by anti-alpha-Gal IgG1 in a rat-to-mouse model. Am J Transplant. 2008;8:32–40.

16. Delikouras A, Hayes M, Malde P, et al. Nitric oxide-mediated expression of Bcl-2 and Bcl-xl and protection from tumor necrosis factor-alpha-mediated apoptosis in porcine endothelial cells after exposure to low concentrations of xenoreactive natural antibody. Transplantation. 2001;71:599–605.
17. Mohiuddin MM, Ogawa H, Yin DP, et al. Antibody-mediated accommodation of heart grafts expressing an incompatible carbohydrate antigen. Transplantation. 2003;75:258–62.
18. Zhang C, Wang L, Zhong S, et al. Over-expression of heme oxygenase-1 does not protect porcine endothelial cells from human xenoantibodies and complement-mediated lysis. J Huazhong Univ Sci Technolog Med Sci. 2013;33:102–6.
19. He KL, Ting AT. A20 inhibits tumor necrosis factor (TNF) alpha-induced apoptosis by disrupting recruitment of TRADD and RIP to the TNF receptor 1 complex in Jurkat T cells. Mol Cell Biol. 2002;22:6034–45.
20. Chen G, Chen S, Chen X. Role of complement and perspectives for intervention in transplantation. Immunobiology. 2013;218:817–27.
21. Wang H, Arp J, Liu W, et al. Inhibition of terminal complement components in presensitized transplant recipients prevents antibody-mediated rejection leading to long-term graft survival and accommodation. J Immunol. 2007;179:4451–63.
22. Dalmasso AP, Benson BA, Johnson JS, et al. Resistance against the membrane attack complex of complement induced in porcine endothelial cells with a Gal alpha(1-3)Gal binding lectin: up-regulation of CD59 expression. J Immunol. 2000;164:3764–73.
23. Chen Song S, Zhong S, Xiang Y, et al. Complement inhibition enables renal allograft accommodation and long-term engraftment in presensitized nonhuman primates. Am J Transplant. 2011;11:2057–66.
24. Tan CD, Sokos GG, Pidwell DJ, et al. Correlation of donor-specific antibodies, complement and its regulators with graft dysfunction in cardiac antibody-mediated rejection. Am J Transplant. 2009;9:2075–84.
25. Gonzalez-Stawinski GV, Tan CD, Smedira NG, et al. Decay-accelerating factor expression may provide immunoprotection against antibody-mediated cardiac allograft rejection. J Heart Lung Transplant. 2008;27:357–61.
26. Brodsky SV, Nadasdy GM, Pelletier R, et al. Expression of the decay-accelerating factor (CD55) in renal transplants-a possible prediction marker of allograft survival. Transplantation. 2009;88:457–64.
27. Parker W, Lin SS, Platt JL. Antigen expression in xenotransplantation: how low must it go? Transplantation. 2001;71:313–9.
28. Sprent J, Kishimoto H. The thymus and central tolerance. Philos Trans R Soc Lond Ser B Biol Sci. 2001;356:609–16.
29. Hogquist KA, Baldwin TA, Jameson SC. Central tolerance: learning self-control in the thymus. Nat Rev Immunol. 2005;5:772–82.
30. Chopek MW, Simmons RL, Platt JL. ABO-incompatible renal transplantation: initial immunopathologic evaluation. Transplant Proc. 1987;19:4553–7.
31. Bannett AD, McAlack RF, Morris M, et al. ABO incompatible renal transplantation: a qualitative analysis of native endothelial tissue ABO antigens after transplant. Transplant Proc. 1989;21:783–5.
32. Metzger TC, Anderson MS. Control of central and peripheral tolerance by Aire. Immunol Rev. 2011;241:89–103.
33. Mueller DL. Mechanisms maintaining peripheral tolerance. Nat Immunol. 2010;11:21–7.
34. Braza F, Dugast E, Panov I, et al. Central role of CD45RA-Foxp3hi memory regulatory T cells in clinical kidney transplantation tolerance. J Am Soc Nephrol. 2015;26:1795–805.
35. Skoberne M1, Beignon AS, Larsson M, et al. Apoptotic cells at the crossroads of tolerance and immunity. Curr Top Microbiol Immunol. 2005;289:259–92.
36. Ruiz P, Maldonado P, Hidalgo Y, et al. Transplant tolerance: new insights and strategies for long-term allograft acceptance. Clin Dev Immunol. 2013;2013:210506.
37. Haanstra KG, Ringers J, Sick EA, et al. Prevention of kidney allograft rejection using anti-CD40 and anti-CD86 in primates. Transplantation. 2003;75:637–43.

38. Pearson TC, Trambley J, Odom K, et al. Anti-CD40 therapy extends renal allograft survival in rhesus macaques. Transplantation. 2002;74:933–40.
39. Adams AB, Shirasugi N, Jones TR, et al. Development of a chimeric anti-CD40 monoclonal antibody that synergizes with LEA29Y to prolong islet allograft survival. J Immunol. 2005;174:542–50.
40. Haanstra KG, Sick EA, Ringers J, et al. Costimulation blockade followed by a 12-week period of cyclosporine A facilitates prolonged drug-free survival of rhesus monkey kidney allografts. Transplantation. 2005;79:1623–6.
41. Scandling JD, Busque S, Dejbakhsh-Jones S, et al. Tolerance and chimerism after renal and hematopoietic-cell transplantation. N Engl J Med. 2008;358:362–8.
42. Scandling JD, Busque S, Dejbakhsh-Jones S, et al. Tolerance and withdrawal of immunosuppressive drugs in patients given kidney and hematopoietic cell transplants. Am J Transplant. 2012;12:1133–45.
43. Scandling JD, Busque S, Shizuru JA, et al. Induced immune tolerance for kidney transplantation. N Engl J Med. 2011;365:1359–60.
44. Leventhal J, Abecassis M, Miller J, et al. Chimerism and tolerance without GVHD or engraftment syndrome in HLA-mismatched combined kidney and hematopoietic stem cell transplantation. Sci Transl Med. 2012;4:124ra128.
45. Kawai T, Sachs DH, Sprangers B, et al. Long-term results in recipients of combined HLA-mismatched kidney and bone marrow transplantation without maintenance immunosuppression. Am J Transplant. 2014;14:1599–611.
46. Kitchens WH. Nonhuman primate models of transplant tolerance: closer to the holy grail. Curr Opin Organ Transplant. 2016;21:59–65.
47. Anderson A, Martens CL, Hendrix R, et al. Expanded nonhuman primate Tregs exhibit a unique gene expression signature and potently downregulate alloimmune responses. Am J Transplant. 2008;8:2252–64.
48. Lei J, Kim JI, Shi S, et al. Pilot study evaluating regulatory T cell-promoting immunosuppression and nonimmunogenic donor antigen delivery in a nonhuman primate islet allotransplantation model. Am J Transplant. 2015;15:273–2749.
49. Bashuda H, Kimikawa M, Seino K, et al. Renal allograft rejection is prevented by adoptive transfer of anergic T cells in nonhuman primates. J Clin Invest. 2005;115:1896–902.
50. Carreras-Planella L, Borràs FE, Franquesa M. Tolerance in kidney transplantation: what is on the B side? Mediators Inflamm. 2016;2016:8491956.
51. Warren DS, Zachary AA, Sonnenday CJ, et al. Successful renal transplantation across simultaneous ABO incompatible and positive crossmatch barriers. Am J Transplant. 2004;4:561–8.
52. Morath C, Zeier M, Döhler B, et al. ABO-incompatible kidney transplantation. Front Immunol. 2017;8:234.
53. Lynch RJ, Platt JL. Accommodation in renal transplantation: unanswered questions. Curr Opin Organ Transplant. 2010;15:481–5.
54. Dehoux JP, Gianello P. Accommodation and antibodies. Transpl Immunol. 2009;21:106–10.
55. Griesemer AD, Okumi M, Shimizu A, et al. Upregulation of CD59: potential mechanism of accommodation in a large animal model. Transplantation. 2009;87(9):1308–17.
56. West LJ, Pollock-Barziv SM, Lee KJ, et al. Graft accommodation in infant recipients of ABO-incompatible heart transplants: donor ABH antigen expression in graft biopsies. J Heart Lung Transplant. 2001;20(2):222.
57. Tang AH, Platt JL. Accommodation of grafts: implications for health and disease. Hum Immunol. 2007;68:645–51.
58. Heslan JM, Renaudin K, Thebault P, et al. New evidence for a role of allograft accommodation in long-term tolerance. Transplantation. 2006;82:1185–93.
59. Jin YP, Jindra PT, Gong KW, et al. Anti-HLA class I antibodies activate endothelial cells and promote chronic rejection. Transplantation. 2005;79:S19–21.
60. Smith RN, Kawai T, Boskovic S, et al. Four stages and lack of stable accommodation in chronic alloantibody-mediated renal allograft rejection in cynomolgus monkeys. Am J Transplant. 2008;8:1662–72.

61. Suhr BD, Black SM, Guzman-Paz M, et al. Inhibition of the membrane attack complex of complement for induction of accommodation in the hamster-to-rat heart transplant model. Xenotransplantation. 2007;14:572–9.
62. Takahashi K. Recent findings in ABO-incompatible kidney transplantation: classification and therapeutic strategy for acute antibody-mediated rejection due to ABO-blood-group-related antigens during the critical period preceding the establishment of accommodation. Clin Exp Nephrol. 2007;11:128–41.
63. Park WD, Grande JP, Ninova D, et al. Accommodation in ABO-incompatible kidney allografts, a novel mechanism of self-protection against antibody-mediated injury. Am J Transplant. 2003;3:952–60.
64. Newell KA, Phippard D, Turka LA. Regulatory cells and cell signatures in clinical transplantation tolerance. Curr Opin Immunol. 2011;23(5):655–9.
65. Adams AB, Newell KA. B cells in clinical transplantation tolerance. Semin Immunol. 2012;24(2):92–5.
66. Kitchens WH, Adams AB. Nonhuman primate models of transplant tolerance: closer to the holy grail. Curr Opin Organ Transplant. 2016;21(1):59–65.

Appendix: The Clinical Guideline of ABO—Incompatible Kidney Transplantation (2017)—The Chinese Society of Organ Transplantation

Yi Wang

Abstract

Organ resource shortage is a huge obstacle for organ transplantation, which can be largely alleviated with the wide application of ABO-incompatible organ transplantation. Although ABO-incompatible kidney transplantation has been performed in many transplant centers, yet there have not been uniform perioperative protocols. In this part, we'll summarize the perioperative protocols of ABO-incompatible kidney transplantation based on a literature review and our clinical experience, hoping to provide a guideline for ABO-incompatible kidney transplantation.

Keywords

ABO-incompatible kidney transplantation · Perioperative protocols · Guideline

Introduction

The expansion of organ resource will be an eternal theme of organ transplantation unless the fundamental solution of organ resource shortage is found. Living-related donor kidney transplantation has been performed in many organ transplantation centers around the world as an effective way to relieve the lack of organ resources.

Y. Wang (✉)
The Second Affiliated Hospital of Hainan Medical University, Haikou City, Hainan Province, China

The Second Affiliated Hospital, University of South China, Hengyang City, Hunan Province, China
e-mail: wayne0108@126.com

Y. Wang (ed.), *ABO-incompatible Organ Transplantation*,
https://doi.org/10.1007/978-981-13-3399-6

The ABO-incompatible kidney transplantation has provided a boon for the patients on the long waiting list.

Early in 1955, Hume et al. firstly reported ABO-incompatible kidney transplantation (ABOi-KT), but a depressing result showed that hyperacute rejection occurred in eight cases of ten patients, which caused acute renal failure [1]. In 1987, Alexandre et al. first reported 26 cases of successful ABOi-KT [2] and established the basic framework of ABOi-KT. According to this report, rejection was significantly reduced due to the procedures of removing the ABO blood group antibodies by repeated preoperative plasmapheresis and performing splenectomy during the operation to inhibit the postoperative immunological rejection caused by the rebound of blood type antibodies.

Early protocols usually suggested performing splenectomy before or during transplantation. But later researches proved that this scheme not only reduced the immune function of recipients, increasing the risk of postoperative infections, causing some side effects such as unexplained indigestion, and even increasing the risk of death, but also had limited inhibition of ABO blood group antibodies [3]. In 2004, Tydén G et al. firstly reported a successful ABOi-KT that used rituximab instead of splenectomy [4]. Up to now, the preoperative use of rituximab and plasmapheresis have been performed in most transplant centers as critical steps in ABOi-KT.

As the world's largest ABOi-KT country, Japan has completed more than 2400 cases of ABOi-KT, accounting for 30% of living kidney transplants [5–7]. According to the statistics by Opelz et al.'s [8], there were 1420 cases of ABOi-KT registered in collaborative transplantation in Europe and Australia during the period from 2005 to 2012, accounting for 4.2% of the total number of live renal transplants. The percentage of ABOi-KT in America is relatively lower, but this figure keeps annually increasing [9]. Since China carried out such transplantation for the first time in December 2006 [10], the number of ABOi-KT cases and qualified transplant centers has been continuously increasing.

ABOi-KT recipients need to eliminate the recipient's natural ABO blood group antibodies before the operation in order to avoid hyperacute rejection (HAR) and accelerated rejection (AR). There are various methods to remove plasma ABO blood group antibodies. Montgomery et al. [11] in America mainly used plasma exchange (PE) or PE combined with intravenous immunoglobulin; Takahashi and others in Japan [12] used double filtration plasmapheresis (DFPP) to remove the antibodies in plasma proteins; and in Sweden, Tyden et al. [13] used blood group antigen adsorption column to specially remove ABO blood group antibodies in the recipients. There is no enough evidence to evaluate which of those treatments is more advantageous [14].

ABOi-KT has had the same or even better prognosis than ABO-compatible kidney transplantation (ABOc-KT) owing to the continuous improvement of perioperative treatment protocols now. According to the report of Takahashi et al. in Japan, since the application of new procedures instead of splenectomy in 2001, among the 1427 cases of ABOi-KT performed in Japan, the graft renal survival rate of ABOi-KT in 1, 3, 5, and 9 years, respectively, was 96%, 93%, 91%, and 83%. This data was similar to ABOc-KT. Montgomery and others studied 738 cases of ABOi-KT in 280 American transplantation centers from 1995 to 2012 and concluded that the 2 weeks after operation was a high-risk period for ABOi-KT, during which the risk of renal allograft loss was higher than ABOc-KT group. They suggested that the 2 weeks after the operation was the critical period for the immune adaptation of ABOi-KT. After 2 weeks, the transplanted kidney successfully established immunological adaptation to the ABO blood group antibodies [15]. Tyden et al. reviewed the data of 60 patients in three centers of Sweden and Germany. According to the 61 months of follow-up after operation, the graft survival rate was 97% in the ABOi-KT group, versus 95% in the contemporaneous 274 cases in ABOc-KT group, which showed no statistical difference between the two groups. Fuchinoue et al. reported among 60 ABOi-KT recipients, the 5-year survival rate was 100%, higher than 88.4% in ABOc-KT group [17]. According to the data above, ABO blood type incompatibility is no longer an independent risk factor for kidney transplantation.

In order to establish a feasible standardized scheme for ABOi-KT, we drew up this guideline for reference based on the international relevant literature and the ABOi-KT experience of China. Since ABOi kidney resource is mainly from living donors around the world, donation after cardiac death (DCD) is rarely used; this guideline also focuses on the ABOi-KT grounded on relative living donors.

Recommendation Level/Evidence Level Standard (Table A.1)

Table A.1 Evidence quality grade and strength of recommendation

Evidence quality grade and strength of recommendation	Definition
Grade of evidence quality	
High A	It is almost impossible to change the reliability of existing efficacy evaluation results by future research
Middle B	Future research may have important implications for the existing efficacy assessment and may change the credibility of the evaluation results
Low C	Future research is likely to have an important implications for the existing efficacy evaluation and is likely to change the credibility of the evaluation results
Very low D	Any assessment of the efficacy is uncertain
Strength of recommendation	
Strong recommendation 1	It is clear that the advantages of the intervention outweigh the disadvantages or opposite
Weak recommendation 2	Pros and cons are uncertain, or evidence quality shows advantages and disadvantages are about equal

Indications and Contraindications of ABOi-KT

Indications

ABOi-KT is suitable for patients with end-stage renal disease (ESRD). The indications and contraindications of ABOi-KT are basically the same as those of ABOc-KT (please refer to Table A.2, or the chapter of "clinical guidelines of living-related kidney transplantation" in *The Clinical Guidelines-Organ transplantation section* published in 2010 by the People's Medical Publishing House). ABOi-KT is especially suitable for those who have difficulty finding ABO blood group-compatible kidney in the short term and, at the same time, are under the following circumstances: (1) hemodialysis has a poor curative effect and/or complications are endangering life and (2) the patient is unable to receive other renal replacement therapy.

The correlation between the titer of ABO blood group antibody in recipients and the outcome is still controversial. Previous studies have reported that higher titer of ABO blood group antibody before transplantation was positively correlated with the antibody mediated rejection (AMR) and the dysfunction of the xenotransplantation [18–20]. Recent studies also revealed that the survival of xenotransplantation had no relationship with the titer of ABO blood group antibody [21, 22], however, higher titer of ABO blood group antibody still meant more times of plasmapheresis and chances of coagulation disorders [22, 23].

Recommendations

1. Before the plasmapheresis, the ABO blood group antibody titer of recipients, including anti-A IgG, anti-A IgM, anti-B IgG, and anti-B IgM, needs to be lower than 1:256 (1-C).
2. The recurrence risk of primary diseases such as focal segmental glomerulosclerosis is relatively high, but can be significantly reduced by plasmapheresis and the use of rituximab (1-B).
3. Patients with glomerular basement membrane disease generally are required to wait till the antibodies vanished. But plasmapheresis and rituximab can reduce and suppress the titer of related antibody, so experienced transplant centers can perform research transplants after informing the patients and their relatives of the related risks (2-C).
4. Patients with type I diabetes combined with renal failure can also take simultaneous pancreas-kidney transplantation even if the blood type does not match (1-B).

Table A.2 Indications for ABOi-KT [24–26]

1.	Glomerulonephritis
2.	Hereditary diseases such as polycystic kidney, nephron consumptive disease, Alport syndrome, etc.
3.	Metabolic diseases such as diabetes, hyperoxaluria, gout, porphyria, etc.
4.	Obstructive nephropathy
5.	Drug-induced renal injury
6.	Systemic diseases: systemic lupus erythematosus, vasculitis, progressive systemic sclerosis, etc.
7.	Hemolytic uremic syndrome
8.	Congenital diseases: such as horseshoe kidney, congenital hypoplasia of kidney
9.	Irreversible acute renal failure
10.	Severe trauma
11.	Double kidney or solitary kidney loss due to trauma

Contraindications (Table A.3)

Recommendations

1. Previous ABOc transplantation history is not an absolute contraindication for ABOi-KT (1-B), but ABOc-KT should be the first choice in patients who have received ABOi organ transplantation (2-C).
2. Patients with positive cross matching could be successfully managed and achieve a good prognosis by plasma exchange, intravenous immunoglobulin infusion, and the use of rituximab to hurdle the blood type and type matching barrier. The 5-year survival rate of highly sensitized patients is lower than that of the non-sensitized patients, but higher than that of the simple dialysis patients. In the absence of other kidney selection, experienced transplant centers can perform research transplants after informing the patients and their relatives of the related risks (2-B).

Table A.3 ABOi-KT contraindications [25, 27]

Absolute contraindications	
1.	Widely disseminated or untreated tumor
2.	Severe mental illness and psychosocial problems
3.	Irreversible multiple organ failure
4.	Irreversible brain damage and other serious neurological damage
5.	Drug abusers
6.	Acute active hepatitis
7.	Severe coagulopathy
8.	Uncontrolled severe infection, active tuberculosis, AIDS (CD4 T cells <200/mL; HIV > 400 copy number/mL)
9.	Various progressive metabolic diseases
10.	Peptic ulcer at active stage
Relative contraindications	
1.	A tumor that has been healed
2.	Chronic liver disease, such as chronic hepatitis B or chronic hepatitis C

(continued)

Table A.3 (*cont.*)

3.	HIV infection
4.	Prestored HLA antibodies were positive for cross matching
5.	History of drug abuse
6.	Serious urinary tract malformation, neurogenic bladder, etc.
7.	Severe malnutrition or cachexia
8.	Evidence of poor compliance
9.	Lack of family and social support
10.	Active infection
11.	ESRD primary disease is in active phase
12.	Patients with primary kidney diseases such as nephron consumptive disease and primary hyperoxaluria combined with abnormal liver function are suggested undergoing combined liver and kidney transplantation
13.	Serious, uncontrollable albuminuria
14.	Abdominal aorta and iliac artery disease

Indications and Contraindications for Donors [24, 27] (Tables A.4 and A.5)

Recommendations

1. HBV and HCV kidney from positive donors could be transplanted into HBV- and HCV-positive recipients under the informed consent principle (1-B).
2. Since ABOi-KT recipients will be treated with plasmapheresis (PE) and double filtration plasmapheresis (DFPP) to remove antibodies including HBsAg, it is recommended that the serum anti-HBS concentration of recipients after plasmapheresis should be detected before HBV- and HCV-positive donor kidney is transplanted to a negative recipient (please refer to the ABOc-KT guideline for the appropriate operation). Only in case of emergency, kidney of HBV- and HCV-positive donor can be transplanted to the negative recipient conforming to the informed consent principle (1-C).

Table A.4 Indications for ABOi-KT donors

1.	Having mental health and completely act autonomously; fully capable of autonomous action; regarding organ donation as a noble act without economic factors involved
2.	18–65 years old
3.	No kidney diseases such as nephritis, nephropathy, infection, stones, tumors, deformities, etc.; the main blood vessels of the kidney to be donated are normal and free of deformity, sclerosis, and significant stenosis; good renal function with creatinine clearance rate > 80 mL/min
4.	No heart, liver, lung relevant diseases; no hypertension, diabetes, systemic lupus erythematosus; no malignant tumor, infectious diseases (such as AIDS, syphilis, hepatitis, etc.); no mental illness; no coagulopathy

The Suitable Antibody Titer of Blood Group on the Day of Operation

Because of the difference between the method of blood group antibody test and plasma treatment scheme, the requirements of ABO antibody titer before the operation are also different among the international transplant centers which range from 1:4 to 1:32. All of them can obtain satisfactory curative effect [12, 22, 28, 29].

Recommendations

Transplantation requirements for A and B blood type antibody titers: adult recipients, IgM $\leq$ 1:16 and IgG $\leq$ 1:16;child recipients, IgM = 1:64 and IgG = 1:64 (1-B)

Table A.5 Contraindications for ABOi-KT donors

Absolute contraindications
1. Widely disseminated or untreated tumor
2. Severe mental illness and psychosocial problems that are difficult to solve
3. Irreversible organ failure
4. Irreversible brain damage and other serious neurological damage
5. Drug abusers
6. Acute active hepatitis
7. The endogenous creatinine clearance rate < 70 mL/min
8. BMI > 35
9. Under 18 years old
Relative contraindications
1. Tumor that has been healed
2. Chronic liver disease, such as chronic hepatitis B or chronic hepatitis C
3. HIV infection
4. History of drug abuse
5. Serious urinary tract malformation, neurogenic bladdcr, ctc.
6. Severe malnutrition or cachexia
7. Evidence of poor compliance
8. Lack of family and social support
9. Active infections
10. Diseases of the abdominal aorta and inferior vena cava
11. The rate of endogenous creatinine clearance was 70–80 mL/min
12. BMI 30–35
13. Other diseases: such as diabetes, hypertension, hyperthyroidism, urinary calculi, etc.

Requirements for Coagulation Function on the Day of Surgery

Preoperative use of rituximab and repeated plasma treatment can deplete the B cells and antibody level of recipients. If albumin supplementation is added to multiple DFPP and plasmapheresis process, the coagulation factor of the recipient may be lost, resulting in hypocoagulability stage.

Recommendations

Coagulation requirements before the surgery:

APTT: 24–26 s (1-B)
TT: 11–21 s (1-B)
FIB:1.2–4 g/L (1-B)
D-dimer: <0.3 mg/L (1-B)

Tissue Matching

The rate of tissue matching and HLA matching is related to graft prognosis [30]. The HLA-A, HLA-B, and HLA-DR are the most important antigens that need detecting in the transplant, and for HLA-DR, it's better to take molecular typing. In order to avoid hyperacute rejection, cross matching is highly necessary. The negative result in cross matched lymphocyte cytotoxicity tests but still positive result in ELISA or more sensitive Luminex analysis indicates that donor-specific antibodies (DSA) are still present in the blood of recipients. The presence of DSA is an independent risk factor, which is positively related to postoperative AMR and graft loss, but has no effect on graft survival [31–33].

Some studies have suggested that the probability of AMR in recipients with O blood group is higher than that in other blood group recipients [22, 34], but the strength of evidence and reproducibility is insufficient [16].

Recommendation

1. The mismatch site of HLA for ABOi-KT donors and recipients should be ≤3 (1-C).
2. The CDC test ≤10% (1-A).
3. Panel reactive antibody (PRA) test <20% (1-C).
4. DSA negative (mean fluorescence intensity of Luminex <1000) (1-B).
5. PRA reflects the probability of the presence of DSA in the recipient. Some recipients with high PRA but DSA negative in CDC and Luminex can still undergo ABOi-KT.

Application of Anti-CD20 Monoclonal Antibodies

CD20 is a marker of B lymphocytes and is expressed in normal human initial B cells and mature B cells. Rituximab is a chimeric murine antihuman CD20 monoclonal antibody that can specifically bind to CD20 antigen. It may perform the function of directly inducing B-cell apoptosis by complement-dependent cytotoxicity (CDC) or eliminating B cells by antibody-dependent cellular cytotoxicity (ADCC). Rituximab was first used in the treatment of B lymphocyte lymphoma. Recently, in a number of literature, it has been reported that it can also effectively prevent humoral rejection [35]. Currently, rituximab has replaced splenectomy as a routine means of ABOi-KT [36, 37]. Cases with anti-CD20 antibodies had better graft survival than non-CD20 plasma treatment protocols, but the statistical significance is still controversial [8, 38, 39].

Recommendations

1. Routine use of rituximab is recommended for ABOi-KT recipients. The following medication options are available. The following dosage regimen can be selected in proportion to CD19 B cells. Appropriate adjustments based on changes in cells proportion during therapeutic process are acceptable (1-C):
   (a) If the proportion of CD19+B cells in recipients ranges from 10% to 15%, rituximab 100 mg, 100 mg, and 100 mg are, respectively, recommended at 4 weeks, 2 weeks, and 24 h before transplantation (estimate the surface area of the recipients as a standard value of 1.73 m^2).
   (b) If the proportion of CD19+B cells in recipients is $\geq$15%, rituximab 200 mg, 100 mg, and 100 mg are, respectively, recommended at 4 weeks, 2 weeks, and 24 h before transplantation (estimate the surface area of the recipients as a standard value of 1.73 m^2).
   (c) If the proportion of CD19+B cells in recipients is $\leq$10%, rituximab 100 mg and 100 mg, are, respectively, recommended at 4 weeks and 2 weeks before transplantation (estimate the surface area of the recipients as a standard value of 1.73 m^2).
2. The use of polyclonal antibodies and monoclonal antibodies such as ATG/OKT3 is feasible when it is necessary.

Plasma Treatment

Preoperative plasma treatment is a critical element to eliminate the anti-A and anti-B blood group antibodies in the blood of recipients as much as possible in order to avoid hyperacute rejection [40]. It mainly includes three aspects: reducing the antibody titer of pre-existing ABO blood group antibody, preventing ABO blood group antibody from rebounding, and adjusting the coagulation function of recipients. There are three methods to remove blood group antibody before ABOi-KT, including plasma exchange (PE), double filtration plasmapheresis (DFPP), and plasma immunosorbent

(IA). Japan mainly uses DFPP, while the USA uses PE plus intravenous gamma globulin (IVIG) [11, 12, 41]. Generally, plasma treatment starts from 7 days before operation, and the subsequent treatment time shall be determined according to the titer of the blood group antigen after the treatment. It must be ensured that the antibody titer reaches the standard before operation [42]. Immunosorbent is a highly selective and specific method that does not affect curative effect of other drugs and coagulation of recipients. But constrained by the costly and rare consumables, it is currently only used by some Nordic countries like Sweden [28].

The plasma treatment scheme within 2 weeks after operation is controversial. Some suggest that the plasma treatment should be preemptive at the fixed time after surgery, depending on or regardless of the antibody titer [11, 28], and others believe that the postoperative antibody titer has no effect on the prognosis and postoperative plasma treatment is unnecessary [12, 22]. Two weeks after transplantation, the titer of the blood group antibody can be ignored with the recipient's immune adaptation established.

Recommendations

1. For recipients who have coagulation disorders combined with severe hypoproteinemia, PE should be chosen as the preoperative plasma treatment and type AB plasma used as replacement fluid (1-B).
2. The coagulation function must be monitored in the period of preoperative plasma treatment, including serum Ca^{2+} concentration, FIB, platelets, PT, APTT, etc. (1-A).
3. Hemodialysis, CRRT, blood perfusion, etc. can be used as the preoperative plasma treatment of ABOi-KT together (unclassified evidence).
4. Pay attention to the prevention of pulmonary edema and heart failure during the preoperative plasma treatment period (1-A).
5. Appropriately use hormones during the preoperative plasma treatment period to reduce side effects caused by transfusion of blood products, such as allergic reactions (2-B).
6. Sodium citrate is a recommended anticoagulant during the preoperative plasma treatment period (2-C).
7. It is recommended to combine large doses of intravenous immunoglobulin (IVIG) for recipients who have a rapid rebound in blood type antibody after preoperative plasma treatment (2-B).
8. DFPP is now commonly used in combination with plasmapheresis to reduce the coagulation dysfunction syndrome and the low protein and hypoperfusion syndrome caused by it (2-B).
9. Antibiotic prophylaxis is recommended after PE (2-C).
10. Hepatitis B immunoglobulin is recommended for patients who require large amounts of fresh frozen plasma (fresh, frozen, plasma, FFP) (such as thrombocytopenic purpura TTP) (2-B).
11. The titer of blood group antibody was monitored within 2 weeks after operation. If the IgG or IgM blood group antibody titer is ≥1:32, perform one to two times of plasma exchange (2-C). No plasma exchange is in need 2 weeks later (1-A).

Preoperative Examination and Preparation of Recipients

The preoperative examination and preparation of recipients of ABOi-KT are exactly the same as that of ABOc-KT (refer to "Relative living renal transplantation" in *Clinical Guidelines Manual of organ transplantation* published by the People's Medical Publishing House) [25].

Preoperative Detection and Postoperative Monitoring of Antibody Titer

The recommended blood type antibody titer detection methods include saline medium colloidal agglutination test, agglutination test, enzyme treatment of red blood cell agglutination, Coombs antiglobulin test and improved Coombs antiglobulin test, and low ionic polybrene test. The same sample may show an obvious difference in the results of the titer of blood type antibody when independently tested in different methods or even the same method in different laboratories. Therefore, in the whole process of ABOi-KT, the titer of blood type antibody should be detected by the same method in the same laboratory.

Recommendations

1. It recommended to detect and monitor anti-A IgG, anti-A IgM, anti-B IgG, and anti-B IgM titer in the preoperative and postoperative ABOi-KT (1-A).
2. The antibody titer needs monitoring at every period during the transplantation like matching time, before and after administration of immunosuppressive agents, before and after receiving rituximab, and before and after PE or/and DFPP.

The Use of Immunosuppressant

We usually begin to use the classic immunosuppressant 1 week before the operation. The drug dosage is usually tacrolimus 0.05–0.1 mg/(kg-D), methylprednisolone 20–80 mg/day, mycophenolate 1–2 g/day, or mycophenolate sodium 1.440 g/day. The use of high-dose methylprednisolone within 3 days after operation is recommended. The dosage is generally 500 mg/day, then gradually goes down, and maintains a low dose until the condition is stable. Thirty days after surgery, ABOi-KT recipients are treated with the same immunosuppressant as ABOc-KT recipients. The withdrawal of hormones remains controversial. Some reports suggest that the withdrawal of hormone 7 or 1 month after ABOi-KT has no effect on graft rejection or graft survival [22, 44].

Recommendations

1. Recipients with high-risk or highly sensitizing factors (high reactive antibody levels, retransplantation, delayed graft function, etc.) are recommended to use anti-thymocyte globulin (ATG) and/or IL-2 receptor monoclonal antibody for induction therapy (1-C).
2. The recommended initial scheme is a triple immune suppress regiment of calcineurin inhibitors (CNI) combined with a kind of antiproliferative drugs and glucocorticoids, using tacrolimus as a first-line drug for CNI.
3. Be careful when you withdraw the hormone. Small dose should be maintained rather than completely deactivated if there is no severe complications (2-B).

Selection and Resection of Donor Kidney

The selection and resection of the donor kidney of ABOi-KT are exactly the same as that of ABOc-KT. Please refer to the chapter of "Relative living renal transplantation" in *Clinical Guidelines Manual of organ transplantation* published by the People's Medical Publishing House [25].

The Monitoring and Treatment of Coagulation Dysfunction

Since the liver function of most ABOi-KT recipients is normal, many transplant centers tend to use albumin as a succedaneum after PE and DFPP, which may lead to thrombocytopenia and loss of coagulation factors. In general, endogenous coagulation and exogenous coagulation can be, respectively, detected by APTT and Pt tests. But the loss of factor XIII may not be detected by these two detection methods [45]. This can cause bleeding within the normal value range of APTT and PT.

Recommendations

1. Use type AB plasma as replacement fluid in PE and DFPP (2-B).
2. The coagulation function must be monitored before the operation, including serum Ca2+ concentration, FIB, platelets, PT, APTT, etc. (1-A). Once there is evidence of bleeding, take the type fresh AB plasma transfusion. If possible, the coagulation factor or prothrombin complex can be supplemented according to the abnormal coagulation function.
3. Pay attention to the possible condition of consumptive coagulation disorder and/or thrombotic microvascular diseases during the plasma treatment, within 24 h after treatment, and within 72 h of transplantation.

4. Plasma Ca ion concentration, routine blood test, and coagulation parameters should be included in preoperative, intraoperative, and postoperative coagulation monitoring (2-B).
5. The bleeding after surgery should be resolved by surgical hemostasis; fresh AB type plasma is used to treat bleeding caused by coagulation factor loss rather than hemostatic agents; when bleeding is due to coagulation disorders that occurs with fibrinolysis, use heparin combined with the transfusion of fresh AB type plasma, cryoprecipitate, and platelets (1-D).
6. Hypothermia can aggravate coagulation dysfunction. Thermal insulation measures such as electric blanket are recommended during the perioperative period to maintain temperature higher than 36 °C (1-D).
7. Keep acid-base balance of internal environment to avoid the coagulopathy aggravated by acidosis (1-D).

Complications and Management

Surgical Complications (Table A.6)

There is no significant difference in the type and incidence of complications between ABOi-KT and ABOc-KT [26, 46]. Factors like multiple plasma treatment before operation, coagulation factors or platelet loss or dysfunction, and application of anticoagulant drugs such as heparin and sodium citrate all can lead to coagulation dysfunction in recipient, which may increase bleeding probability according to some reports. The use of rituximab reduces the number of plasma treatments and decreases the tendency to bleed. For patients with normal preoperative coagulation function, adjusted dose of anticoagulation according to the postoperative coagulation has better long-term effect than no use of anticoagulation [49]. The other complications and surgical treatment should follow the "clinical guidelines for diagnosis and treatment of living relative kidney transplantation."

Table A.6 Common surgical complications of ABOi-KT

Complication
Bleeding
Thrombopoiesis
Transplant renal artery stenosis
Spontaneous rupture of renal allograft
Arteriovenous fistula
Urinary fistula
Ureteral obstruction
Epididymitis
Hydrocele testis

Recommendations

1. If the coagulation function is normal, 6000 iu LMWH should be given two times a day for 3–7 days after surgery. Oral antiplatelet drugs, such as aspirin, are given until the condition is stable (1-B).
2. If the patient's low coagulation state leads to the formation of local hematoma, the hematoma cannot be removed actively (2-B).

Rejection

The occurrence of rejection should be taken into consideration if the patient's blood creatinine level increases and urine output reduces. Biopsy of transplanted kidney is the gold standard for the diagnosis of rejection. The incidence of rejection in ABOi-KT was not significantly different from that of ABOc-KT [6]. Forty-eight hours to 2 weeks after operation is the critical period for high incidence of ABOi-KT rejection, during which improper treatment may lead to an increase in the incidence of ABOi-KT rejection [9]. C4D staining has no guiding significance in the diagnosis of humoral rejection of ABOi-KT [50].

Hyperacute Rejection (HAR)

HAR rarely occurs due to preoperative HLA matching, cross matching tests, DSA testing, preoperative plasma treatment, and removal of blood group antibodies.

Recommendation

HAR currently lacks effective treatment and requires immediate removal of the graft as soon as the diagnosis is made.

Accelerated Rejection

Accelerated acute rejection usually occurs in 48 h to 7 days after surgery.

Recommendations

1. If accelerated rejection occurs, we recommend the use of plasma exchange (PE) combined with large dose of immunoglobulin (IVIG) and the increase of rituximab dose to 375 mg/m^2. A salvage splenectomy should be performed if necessary (1-C).
2. The immunosuppressive regimen should be adjusted in time so as to avoid acute rejection (1-B).
3. For very few patients, if treatments are ineffective, the transplanted kidney should be removed as soon as possible (2-C).

Acute Rejection

Acute rejection can occur at any stage after surgery, but usually within 3 months after surgery. The delayed acute rejection usually occurs when the immunosuppressive agent is stopped or reduced or combined with infections.

Recommendations

1. Doppler color ultrasonography is an ideal noninvasive diagnostic tool (1-A).
2. Corticosteroids are recommended as an initial drug for acute cellular rejection. If acute rejection occurs continuously in the short term, the dose should be controlled within 5 g (1-D).
3. For patients with acute cellular rejection and relapsed acute cellular rejection, if hormonal treatment is ineffective, lymphocyte clearing antibodies, including anti-lymphocyte immunoglobulin (ALG), anti-thymocyte globulin (ATG), and anti-CD3 monoclonal antibodies, are recommended.
4. One or more regimens united or not united with hormone are recommended for the treatment of antibody-mediated acute rejection:plasmapheresis, intravenous administration of large doses of immunoglobulin (IVIG), proteasome inhibitors, and lymphocyte clearance antibodies (2-C).
5. The immunosuppressive regimen should be adjusted in the course of treatment (2-C).

Chronic Rejection

There is no specific drug for chronic rejection at present. It can only be prevented by reducing the preoperative HLA matching, reducing the ischemia reperfusion injury of renal supply, and preventing infections. If the elevated creatinine levels and proteinuria are founded during the regular follow-up, recipients should be admitted to hospital as soon as possible.

Recommendation

It is recommended to strengthen immunosuppressive therapy if the immune response is very active, such as adding mTOR pathway inhibitors. If the treatment fails, the immune aid should be discontinued, and blood treatment should be resumed before a second kidney transplant (2-B).

Infections

The ABOi-KT has a higher risk of infection due to multiple plasma treatment and the use of rituximab and potent immunosuppressive agents. Some studies have confirmed that ABOi-KT recipients have a higher risk of pneumonia and infections of cytomegalovirus (CMV), herpes simplex virus (HSV), herpes zoster virus (VZV), and multi-tumor virus (BKV) than ABOc-KT recipient [51, 52]. But there is no enough evidence indicating that rituximab increases the risk of infection [53]. Nonstandard handling of plasma treatment may increase the risk of infections. However, the low immunoglobulin and low complement status of recipients may be the major causes of increased infection risk [54–56].

Whether or not to reduce the dose of immunosuppressive drugs depends on the integrated assessment of the patient's immune status and infection. The activation of latent virus infection and recurrence of tuberculosis may indicate excessive immunosuppression. Corticosteroid dosage should be reduced when a bacterial infection occurs, and tacrolimus dosage should be reduced if viral infection is detected. When neutrophils and immunoglobulin levels are low, the use of GM-CSF and infusion of gamma globulin should be considered first.

For specific measures, please refer to "living-related kidney transplantation clinical guidelines."

Recommendations

1. The incidence of CMV infection is high. Its clinical manifestations are fever of unknown origins, decrease in white blood cells and platelets, malaise, and mild liver and kidney dysfunction. It is recommended to make a diagnosis by detecting the number of CMV copies in the blood plasma through quantitative PCR (1-B).
2. Prophylactic ganciclovir or valganciclovir and the CMV hypersensitive immune globulin if necessary are recommended, except in transplant between CMV-negative donors and recipients (2-C).

Complications of Other Systems

Compared with ABOc-KT, the incidence of complications in ABOi-KT, of digestive system, cardiovascular system, metabolic system, motor system, reproductive system, etc., is not significantly increased.

Tumor

Extensive use of immunosuppressive agents after transplantation can lead to a marked increase in the incidence of cancer, about 100 times as much as the average age normal group. However, there is no difference in occurrence ratio between ABOi-KT and ABOc-KT [57]. Deactivation or reduction of CNI or replacement of mTOR inhibitors is the basis for the treatment of postoperative tumors.

Recommendations

1. When the recipient has rapid or recurrent squamous cell carcinoma or skin cancer occurs all over the body, immunosuppressive agent should be changed or deactivated (2-A).
2. Some skin changes can recover after use chlorambucil or cyclophosphamide instead of azathioprine, but this method often leads to graft rejection (2-D).

Postoperative Management and Follow-Up

ABOi-KT follow-up was similar to ABOc-KT. As the immunological adaptation will be established 2 weeks after operation, blood type antibody titer monitor is no longer necessary.

Recommendations

Regular follow-up to encourage patients to build a healthy lifestyle, do moderate exercise, have a reasonable diet, and lose weight as needed. Assess the patient's depression and anxiety (not graded).

Conclusion

ABOi-KT have been routinely carried out in Japan and Europe and America, and there is no difference in the graft survival and prognosis of patients between ABOi-KT and ABOc-KT, or ABOi-KT is even better than ABOc-KT. Recently, ABO-incompatible donor grafts have been successfully extended to Donation After Cardiac Death (DCD) [58, 59]. Therefore, the popularization of this extension can relieve the shortage of transplant organs to a certain extent. Following ABOi-KT, ABOi heart transplantation, ABOi liver transplantation, and so on, all have been successfully carried out [60]. The use of plasma processing techniques has improved the prognosis of HLA highly sensitized patients, and made a major step forward in kidney transplantation over HLA barriers [61].

However, there are still some problems to be solved and some mechanisms to be further studied for ABOi-KT. The treatment cost/benefit needs to be further optimized. In addition, different transplantation centers still have different plasma treatment schemes and different antibody titer standards. The use of rituximab and its dosage and the course of treatment are also varied. Although there are various researches on the mechanism of immune adaptation, the core and key reasons have not been clear. The further interpretation of immune adaptation mechanisms will help to optimize the treatment options and provide the basis for individualized application of treatment protocols.

Declaration

There is no conflict of interest between the publication of this guideline and any company, institution, or individual.

References

1. Hume DM, Merrill JP, Miller BF, et al. Experiences with renal homotransplantation in the human: report of nine cases. J Clin Invest. 1955;34:327–82.
2. Alexandre GP, Squifflet JP, De Bruyere M, et al. Present experiences in a series of 26 ABO-incompatible living donor renal allografts. Transplant Proc. 1987;19:4538–42.
3. Tanabe K, Ishida H, Inui M, et al. ABO-incompatible kidney transplantation: long-term outcomes. Clin Transpl. 2013:307–12.
4. Sonnenday CJ, Warren DS, Cooper M, et al. Plasmapheresis, CMV hyperimmune globulin, and anti-CD20 allow ABO-incompatible renal transplantation without splenectomy. Am J Transplant. 2004;4:1315–22.
5. Tyden G, Kumlien G, Fehrman I. Successful ABO-incompatible kidney transplantations without splenectomy using antigen-specific immunoadsorption and rituximab. Transplantation. 2003;76:730–1.
6. Takahashi K, Saito K. ABO-incompatible kidney transplantation. Transplant Rev (Orlando). 2013;27:1–8.
7. Aikawa A, Saito K, Takahashi K. Trends in ABO-incompatible kidney transplantation. Exp Clin Transplant. 2015;13(Suppl 1):18–22.
8. Opelz G, Morath C, Susal C, et al. Three-year outcomes following 1420 ABO-incompatible living-donor kidney transplants performed after ABO antibody reduction: results from 101 centers. Transplantation. 2015;99:400–4.
9. Montgomery JR, Berger JC, Warren DS, et al. Outcomes of ABO-incompatible kidney transplantation in the United States. Transplantation. 2012;93:603–9.
10. Wang Y, Luo Z, Gui P, et al. A case report of ABO-incompatible kidney transplantation without splenectomy in China. Chin J Organ Transpl. 2007;28(11)::694–5.
11. Segev DL, Simpkins CE, Warren DS, et al. ABO incompatible high-titer renal transplantation without splenectomy or anti-CD20 treatment. Am J Transplant. 2005;5:2570–5.
12. Tanabe K. Japanese experience of ABO-incompatible living kidney transplantation. Transplantation. 2007;84:S4–7.
13. Genberg H, Kumlien G, Wennberg L, et al. Isoagglutinin adsorption in ABO-incompatible transplantation. Transfus Apher Sci. 2010;43:231–5.
14. Lo P, Sharma A, Craig JC, et al. Preconditioning therapy in ABO-incompatible living kidney transplantation: a systematic review and meta-analysis. Transplantation. 2016;100(4):933–42.
15. Galili U. Xenotransplantation and ABO incompatible transplantation: the similarities they share. Transfus Apher Sci. 2006;35:45–58.

16. Tyden G, Donauer J, Wadstrom J, et al. Implementation of a protocol for ABO-incompatible kidney transplantation—a three-center experience with 60 consecutive transplantations. Transplantation. 2007;83:1153–5.
17. Fuchinoue S, Ishii Y, Sawada T, et al. The 5-year outcome of ABO-incompatible kidney transplantation with rituximab induction. Transplantation. 2011;91:853–7.
18. Shimmura H, Tanabe K, Ishikawa N, et al. Role of anti-A/B antibody titers in results of ABO-incompatible kidney transplantation. Transplantation. 2000;70:1331–5.
19. Gloor JM, Lager DJ, Moore SB, et al. ABO-incompatible kidney transplantation using both A2 and non-A2 living donors. Transplantation. 2003;75:971–7.
20. Chung BH, Lim JU, Kim Y, et al. Impact of the baseline anti-A/B antibody titer on the clinical outcome in ABO-incompatible kidney transplantation. Nephron Clin Pract. 2013;124:79–88.
21. Shimmura H, Tanabe K, Ishida H, et al. Lack of correlation between results of ABO-incompatible living kidney transplantation and anti-ABO blood type antibody titers under our current immunosuppression. Transplantation. 2005;80:985–8.
22. van Agteren M, Weimar W, de Weerd AE, et al. The first fifty ABO blood group incompatible kidney transplantations: the Rotterdam experience. J Transpl. 2014;2014:913902.
23. Won D, Choe W, Kim HJ, et al. Significance of isoagglutinin titer in ABO-incompatible kidney transplantation. J Clin Apher. 2014;29:243–50.
24. Mital D, Hammes E. Indications for renal transplantation. In: Saclarides JT, Myers AJ, Millikan WK, editors. Common surgical diseases: an algorithmic approach to problem solving. New York: Springer; 2015. p. 239–42.
25. Chinses Medical Association. Guidelines for living donor transplantation between relatives. Guidelines for clinical diagnosis and treatment-organ transplantations. Beijing: People's Medical Publishing House (PMPH); 2010.
26. Gohh RY, Yango AF, Morrissey PE, et al. Preemptive plasmapheresis and recurrence of FSGS in high-risk renal transplant recipients. Am J Transplant. 2005;5:2907–12.
27. Andrews P, Burnapp L, Manas D, et al. Summary of the British Transplantation Society/ Renal Association U.K. Guidelines for living donor kidney transplantation. Transplantation. 2012;93:666–73.
28. Tyden G, Kumlien G, Genberg H, et al. The Stockholm experience with ABO-incompatible kidney transplantations without splenectomy. Xenotransplantation. 2006;13:105–7.
29. Wilpert J, Fischer KG, Pisarski P, et al. Long-term outcome of ABO-incompatible living donor kidney transplantation based on antigen-specific desensitization. An observational comparative analysis. Nephrol Dial Transplant. 2010;25:3778–86.
30. Opelz G. Strength of HLA-A, HLA-B, and HLA-DR mismatches in relation to short- and long-term kidney graft survival. Collaborative transplant study. Transpl Int. 1992;5(Suppl 1):S621–4.
31. Lefaucheur C, Loupy A, Hill GS, et al. Preexisting donor-specific HLA antibodies predict outcome in kidney transplantation. J Am Soc Nephrol. 2010;21:1398–406.
32. Thammanichanond D, Ingsathit A, Mongkolsuk T, et al. Pre-transplant donor specific antibody and its clinical significance in kidney transplantation. Asian Pac J Allergy Immunol. 2012;30:48–54.
33. Hirai T, Kohei N, Omoto K, et al. Significance of low-level DSA detected by solid-phase assay in association with acute and chronic antibody-mediated rejection. Transpl Int. 2012;25:925–34.
34. Toki D, Ishida H, Horita S, et al. Blood group O recipients associated with early graft deterioration in living ABO-incompatible kidney transplantation. Transplantation. 2009;88:1186–93.
35. Barnett AN, Hadjianastassiou VG, Mamode N. Rituximab in renal transplantation. Transpl Int. 2013;26:563–75.
36. Gloor J, Stegall M. ABO-incompatible kidney transplantation with and without splenectomy. Transplantation. 2006;82:720.
37. Genberg H, Kumlien G, Wennberg L, et al. ABO-incompatible kidney transplantation using antigen-specific immunoadsorption and rituximab: a 3-year follow-up. Transplantation. 2008;85:1745–54.

38. Kohei N, Hirai T, Omoto K, et al. Chronic antibody-mediated rejection is reduced by targeting B-cell immunity during an introductory period. Am J Transplant. 2012;12:469–76.
39. Montgomery RA, Locke JE, King KE, et al. ABO incompatible renal transplantation: a paradigm ready for broad implementation. Transplantation. 2009;87:1246–55.
40. Tobian AA, Shirey RS, Montgomery RA, et al. ABO antibody titer and risk of antibody-mediated rejection in ABO-incompatible renal transplantation. Am J Transplant. 2010;10:1247–53.
41. Tanabe K. Double-filtration plasmapheresis. Transplantation. 2007;84:S30–2.
42. Zschiedrich S, Kramer-Zucker A, Janigen B, et al. An update on ABO-incompatible kidney transplantation. Transpl Int. 2015;28:387–97.
43. Muramatsu M, Gonzalez HD, Cacciola R, et al. ABO incompatible renal transplants: good or bad? World J Transplant. 2014;4:18–29.
44. Galliford J, Charif R, Chan KK, et al. ABO incompatible living renal transplantation with a steroid sparing protocol. Transplantation. 2008;86:901–6.
45. Focosi D. Acquired factor XIII deficiency after desensitization as a potential contributor to postoperative bleeding: more than meets the eye. Transpl Int. 2015;28:246–7.
46. Humar A, Matas AJ. Surgical complications after kidney transplantation. Semin Dial. 2005;18:505–10.
47. Kim MH, Jun KW, Hwang JK, et al. Risk factors for postoperative bleeding in ABO-incompatible kidney transplantation. Clin Transplant. 2015;29:365–72.
48. de Weerd AE, van Agteren M, Leebeek FW, et al. ABO-incompatible kidney transplant recipients have a higher bleeding risk after antigen-specific immunoadsorption. Transpl Int. 2015;28:25–33.
49. Takahashi K, Saito K, Takahara S, et al. Excellent long-term outcome of ABO-incompatible living donor kidney transplantation in japan. Am J Transplant. 2004;4:1089–96.
50. Haas M, Rahman MH, Racusen LC, et al. C4d and C3d staining in biopsies of ABO- and HLA-incompatible renal allografts: correlation with histologic findings. Am J Transplant. 2006;6:1829–40.
51. Habicht A, Broker V, Blume C, et al. Increase of infectious complications in ABO-incompatible kidney transplant recipients—a single centre experience. Nephrol Dial Transplant. 2011;26:4124–31.
52. Lentine KL, Axelrod D, Klein C, et al. Early clinical complications after ABO-incompatible live-donor kidney transplantation: a national study of medicare-insured recipients. Transplantation. 2014;98:54–65.
53. Kelesidis T, Daikos G, Boumpas D, et al. Does rituximab increase the incidence of infectious complications? A narrative review. Int J Infect Dis. 2011;15:e2–16.
54. Kaplan A. Complications of apheresis. Semin Dial. 2012;25:152–8.
55. Moriya Y, Yamaji K, Kanai Y, et al. The effectiveness of intravenous human immunoglobulin treatment after plasmapheresis in restoring serum immunoglobulin levels: a preliminary study. Ther Apher. 2002;6:154–8.
56. Biglarnia AR, Nilsson B, Nilsson Ekdahl K, et al. Desensitization with antigen-specific immunoadsorption interferes with complement in ABO-incompatible kidney transplantation. Transplantation. 2012;93:87–92.
57. Hall EC, Engels EA, Montgomery RA, et al. Cancer risk after ABO-incompatible living-donor kidney transplantation. Transplantation. 2013;96:476–9.
58. Masterson R, Hughes P, Walker RG, et al. ABO incompatible renal transplantation without antibody removal using conventional immunosuppression alone. Am J Transplant. 2014;14:2807–13.
59. Stewart ZA, Locke JE, Montgomery RA, et al. ABO-incompatible deceased donor liver transplantation in the United States: a national registry analysis. Liver Transpl. 2009;15:883–93.
60. Koestner SC, Kappeler A, Schaffner T, et al. Histo-blood group type change of the graft from B to O after ABO mismatched heart transplantation. Lancet. 2004;363:1523–5.
61. Montgomery RA, Lonze BE, King KE, et al. Desensitization in HLA-incompatible kidney recipients and survival. N Engl J Med. 2011;365:318–26.

MIX
Papier aus verantwortungsvollen Quellen
Paper from responsible sources
FSC® C105338

If you have any concerns about our products,
you can contact us on
ProductSafety@springernature.com

In case Publisher is established outside the EU,
the EU authorized representative is:
Springer Nature Customer Service Center GmbH
Europaplatz 3, 69115 Heidelberg, Germany

Printed by Libri Plureos GmbH
in Hamburg, Germany